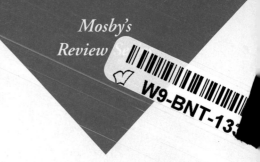

Mosby's
Review Se

W9-BNT-133

MEDICAL-SURGICAL
NURSING

Mosby's Review Series

MEDICAL-SURGICAL NURSING

Paulette D. Rollant, PhD, MSN, RN, CCRN
President, Multi-Resources, Inc.
Grantville, Georgia

Deborah A. Ennis, RN, MSN, CCRN
Professor of Nursing
Harrisburg Area Community College
Harrisburg, Pennsylvania

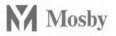 Mosby

St. Louis Baltimore Boston Carlsbad Chicago Naples New York Philadelphia Portland
London Madrid Mexico City Singapore Sydney Tokyo Toronto Wiesbaden

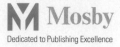

Mosby
Dedicated to Publishing Excellence

A Times Mirror
Company

Vice-President and Publisher: Nancy L. Coon
Senior Editor: Susan R. Epstein
Associate Developmental Editor: Laurie K. Muench
Project Manager: Carol Sullivan Weis
Designer: Sheilah Barrett
Manufacturing Supervisor: Karen Lewis
Cover Illustrator: Susan Swan

Printed in the United States of America
Composition by Shepherd, Inc.
Printing/binding by R.R. Donnelly

Mosby–Year Book, Inc.
11830 Westline Industrial Drive
St. Louis, MO 63146

International Standard Book Number 0-8151-7249-4

95 96 97 98 99 / 9 8 7 6 5 4 3 2 1

▼ ▼ ▼ ▼ ▼ ▼ ▼ ▼ ▼   ▼ ▼ ▼

Patricia T. Ketcham, RN, BSN, MSN
Undergraduate Program Director/Assistant Professor
Oakland University School of Nursing
Rochester, Michigan

Julia R. Popp, RN, BSN, MSN, CNS
Nursing Instructor
Owens Community College
Toledo, Ohio

REVIEWERS

To Dan, Mom, Dad, Joanne, Joe, Alan, and Amy
Paulette Rollant

To Bill
Deborah Ennis

HOW CAN *MOSBY'S REVIEW SERIES* BE USED?

Mosby's Review Series is designed to help you obtain the most from your preparation and study time for your nursing exams. These books should be used to review essential concepts, theory, and content prior to nursing courses, challenge, certification, or licensing examinations. The review series can be used to prepare for clinical experiences and as a quick reference when providing care of clients. Mosby's Review Series consists of five books:

> *Maternity Nursing*
> *Medical-Surgical Nursing*
> *Mental Health Nursing*
> *Pediatric Nursing*
> *Nursing Pharmacology*

The series is designed to highlight important information related to the specific content. It is not meant to provide a comprehensive, in-depth coverage of the selected area of nursing. The reference list at the end of each book is a compilation of resources used to develop these books. These references as well as other texts should be consulted when a more comprehensive discussion of a particular topic is desired. Use these books to jog your memory, to reinforce what you know, to guide you to identify what you don't know, and to lead you to appropriate sources for more details. If you are in a formal education setting, these books are not intended to be considered as a substitute for attending classes or completing required reading assignments.

Used correctly these books can help you:
1. Increase your ability to prioritize in clinical situations while using the nursing process.
2. Increase your ability to remember essential content.
3. Increase your productivity in studying to leave some time for you and your family.
4. Apply new behaviors for improvement of your testing skills.
5. Evaluate your strengths and weakness related to content areas or testing situations.

WHAT IS UNIQUE ABOUT *MOSBY'S REVIEW SERIES?*

1. Computer disks of exams
2. Comprehensive rationales
3. Test-taking tips
4. Chapter format
5. References for further reading

Computer Disk

Each book in the series has a comprehensive exam on computer disk. For your convenience, the exam is also included in the book. The answers for the comprehensive exams, like the end of the chapter questions, include the answers, comprehensive rationales, and test-taking tips.

Comprehensive Rationales

These include answers and rationales for each option in each test question.

Test-Taking Tips

These tips aid in your decision-making and facilitate the development of your logical thinking for the selection of the correct answers, especially if you have narrowed your choice to two options.

Chapter Format

Each chapter contains an easy-to-follow format divided into five sections:

Study Outcomes: provides an advanced organizer approach to what is in each chapter

Key Terms: includes the most common difficult terms to recall

Content Review: is organized and structured by the nursing process to help you identify what is most important

▼ All information within each heading is prioritized
▼ Nursing diagnoses are prioritized
▼ Goals are client-centered
▼ Client teaching content is focused for in-hospital and at-home clinical settings
▼ Home care content is included
▼ Older adult alerts are included where applicable
▼ Evaluation criteria includes decision-making tools concerning which actions to take when client's clinical status shows improvement or deterioration
▼ Many tables, charts, and figures contrast, cluster, and simplify information for ease of remembering

Review Questions: stand-alone, 4-option multiple choice

Answers, Rationales, and Test-Taking Tips:

▼ Comprehensive rationales: given for each option to explain why it is correct or incorrect

▼ Test-taking tips: give strategies to use in situations such as when options are narrowed to two or when you have no idea of a correct answer

References
Current references are suggested for further study if more in-depth discussion is needed.

WHAT'S IN *MOSBY'S REVIEW SERIES: MEDICAL-SURGICAL NURSING?*

Mosby's Review Series: Medical-Surgical Nursing is organized in a head-to-toe systems approach with the initial sequence of content for: the neurological, the cardiac with vascular and hematology, and the respiratory systems. Following this section are the elimination systems of gastrointestinal, renal, and urinary. The hormonal systems of the reproductive and the endocrine are then covered. Lastly, the musculoskeletal, integumentary, and immune systems are discussed. This sequence will enhance the ability to recall content, especially if the reader's developed study plan is similar in sequence. Content in each chapter is formatted in the outline of the nursing process, which includes acute and home care focuses. The most common pathological disorders are included in each given major system.

ACKNOWLEDGMENTS

I express my heartfelt gratitude to those who have endured with me throughout this publication opportunity for a nursing review series: an adventure from idea to reality.

I especially want to thank the following people:

Beverly Copland, who thought that I had the potential to complete this project and who eagerly gave me tons of strong support in the initial and ongoing book development phases.

Laurie Muench, who picked up the ball in the middle of manuscript preparation and persisted with me through the process to completion of book publication. The response "OK . . . when *can* I expect it?" provided silent encouragement and sometimes comic relief when my mental and physical energies ran quite low. Laurie's thoughtfulness and guidance to help me set priorities were invaluable! I am very grateful and fortunate to work with Laurie.

Suzi Epstein, who was full of enthusiasm and total support from the birth of the idea for a nursing review series to the final publication of the books. Suzi's creativity and suggestions provided essential building blocks in the overall development of the series.

My *coauthors,* for their enormous efforts to produce manuscript content in a short period of time. Their nursing expertise was helpful for the development of the unique aspects of each book.

My wonderful husband, *Dan,* for his patience, humor, support, and love. His faith in my abilities has sustained my energies and maintained my sense of self.

My parents, *Joseph* and *Mildred Demaske,* for their love, encouragement, and prayers.

Paulette D. Rollant

I want to thank the following people:

Bill, for his love and his never-ending confidence and support.

Heather and *Megan,* for never complaining when Mom was busy writing her book.

Mom and *Dad,* for encouraging me to go for the degree(s)—I wouldn't be where I am today without them.

Last, but not least, *Paulette,* for believing in me!

Deborah A. Ennis

CONTENTS

HOW CAN I USE THIS BOOK?

This book is designed to work for you—at your convenience. Read the following guidelines first to help save you time and energy during test preparation. The chapters are designed for short, quick intervals of review. Carry this book with you to catch the times when you are stuck and have nothing to do.

The directions will help you to:

- ▼ **Maximize your individual performance in review and testing situations.**
- ▼ **Identify your personal priorities in preparation for testing.**
- ▼ **Sharpen your thinking and discrimination skills for testing.**

DIRECTIONS ON HOW TO REVIEW

I. Identify your routine for reviewing: the best days, the best time of day

    A. Write the days and times on the inside front cover of this book and on your personal calendar and the calendar at home. This communicates to your family or support systems that you will be unavailable to them at these times. It is also a nice reminder every week to yourself that this is important to you.

    B. Refer to section V for specific directions on how to develop your routine

II. Scan the table of contents

    A. Put a check mark in front of the content with which you are comfortable

    B. Circle the content in which you think you are weak

    C. Prioritize the weak content with #1 being the weakest content area. Put these numbers in front of your circles.

    D. Prioritize the strongest content areas in the same manner

III. When you are feeling a high-energy day

    A. Go to the #1 chapter of the weakest content area for review

IV. When you are having a low-energy day

    A. Go to the #1 chapter of the strongest content area for review

V. General guidelines for the development of a routine for reviewing
    A. Develop a system of review that meets your needs
    B. Set aside time when you are least tired or stressed both mentally and physically
    C. Limit your review time to a maximum of 90 minutes for the most effective, efficient retention of reviewed content
    D. If possible, relax and take a nap after reviewing to further place the information into long term memory. Some research reveals that sleeping for 2 to 3 hours after studying results in a 70 to 80% retention rate of content into long term memory in contrast to 30 to 40% retention when you are active after studying.
    E. Use at least one relaxation technique *at the onset* and *at the end* of your review time. Deep breathing that is slow with a concentration on the air movement going in and out is one of the best ways to relax physically and mentally.
    F. Use at least one relaxation technique *during* the time you review.
    G. If your time is limited, use 10 to 15 minute intervals to review small portions of the content. For example, you may want to review the different aspects of hypertension in one study session.
    H. Use a theme per week or per day approach. For example, if there is enough time between your test and when you begin to study, every Monday review something on sodium from the book. Then at work find clients with sodium imbalances, review their charts, and discuss their situations with colleagues or with the clients' physicians. Continue with themes for the day such as:
        1. Tuesdays are potassium
        2. Wednesdays are calcium
        3. Thursdays are magnesium
        4. Fridays are acidosis situations
        5. Saturdays are alkalosis days
        6. Sundays are fun days. Don't forget to keep one day to relax and have fun. This allows your mind to work for retention and reorganization of the content that you reviewed during the week.
        7. Weekly themes also might be of help. Do one system per week such as pulmonary, endocrine and so forth.

DIRECTIONS ON HOW TO USE THIS BOOK FOR SUCCESS

I. Suggested study sequence #1 for each chapter
    A. Read the objectives
    B. Complete the key terms

     C.   Complete the content review
     D.   Complete the review questions
     E.   Review the answers, rationales, test-taking tips
II.   Suggested study sequence #2 for each chapter
     A.   Complete the review questions
     B.   Review the answers, rationales, test-taking tips
     C.   Review the missed content areas
     D.   Review the unfamiliar and the familiar content areas
     E.   Complete the key terms
     F.   Complete the objectives to evaluate your level of understanding
III. Suggested study sequence #3 *after* doing #1 or #2 suggested sequence
     A.   Complete the comprehensive exam in the book
     B.   Correct comprehensive exam answers with review of the rationales and test-taking tips
     C.   List content areas missed, then cluster them in terms of similar content
     D.   Prioritize these clusters with #1 being the least familiar content
     E.   Review additional content as directed by the questions you missed
IV. Suggested study sequence #4 *before* doing #1 or #2 suggested sequence
     A.   Complete the comprehensive exam in the book
     B.   Correct comprehensive exam answers with review of the rationales and test-taking tips
     C.   List content areas missed, then cluster them in terms of similar content
     D.   Prioritize these clusters with #1 being the least familiar content
     E.   Implement either sequence #1 or #2
     F.   Complete the computer comprehensive exam. Note that even though the questions are the same as in the book, you should evaluate how your reading of the questions and options differed as related to perception and consistent ability to identify key words, terms, age, and developmental needs.
     G.   Review content as needed and directed from your missed questions on your exam
V.   Suggested techniques for use of the objectives during your review
     A.   Read the objectives to have them guide you where to start
     B.   Put a check next to the ones in which you feel the weakest
     C.   Prioritize them with #1 being the weakest
     D.   Review the weakest content first or on high-energy days
     E.   Review the most familiar content last or on low-energy days
VI. Suggested techniques for the use of the key terms, the content review section, and the exams
     A.   Key terms—suggested study techniques
          1.   Use a 3 x 5 index card to cover the definitions of the key terms
          2.   State your definition out loud

3. Uncover the definition and read the given definition out loud (speaking the content as well as seeing the content will enhance your retention)

4. Write key notes in terms of a few words on a 3 x 5 card for the information you have difficulty recalling

5. Carry the card with you for a few days to review this content again. Suggestion: put the card on your sunvisor in the car and review it at the stoplight or if stopped in traffic.

B. Content review—suggested study techniques

1. Use a 3 x 5 card to cover the content under a major heading

2. State out loud what 3 or 4 important aspects of the content under the major heading might be or ask yourself a few questions about that content heading. Try to state the items in order of priority.

3. Uncover the content under the major heading. Check your information against that given in the book. See what you forgot or added that may or may not be important.

4. Write key notes in terms of a few words on a 3 x 5 card for the information you have difficulty recalling

5. Carry the card with you for a few days to review this content again. Suggestion: carry the card with you to review whenever you get 5 to 10 minutes free.

6. When you practice prioritizing the content you will enhance your critical thinking skills

C. Exam review—suggested study techniques

1. For all tests read all the rationales and test-taking tips for missed and correct questions. These often contain pearls of wisdom on how to remember or get a better understanding of the content.

2. Remember to do a relaxation exercise before you begin your questions and repeat the exercise about every 25 questions

3. When you miss a question ask yourself
   a. Did I not know the content?
   b. Did I misread the question or option(s)?

4. If you miss questions because of a knowledge deficit
   a. Make a list on a 3 x 5 card for 3 to 4 days
   b. Group or cluster the content according to the steps in the nursing process, the content area, or a system
   c. Look up that content
   d. Do not look up content after every practice test. A better approach is to cluster the content and look it all up every

3 to 4 days. With this approach you will have better retention into long term memory and the best recall at a later time.

    e.   Try to identify new ways to approach reading questions and their options

5.   If you misread the question or the option(s)

    a.   Try to identify what key words, timeframes, ages, and developmental stages that you may have overlooked

    b.   Try to identify new ways to approach reading the questions and their options

    c.   Practice, practice, and practice doing questions

    d.   Practice, practice, and practice doing relaxation before you begin the practice exam, after every 10 to 20 questions, and then at the end of the exam to refresh your thinking and diminish your tenseness or tiredness.

6.   Be sure to do a practice exam with the exact number of questions as your real exam. Note after this exam when you were the most tired, anxious, or nervous. Plan to do a relaxation exercise at these times during the real exam.

7.   Your success is directly correlated to your degree of effort to review content as well as relax during the review and exam processes.

SUMMARY

It is hoped that after you have completed your review with the use of this book as your major tool that you have:

▼ Maximized your individual performance in review and testing situations.

▼ Identified your personal priorities in preparation for testing.

▼ Sharpened your thinking and discrimination skills for testing.

Let this book work for you to make it easy, enjoyable, and effective to review at times that are convenient for you. The short, condensed, and prioritized chapter content may spark new ways to develop your skills in critical thinking and content recall.

It is feedback from students, graduates, and practitioners in nursing that prompted the development and publication of this book. We welcome your comments. We wish you a successful career in the nursing profession and hope that *Mosby's Nursing Review Series* has made that success a little easier to obtain!

Essential Elements for Nursing

STUDY OUTCOMES

After completing this chapter, the reader will be able to do the following:

▼ Identify essential elements common to all nursing specialties.
▼ Discuss the priority content for each essential element.
▼ Incorporate the essential elements into nursing practice.

KEY TERMS

Client education	Process of meeting the client's needs for the acquisition of skills, knowledge, or attitudes to deal with a pathological condition in the arenas of primary, secondary, or tertiary health promotion as based on the prior skills, knowledge, and attitudes of the client.
Nursing process	Process used as the basis of nursing practice. It includes five steps: (1) assess, (2) select nursing diagnosis, (3) plan, (4) intervene, and (5) evaluate.

CONTENT REVIEW

ESSENTIAL ELEMENTS IN NURSING

I. The essential elements
  A. Nursing process
  B. Client education

II. Nursing incorporates these common essential elements irrespective of the level, environment, or client population

III. The nursing process is the priority common thread throughout nursing practice

IV. Client education facilitates clients' behavior changes in areas of primary (preventive), secondary (early diagnosis), and tertiary (restorative, rehabilitative) health promotion

NURSING PROCESS

I. The nursing process has five steps
  A. Assess
  B. Select nursing diagnosis
  C. Plan
  D. Intervene
  E. Evaluate

1. Nurses follow the nursing process sequence in any initial client contact
2. Evaluation of the interventions occurs to determine effectiveness or ineffectiveness
3. If effective results, the client-nurse relationship either terminates or new priorities are set for new client problems
4. If ineffective results, nurses select the appropriate step(s); at this point in the evaluation process, the sequence of steps is a creative process by nurses as dictated by client need
5. If a client has unexpected changes during care, nurses typically do further assessment of the situation before implementing actions
6. Use of these steps is a dynamic, client-centered process
7. Communication is essential in all phases of the nursing process

II. The initial assessment process
A. Includes subjective and objective information
B. Subjective information: elicited by questions such as
   1. What is the one item that made you decide to seek help?
   2. What is your major problem today?
   3. When did this start? How long did it last? What relieved it?
   4. Do I need to know any other information that can help me better care for you?
C. Objective information: elicited through the senses
   1. Inspection: done initially for the client's respiratory rate, breathing effort, color, and position
   2. Inspection and touch: a handshake of the client elicits
      a. Demonstration of respect for the client; reduction of client's anxiety
      b. Level of consciousness and the motor ability/strength of client to initiate an appropriate response
      c. Pulse assessment for rate and regularity if two-handed technique is used
      d. Skin assessment for temperature, color, texture, and moisture
   3. Smell for odors: done simultaneously with inspection
   4. Hearing: asking the initial questions, then auscultating elicits
      a. Specific information about the client's perception of the problem
      b. Information about the client's emotional reaction to the situation by noting the tone and inflection of the speech
      c. Degree of influence from others based on whether they answer or clarify client's answers to questions

        d.   Auscultation typically includes the lungs, heart sounds, bowel sounds, and then any vascular sounds such as the carotid arteries or arterio-venous (A-V) fistulas

    5.   Touch: commonly the approaches to other touch techniques such as percussion or palpation are completed by starting with the problem system then moving to the respiratory, cardiac, and neurological systems followed by the other systems

D. **In emergency situations, objective information may take precedent over subjective information**
    1.   Airway, breathing, and circulation, the ABCs, may dictate assessment priorities
    2.   Deferment of the history and physical assessment of all body systems may take a secondary focus, with priority actions aiming to support the cardiac and respiratory systems

E. **Subjective information is best obtained from the client, the primary source, or from secondary sources such as the caretaker, family, or friends**

F. **History can be obtained from prior documentation to expedite the initial contact and conserve client energy**

G. **Results of the client's assessment act as the foundation for selecting priority nursing diagnoses and the development of an appropriate plan of care**

H. **In acute- and home-care settings, nurses may limit priorities to two nursing diagnoses for a more realistic, attainable, efficient, and effective approach to client care**

III. The selection of nursing diagnoses

A. **Nursing diagnoses**
    1.   Are clinical judgments about responses of an individual or family to actual or potential threats to health or life situations
    2.   Provide the basis for the selection of nursing interventions or referrals to achieve positive outcomes for evaluation
    3.   Are designed with a three-part statement; however, in clinical practice the first part is consistently used, but the other parts may not be required as part of the documentation
        a.   The three parts, also referred to as the PES format, are
            (1)   P = health problem, stated as a nursing problem
            (2)   E = etiological or related factors
            (3)   S = the defining characteristics or cluster of signs/symptoms as identified from the assessment data
        b.   The words *related to* connect the health problem and the etiological factors

      c. The words *as manifested by* connect the etiological factors and the signs/symptoms

      d. Example: urinary elimination—altered *related to* loss of muscle tone *as manifested by* incontinence, nocturia, dribbling.

      e. A health problem may be an actual or risk for (formerly potential or high-risk) problem

B. Process to the selection of nursing diagnoses

    1. Assessment data are analyzed and interpreted for priorities in relation to time, for an actual or high-risk problem with respect to what interventions are accountable by nursing

      a. In acute care: what needs to be accomplished

        (1) In the next 30 to 60 minutes?

        (2) In the next 8 hours?

        (3) In the next 24 hours?

        (4) By discharge from the facility?

      b. In other settings such as clinic, home, and outpatient care

        (1) What was the priority in the last few visits?

        (2) What necessitated this visit?

        (3) What has changed to require a reorganization of the priorities?

    2. A diagnostic label is selected with or without the phrases *related to* and *as manifested by;* institutional documentation policies guide the specific format for each agency

    3. In most situations, one or two priority nursing diagnoses are appropriate

    4. The ABCs are appropriate to use as a guide for setting priorities

IV. The planning process

A. Blueprint for nursing actions, also called nursing orders or planned nursing interventions, which are

    1. Based on the priorities collected or clustered from the assessment data

    2. Selected in reference to time and resources available

    3. Safe for the client and the nurse

    4. Commonly a combination of independent, interdependent, and dependent actions

B. Involves goal setting for achievement of client outcomes

C. May be done cooperatively if client is able to participate

D. Commonly involves some component of education for a client knowledge deficit

    E. Commonly dictates client outcomes, which need to be
1. Achieved in a set amount of time
2. Objective
3. Realistic
4. Observable or measurable for changes in client's activity, behavior, or physical state
5. Used as a standard of measure in the evaluation process
6. Examples
    a. Client outcome: within 48 hours the client will sleep through the night without the need to void
    b. Planned interventions
      (1) Provide use of the bedside commode before bedtime
      (2) Give no liquids after 8:00 P.M.

V. The intervention process
A. Actual execution of the planned nursing actions
B. Incorporates supervision, coordination, or evaluation of the delivery of care
C. Includes the recording and exchange of information among different disciplines

VI. The evaluation process
A. Based on client outcomes as identified from the planning process
B. Determination of the degree of effectiveness or ineffectiveness of the interventions taken to achieve the stated outcomes
C. Ongoing throughout the client-nurse relationship
D. Often performed concurrently with other phases of the nursing process rather than as a distinctly individual step
E. May result in the client's reassessment to reorder priorities and set new outcomes, especially if the stated time frame has been exceeded
F. Requires documentation of the date when revisement or resolution of the health problem occurred; may be documented as ongoing
G. Requires timely, accurate, and objective documentation and communication
H. Includes identification of the client's level of knowledge and degree of willingness to change behaviors, skills, knowledge, or attitudes in any of these areas
1. Diet
2. Activity

    3. Environment
    4. Equipment
    5. Medications: knowledge of
       a. Expected side effects
       b. Side effects that are treatable
       c. Side effects to report to the physician and within what time frame
       d. Length for the course of treatment

CLIENT EDUCATION

I. Client education: the process

  A. **Integral part of nursing care on either a formal or informal basis**
  B. **Incorporates the use of the nursing process**
  C. **Requires the use of teaching and learning principles**
  D. **Varies with clients according to their life experiences, present situation, and age**
  E. **Includes six main steps**
    1. Assessment of client education needs or wants
    2. Identification of priorities
    3. Identification of client goals or outcomes: what is needed
       a. Behavior changes
       b. Skill acquisition
       c. Cognitive or attitude changes
    4. Development of a teaching plan
       a. Development of learner objectives
       b. Determination of the content required for the given situation
       c. Determination of the resources and how to use them
          (1) Identify the available referral support agencies
          (2) Identify the materials available for teaching/learning activities
          (3) Investigate whether there is money available for materials, courses, transportation to and from education classes
          (4) Estimate the amount of time available versus the amount of time needed to implement the teaching plan
          (5) Decide whether the nurse will initiate and complete the education or refer to another support service for the education
       d. Determination of sequence and presentation approach of the content

5. Implementation of the teaching plan over a stated time frame
6. Evaluation of outcomes with revisions or reteaching as needed

II. Client assessments for education

A. Client's knowledge base. What does the client know? What does he or she want to know? Respect that some clients desire no information and document that response.

B. Readiness
1. Emotional
   a. Which stage of loss does client exhibit?
      (1) Denial
      (2) Anger
      (3) Bargaining
      (4) Depression
      (5) Acceptance
   b. If clients are in denial or anger, education will probably be ineffective; document stage of loss
2. Motivational: intrinsic motivation, stimulated from within the learner, is preferred to extrinsic motivation, stimulated from outside the learner
3. Experiential climate
   a. Values associated with social roles
   b. Personal resources and support systems
      (1) Family, friends
      (2) Finances for medications, equipment
      (3) Environmental factors: indoor plumbing, electricity
      (4) Prior and currect exposure to interactions with the healthcare system and providers
      (5) Availability of healthcare services, time versus distance with available transportation
   c. Developmental stage
4. Physical
   a. Clinical status is stable or improved
   b. Functional abilities
      (1) Hearing, attention span, listening
      (2) Vision
      (3) Touch and manual dexterity
      (4) Reading, level of highest education
      (5) Endurance
      (6) Short-term memory
         (a) Limited in its capacity
         (b) Enhanced if distractions are avoided

            (c) Enhanced if opportunities are given for repeating or rehearsing the information

        (7) Long-term memory

            (a) Unlimited in its capacity and duration

            (b) Influenced by the rate at which new information is introduced: the best approach is to introduce one new item every 4 to 5 seconds

            (c) Enhanced by 20 to 90% if material is incorporated into a story or real-life situation

  5. Signs of client's readiness

    a. Beginning behaviors of adaption to the original problem

    b. Exhibits awareness of the health problem and its implications

    c. Asks direct questions

    d. Presents clues that suggest client is seeking information

    e. Begins to ask questions about how to handle situations at home

    f. Indicators during a teaching session

        (1) Client is physically comfortable; basic needs are met

        (2) Client readily gives attention; eye contact is made

        (3) Client turns off television or asks visitors to leave

III. Special needs of clients for their education

  A. Interventions for low-literacy clients

    1. Give only simple (basic) information

    2. Present no more than three new points at a given time

    3. Give the most important information first and last

    4. Sequence information in the way the client will use it

    5. Give information the client can use immediately

    6. Use the same words when meanings are the same (e.g., medicine or drug, not both words)

    7. Use small, simple words and short sentences; introduce no more than five new words in one session

    8. Present information at the fifth-grade level or lower

    9. Be concrete and time specific. Example: take two pills at 4:00 P.M.

   10. Ask the client to repeat the information or the skill

   11. Use humor appropriately; be creative

   12. Avoid long explanations

   13. Reward frequently—even for small accomplishments

  B. Interventions for older clients

    1. Priority evaluations

      a. Establish the degree of functional losses

          b. Identify the degree of social support; lack of social support may be an important determinant in the decreased compliance of older adults

          c. Identify their habit structures

          d. Have an evaluation completed by social services or the business office for the availability of monies

  2. Clients with impaired hearing

          a. Use low-pitched voice

          b. Face client when speaking

          c. Use clear, concise terms

  3. Clients with impaired vision

          a. Use large print and a magnifying glass

          b. Black on white or black on yellow paper may be easier for the older clients to read

          c. Provide adequate lighting

          d. Have client use prescription glasses

  4. Clients with limited endurance

          a. Keep sessions short (10 to 15 minutes)

          b. Schedule the teaching session at a time of day when clients are comfortable and their energy levels are higher

          c. Break down the information into small steps

          d. The initial session should have only survival-level information

  5. Clients with memory loss

          a. Provide repeated exposure to same message

          b. Provide cues: visual, verbal, written

          c. Question frequently

          d. Use advanced organizers: "I'm going to tell you 2 ways to give your insulin," "I've told you how to give your insulin by using two methods."

IV. Learning theory

  A. Learning theory for adults

    1. Adult learner is defined as a self-directed, independent person who becomes ready to learn when the need to know or perform is experienced

    2. Adult education is learner centered

    3. Adult education is dynamic, interactive, and cooperative

    4. The responsibility for success of adult learners is shared by all participants

    5. Adult learners

          a. Like to participate in identification of their learning needs, formulation of learning objectives, and evaluation of learning

      b. Expect a climate of mutual respect
      c. Enter the learning situation with a life-centered, task-centered, or problem-centered approach
      d. Are motivated internally to learn in order to increase self-esteem, self-confidence, or seek a better quality of life
      e. See the educator as a facilitator rather than a director of the activity

B. Learning theory for children
1. Learning programs for children are more subject centered
2. Design of learning experiences is topic centered
3. Learning may be more of an external process with emphasis on externally sanctioned approvals for learning such as stars, happy-face stickers
4. Objective, content development, and evaluation process are teacher controlled

C. Factors that interfere with learning
1. Nervousness, anxiety, fear
2. Too much content at one session
3. Unfamiliar terms
4. Complexity of the task
5. Limited time with too much content, results in rushing
6. Background noise or other distractions
7. Fear of the task or information
8. Frequent interruptions
9. Inability of an educator to listen to the client
10. Absence of silence
11. Left-handed student's learning skills with right-handed educator
12. Client is not healthcare oriented; healthcare educator is
13. Stage of development; older adults may have the attitude that they have lived more or less successfully with their present habits and there is no reason to change now

V. Tools for teaching
A. Types of teaching
1. One to one
2. Group
      a. Homogeneous clients for a topic
      b. Heterogeneous clients for a topic
3. Programmed instruction
4. Guided independent study
5. Lecture

      6. Role playing
      7. Simulation
      8. Case method
      9. Demonstration/return demonstration
     10. Computerized instruction

B. Media for teaching
      1. Printed materials: pamphlets, books, crossword puzzles, study guides
      2. Pictorial materials: coloring books, videotapes, cartoons, flowcharts, slides, posters, overhead transparencies, computer simulations
      3. Visual representations: models, actual equipment
      4. Auditory: lectures, paired and small-group discussion, one-to-one interaction, role playing, cassette tapes, simulations
      5. Tactile, kinesthetic: practice with real or simulated items, manipulating or constructing models, playing games, completing worksheets, drawing, preparing charts, bulletin boards, developing a calendar of activities

C. Factors to consider in the selection of media/support materials
      1. Items readily available within acceptable costs
      2. Suitability: for the purpose of the teaching, to the environment in which the teaching will take place, for the availability of ancillary equipment
      3. Language: appropriate, understandable, and useful to the audience
      4. Materials: accurate and relevant to the intended age group and culture
      5. Print size: readable for the intended age group
      6. Illustrations: accurate and related to the intended audience

D. Nurse as a tool of teaching: the nursing professional should
      1. Show interest, empathy, and enthusiasm
      2. Practice expert listening skills; listen between the lines not only to what clients say, but how they say it
      3. Note clients' verbal and nonverbal communication that occurs; be aware of your own communication style
      4. Take a break when the client indicates a need; vary the schedule
      5. Be creative
      6. Keep language simple
      7. Allow enough time for demonstrations and return demonstrations
      8. Summarize at the end with encouragement for any progress, no matter how small

E. Evaluation tips for achievement of education outcomes
   1. Evaluation is an ongoing process throughout the entire teaching session
   2. If periodic reassessment of learning indicates no progress, try a different approach
   3. Ask open-ended questions along with specific questions
   4. Ask clients to evaluate themselves
F. Intervention tips for different age groups
   1. Pediatrics: the play approach works best with dolls or models; coloring, comic, or storybooks
   2. Teenagers and persons in their 20s: use peer speakers, entertainment, and peer groups and keep in mind that body image and independence are a priority for these age groups
   3. Persons in their 30s to mid-40s: written materials work well with follow-up time to answer questions or clarify information
   4. Persons from mid-40s to early 60s: a few long, single sessions to discuss how the effects of the health problem will interfere with attainment of or plans for lifelong goals
   5. Persons over mid 60s: use short, frequent, one-to-one meetings with material in larger print and keep in mind that maintaining functional abilities is a priority

SUMMARY

A working knowledge of the content in Chapter 1, the essential elements for nursing, will enhance the application of the remainder of the content in the review series. Most nursing professionals incorporate the two elements into their practice, which is based on the changing needs of clients who pursue the acquisition of healthcare services and actions to prevent pathological deterioration of the body. The nursing process and client education are intertwined in the areas of primary (preventive), secondary (early diagnosis), and tertiary (restorative, rehabilitative) health promotion.

NANDA-APPROVED NURSING DIAGNOSES

Activity intolerance
Activity intolerance, risk for
Adaptive capacity, decreased: intracranial
Adjustment, impaired
Airway clearance, ineffective
Anxiety
Aspiration, risk for

Body-image disturbance
Body temperature, altered, risk for
Bowel incontinence
Breastfeeding, effective
Breastfeeding, ineffective
Breastfeeding, interrupted
Breathing pattern, ineffective
Cardiac output, decreased
Caregiver role strain
Caregiver role strain, risk for
Communication, impaired verbal
Community coping, ineffective
Community coping, potential for enhanced
Confusion, acute
Confusion, chronic
Constipation
Constipation, colonic
Constipation, perceived
Coping, defensive
Coping, family: potential for growth
Coping, ineffective family: compromised
Coping, ineffective family: disabling
Coping, ineffective individual
Decisional conflict (specify)
Denial, ineffective
Diarrhea
Disuse syndrome, risk for
Diversional activity deficit
Dysreflexia
Energy field disturbance
Environmental interpretation syndrome: impaired
Family processes, altered
Family processes, altered: alcoholism
Fatigue
Fear
Fluid volume deficit
Fluid volume deficit, risk for
Fluid volume excess
Gas exchange, impaired
Grieving, anticipatory
Grieving, dysfunctional
Growth and development, altered

Health maintenance, altered
Health-seeking behaviors (specify)
Home maintenance management, impaired
Hopelessness
Hyperthermia
Hypothermia
Incontinence, functional
Incontinence, reflex
Incontinence, stress
Incontinence, total
Incontinence, urge
Infant behavior, disorganized
Infant behavior, disorganized: risk for
Infant feeding pattern, ineffective
Infection, risk for
Injury, perioperative positioning: risk for
Injury, risk for
Knowledge deficit (specify)
Loneliness, risk for
Management of therapeutic regimen, community: ineffective
Management of therapeutic regimen, families: ineffective
Management of therapeutic regimen, individuals: effective
Management of therapeutic regimen, individuals: ineffective
Memory, impaired
Mobility, impaired physical
Noncompliance (specify)
Nutrition, altered: less than body requirements
Nutrition, altered: more than body requirements
Nutrition, altered: risk for more than body requirements
Oral mucous membrane, altered
Pain
Pain, chronic
Parent/infant/child attachment altered, risk for
Parental role conflict
Parenting, altered
Parenting, altered, risk for
Peripheral neurovascular dysfunction, risk for
Personal identity disturbance
Poisoning, risk for
Posttrauma response
Powerlessness
Protection, altered

Rape-trauma syndrome
Rape-trauma syndrome: compound reaction
Rape-trauma syndrome: silent reaction
Relocation stress syndrome
Role performance, altered
Self-care deficit, bathing/hygiene
Self-care deficit, dressing/grooming
Self-care deficit, feeding
Self-care deficit, toileting
Self-esteem disturbance
Self-esteem, chronic low
Self-esteem, situational low
Self-mutilation, risk for
Sensory/perceptual alterations (specify) (visual, auditory, kinesthetic,
    gustatory, tactile, olfactory)
Sexual dysfunction
Sexuality patterns, altered
Skin integrity, impaired
Skin integrity, impaired, risk for
Sleep pattern disturbance
Social interaction, impaired
Social isolation
Spiritual distress (distress of the human spirit)
Spiritual well-being, potential for enhanced
Suffocation, risk for
Swallowing, impaired
Thermoregulation, ineffective
Thought processes, altered
Tissue integrity, impaired
Tissue perfusion, altered (specify type) (renal, cerebral,
    cardiopulmonary, gastrointestinal, peripheral)
Trauma, risk for
Unilateral neglect
Urinary elimination, altered
Urinary retention
Ventilation, inability to sustain spontaneous
Ventilatory weaning process, dysfunctional
Violence, risk for: self-directed or directed at others

▼ ▼ ▼ ▼ ▼ ▼ ▼ ▼ ▼ ▼   ▼ ▼ ▼

The Neurosensory System

STUDY OUTCOMES

After completing this chapter, the reader will be able to do the following:

▼ Identify major anatomic components and functions of the neurosensory system.

▼ Identify assessment findings of clients with alterations of the neurosensory system.

▼ Choose appropriate nursing diagnoses for clients with a neurosensory disorder.

▼ Implement appropriate nursing interventions for clients with a neurosensory disorder.

▼ Evaluate progress of clients with a neurosensory disorder for establishment of new nursing interventions based on evaluation findings.

KEY TERMS

Equilibrium	Body's orientation in space.
Nerve impulse	Depolarization and repolarization of a neuron generated by a chemical or physical stimuli.
Neurotransmitter	Chemical secreted by the neuron axon terminals, responsible for transmission of nerve impulses across synapses or spaces between either the neurons, neurons and muscle fibers, or neurons and glandular cells.
Proprioception	An individual's ability to sense body position and movement.
Reflex	Protective, learned response to a change in the pattern or frequency of sensory impulses that reach the spinal cord, such as pain.

CONTENT REVIEW

I. **The neurosensory system is responsible for receiving and transmitting information from all areas of the body and from external stimuli, for the purpose of controlling functions of the body**

II. **Structure and function**
   A. Central nervous system
      1. Protective structures
         a. Skull
         b. Meninges—membranes covering brain and spinal cord
            (1) Dura mater
            (2) Arachnoid
            (3) Pia mater
      2. Cerebrum—80% of the brain's bulk; right and left hemisphere, each with four lobes, connected by the corpus callosum
         a. Frontal lobes
            (1) Personality
            (2) Learning, problem solving
            (3) Moral behavior
            (4) Motor activity
            (5) Broca's area—speech (on dominant side)
            (6) Parietal lobes
            (7) Interprets sensory information—position sense, touch

    b. Temporal lobes
        (1) Hearing
        (2) Taste
        (3) Smell
        (4) Wernickes's area—comprehension of written and spoken language
    c. Occipital lobes—receives and interprets visual stimuli
  3. Cerebellum—two lateral hemispheres, separated by the vermis (worm-like middle lobe of the cerebellum)
    a. Coordinating movement
    b. Equilibrium
    c. Muscle tone
    d. Proprioception
  4. Brainstem
    a. Midbrain—relays information about muscle movement to other areas of the brain; cranial nerves III, IV originate here
    b. Pons—relays information to brain centers and lower spinal areas; cranial nerves V, VI, VII, VIII originate here
    c. Medulla oblongata—reflex center for involuntary functions (breathing, sneezing, swallowing, coughing, salivation, vomiting); cranial nerves IX, X, XI, XII originate here
  5. Cerebral ventricular system—four interconnecting ventricles that produce and circulate cerebrospinal fluid
  6. Diencephalon
    a. Thalamus—relay from the spinal cord and the cerebral cortex
    b. Hypothalamus
        (1) Regulates body temperature
        (2) Hunger, thirst
        (3) Generates autonomic nervous system responses
        (4) Controls pituitary gland hormonal secretions
    c. Epithalamus—contains the pineal gland, believed to be important in physical growth and sexual development

B. Spinal cord
  1. Protective structure—33 spinal vertebrae, divided into five regions: cervical, thoracic, lumbar, sacral, coccygeal
    a. Thirty-one segments with pair of spinal nerves from each segment
        (1) Cervical (8)—supplies neck, upper extremities, diaphragm, intercostal muscles
        (2) Thoracic (12)—supplies thoracic and abdominal areas

(3) Lumbar (5)—supplies lower extremities
(4) Sacral (5)—supplies lower extremities, urinary and bowel control
(5) Coccygeal (1)—supplies perineum
b. Anterior portion of the cord—descending motor tracts
c. Posterior portion of the cord—ascending sensory tracts
d. Lateral columns—preganglionic fibers for the autonomic nervous system

C. **Peripheral nervous system**
1. Cranial nerves—12 pairs that arise from the brain
2. Spinal nerves—31 pairs that arise from the spinal cord

D. **Autonomic nervous system**
1. Parasympathetic (craniosacral)—controls normal bodily functions
2. Sympathetic (thoracolumbar)—controls stress response

E. **Eye—produces vision when light is transmitted through the cornea and lens, to the retina, which is then transmitted to the optic nerve and finally to the occipital lobe of the brain**
1. Exterior structures
a. Cornea—clear fibrous covering of the eye
b. Sclera—outer layer of the eye
c. Eye muscles (6)—allow movement of the eye
d. Lacrimal glands—secrete tears to lubricate eyes; drains into the lacrimal ducts
2. Interior structures
a. Iris—muscle responsible for dilation and constriction of pupil; adds color to the eye
b. Lens—focuses images on retina
c. Aqueous humor—refraction medium for light; gel found in the anterior chamber
d. Vitreous humor—refraction medium for light; gel found in the posterior chamber
e. Chorioid—black, second layer of the eye
f. Retina—inner, photosensitive layer of the eye

F. **Ear—responsible for hearing and balance**
1. External structures
a. Pinna—flap of cartilage that collects sound waves and transmits them into the canal
b. Auditory meatus (external ear canal)—conducts sound waves toward the tympanic membrane; ceruminous glands in canal produce cerumen (wax) to protect the canal from small particles

      c. Tympanic membrane—pearl grey membrane found at the end of the auditory meatus; conducts sound waves to middle ear

  2. Middle ear

      a. Ossicles—three small bones: the malleus, the incus, and the stapes, vibrate and transmit sound to inner ear

      b. Eustachian tube—connection between inner ear and nasopharynx; equalizes pressure between middle ear and atmospheric pressure

  3. Inner ear

      a. Cochlea—spiral tube that contains the receptors for sound

      b. Controls balance

III. Targeted concerns

  A. Pharmacology: priority drug classifications

    1. Osmotic diuretics—increase osmotic pressure in the vascular space

      a. Expected effects—diuresis; decreases increased intracranial pressure

      b. Commonly given drugs

        (1) Mannitol (Osmitrol)

        (2) Urea (Ureaphil)

      c. Nursing considerations

        (1) Mannitol easily crystallizes—warm before infusing, then cool to body temperature before administering

        (2) In-line filter should be used to administer mannitol

        (3) Monitor blood pressure and pulse hourly for changing blood volume

          (a) Increased BP—indicative of fluid overload, which is transient

          (b) Decreased BP—indicative of dehydration

          (c) Tachycardia, which can be indicative of fluid overload or dehydration

        (4) Evaluate for signs of dehydration (decreased central nervous pressure (CVP) or skin turgor)

    2. Anticholinesterase drugs—prevent destruction of acetylcholine by inhibiting acetylcholinesterase

      a. Expected effect—decreases the symptoms of myasthenia gravis

      b. Commonly given drugs

        (1) Edrophonium choloride (Tensilon)—for diagnostic tests only

        (2) Pyridostigmine bromide (Mestinon)

        (3) Neostigmine bromide (Prostigmine Bromide)

   c. Nursing considerations

        (1) Parenteral atropine should be available for the advent of cholinergic crisis

        (2) Give 30 minutes before meals

3. Anticonvulsants—increase cerebral cortex threshold to reduce its response to stimuli

   a. Expected effect—depresses seizure activity

   b. Commonly given drugs

        (1) Phenobarbital (Luminal)

        (2) Phenytoin (Dilantin)

        (3) Carbamazepine (Tegretol)

        (4) Valproic acid (Depakene)

   c. Nursing considerations

        (1) Blood, renal, and liver studies must be monitored at specific intervals identified by physician for long-term use

        (2) Dilantin IV push must be given slowly, *only* into normal saline

        (3) Depakene must be given with food to avoid GI distress

4. Antidyskinetic drugs—increase the release of dopamine in the brain

   a. Expected effect—reduces the effects of Parkinson's disease

   b. Commonly given drugs

        (1) Levodopa (Larodopa)

        (2) Carbidopa/Levodopa (Sinemet)

        (3) Amantadine (Symmetrel)

   c. Nursing considerations

        (1) The physician may have to adjust dose of Symmetrel if effectiveness decreases (i.e., if tremors reappear)

        (2) Postural hypotension may be a problem

        (3) Caution client to avoid alcohol while taking medication

5. Cycloplegic or mydriatic ophthalmic agents—cause paralysis of the ciliary muscles of the eye

   a. Expected effect—dilates the pupil

   b. Commonly given drugs

        (1) Atropine sulfate

        (2) Scopolamine hydrobromide

   c. Nursing considerations

        (1) Inform clients they will be photophobic for the length of time the drugs are effective; advise physician if effect is longer than one week

        (2) Inform clients they will be unable to focus on near objects for as long as 24 hours

6. Miotic ophthalmic agents—cause contraction of the sphincter muscle of the iris; vasodilate vessels where the intraocular fluid leaves the eye

    a. Expected effect—pupillary constriction; treats glaucoma

    b. Commonly given drugs

        (1) Pilocarpine hydrochloride (Pilocar)

        (2) Carbachol (Carbacel)

        (3) Physostigmine salicylate (Eserine)

    c. Nursing considerations

        (1) Teach client correct method for eye drop administration: head tilted back, pull down on lower lid, place drop in cup of lower lid

        (2) Client should not touch tip of eye dropper to the eye

        (3) Client should be periodically evaluated for intraocular pressure changes

7. Beta blocking ophthalmic agents—decrease intraocular pressure by decreasing aqueous formation

    a. Expected effect—treats glaucoma

    b. Commonly given drugs

        (1) Timolol maleate (Timoptic)

        (2) Betaxolol hydrochloride (Betoptic)

    c. Nursing considerations

        (1) Some agents in this group are contraindicated in the client with chronic obstructive pulmonary disease (COPD) also called chronic airflow limitation (CAL)

        (2) Same precautions as in the previous group

8. Carbonic anhydrase inhibitors—inhibit the enzyme necessary for the formation of aqueous humor

    a. Expected effect—decreases intraocular pressure

    b. Commonly given drugs

        (1) Acetazolamide (Diamox)

        (2) Ethoxzolamide (Cardase)

    c. Nursing considerations

        (1) Assess for hypokalemia

        (2) Give with food

        (3) Avoid IM injections because of the extreme pain caused by injection of the medication

9. Antiinfectives ophthalmic agents—prevent bacterial cell wall synthesis

    a. Expected effect—attacks bacterial infection of the eye

      b. Commonly given drugs
- (1) Bacitracin ophthalmic ointment (Baciguent)
- (2) Neomycin sulfate (Myciguent)
- (3) Sulfacetamide sodium (Bleph-10)

      c. Nursing considerations
- (1) Remove exudate from the eye before instilling medication to enhance action
- (2) Instruct client on correct instillation of ointment into the eye—inner to outer canthus

B. Procedures

1. Lumbar puncture (spinal tap)—collects and evaluates CSF; measures pressure around spinal cord
2. X-rays of the skull, vertebral column—evaluate for abnormalities
3. CT scan—evaluates for bony and soft tissue abnormalities using cutaway views of the area
4. MRI scan—evaluates bony and soft tissue abnormalities using a magnetic force
5. Positron Emission Tomography (PET scan)—using radioactive substance, scans brain for structure and function
6. Cerebral arteriogram—radiopaque dye administered; arteries that feed the brain are visualized with x-rays
7. Electroencephalogram (EEG)—evaluates the electrical activity of the brain
8. Electromyography (EMG)—records nerve conduction in skeletal muscle
9. Evoked potentials—records brain activity in response to stimuli such as visual, auditory, or somatosensory
10. Snellen test (eye chart)—evaluates client visual acuity
11. Ophthalmoscopic exam—evaluates the inner structures of the eye
12. Intraocular pressure—measure intraocular pressure
13. Audiogram—evaluates hearing

C. Psychosocial

1. Anger—common in the client with limiting degenerative neurosensory disorders
2. Denial—common in the client with degenerative changes due to neurosensory disorders
3. Anxiety—common in the client unable to discern changes that will occur due to a neurosensory disorder
4. Immobility—very common in the client with neurologic impairment
5. Lifestyle changes—common in the client with neurosensory impairment due to decreased mobility

D. Health history—question sequence
1. What symptoms are you having that made it necessary for you to seek assistance?
2. When did your symptoms begin and how have they progressed?
3. What medical problems have you been treated for in the past and presently?
4. Is there a history of neurological or sensory disorders in your family?
5. Have you ever been hospitalized or had surgery? What for and when?
6. What medications are you presently taking, both prescriptions and over-the-counter medications?
7. Have you found it necessary to make changes in your daily routine?
8. What is your occupation?
9. Are there any toxic substances that you have been exposed to at your place of work or in your home?
10. Do you ever black out? If yes, how often and how long are you unconscious?
11. Do you feel, see, or hear anything unusual before you black out?
12. Would you ever consider yourself moody?
13. Do you ever have difficulty walking?
14. Do you ever feel strange sensations in your arms and legs, or anywhere else in your body?

E. Physical exam—appropriate sequence
1. Airway, breathing, circulation—vital signs
2. Pupillary response
3. Level of consciousness, orientation, mood, affect, memory, intellectual level, speech
4. Inspect head, neck and spine, eyes, ears, nose
5. Skull and spine palpation
6. Inspect muscle size, tone and strength in all major muscle groups
7. Inspect gait
8. Evaluate ability to feel touch and pain
9. Evaluate reflexes
10. Evaluate cranial nerves (Table 2-1)

IV. Pathophysiologic disorders

A. Cerebral vascular accident (CVA)
1. Definition—sudden disruption of blood supply to the brain, leading to ischemia and eventual necrosis of part of the brain

Table 2-1. Cranial Nerve Evaluation Procedures

Cranial Nerve	How to Assess
I Olfactory	Identify common smells
II Optic	Observe eye abnormalities, test vision
III Oculomotor	Test pupillary size and reaction; ptosis?
IV Trochlear	Client's eyes follow object in all directions
V Trigeminal	Clamp jaws, open jaws widely and back and forth; feels touch to face; sterile wisp of cotton to cornea causes blink
VI Abducens	Move eyes back and forth
VII Facial	Smile, frown, raise forehead and eyebrows, taste of different types of foods
VIII Acoustic	Auditory acuity
IX Glossopharyngeal	Uvula, palate rise symmetrically when client says "Ah"
X Vagus	Cough, speak
XI Spinal Accessory	Elevate shoulders, turn head to one side and the other, back and forward
XII Hypoglossal	Stick out tongue, move side to side

    2. Pathophysiology

       a. Ischemic—decreased blood flow to the brain tissue causes infarcted areas which will become edematous as a result of the infarct; if the infarcted areas are large enough the cerebral edema may increase to the point of displacing the brain and forcing it through the foramen magnum, causing death

       b. Hemorrhagic—neurons are damaged at the site of the hemorrhage; intracranial pressure is a result of the tissue edema from the injury and from the space occupying blood that has been spilling into the brain area and displacing brain; this type of CVA can also result in brain displacement through the foramen magnum, causing death

    3. Etiology

       a. Ischemic—thrombosis, embolism, decreased blood flow due to arteriosclerotic changes of the arteries

       b. Hemorrhagic—intracerebral hemorrhage usually from damage to the vessels as a result of long-term hypertension; subarachnoid hemorrhage as a result of a rupture of an intracranial aneurysm

    4. Incidence—third leading cause of death in the United States

5. Assessment
   a. Ask the following questions
      (1) Do you ever have periods of time when you feel weak?
      (2) Do you ever have difficulty speaking?
      (3) Have you ever had a period of time when your vision was impaired?
   b. Four stages of clinical manifestation
      (1) Transient Ischemic Attack (TIA)
         (a) Warning of impending CVA
         (b) Weakness
         (c) Aphasia—impaired language function
            (i) Expressive—(motor) words cannot be formed or spoken
            (ii) Receptive—(sensory) language cannot be understood
         (d) Drop-attack—drop to the floor for no apparent reason
         (e) Symptoms gone sometimes after minutes or within 24 hours
      (2) Reversible Ischemic Neurologic Deficit (RIND)
         (a) Similar to TIA but symptoms last longer than 24 hours
         (b) Risk of CVA is greatly enhanced at this stage
      (3) Stroke in evolution
         (a) Increasing neurologic deficits over a period of days
         (b) Clinical worsening, decreasing level of consciousness
      (4) Stroke
         (a) Right- or left sided weakness (hemiparesis) or paralysis (hemiplegia); deficit on opposite side of infarct
         (b) Aphasia (receptive most common in left lesions)
         (c) Left neglect—seen in right lesions; physical neglect of left side of the body
   c. Abnormal diagnostic tests
      (1) CT scan—identifies cause of CVA, placement in brain, and possible shift in brain contents
      (2) MRI—same as CT scan
      (3) Arteriography—identifies site of aneurysms, stenosis, and vessel abnormalities

6. Expected medical interventions
   a. Oral anticoagulation to prevent further intraarterial clot formation
   b. Aspirin or Persantine administration to decrease clot formation
   c. Measures to maintain BP at acceptable levels; drug therapy to raise or lower BP as needed
   d. Anticonvulsants to prevent seizures related to cerebral edema
   e. Mannitol to decrease cerebral edema
   f. Corticosteroids (Dexamethasone) to decrease cerebral edema
   g. Amicar, an antifibrinolytic agent, used to prevent rebleeding in the case of an aneurysm
7. Nursing diagnoses
   a. Ineffective airway clearance related to decreased neurologic status
   b. Altered physical mobility related to effects of hemiparesis or hemiplegia secondary to CVA
   c. Impaired verbal communication related to altered cerebral function
   d. Risk for injury related to altered mobility and/or seizures
8. Client goals
   a. Airway will remain clear as evidenced by clear upper airway sounds and respiratory rate of 16 to 20 breaths per minute
   b. Mobility will improve when clients begin to help turn themselves in bed and complete half of their ROM as active exercise
   c. Client will verbalize one new word per week
   d. Client will not be injured during hospitalization
9. Nursing interventions
   a. Acute care
      (1) Measures to reduce increased intracranial pressure include the following
         (a) HOB increased 15 to 30 degrees
         (b) Keep head and neck in alignment; avoid neck flexion
         (c) Avoid Valsalva's maneuver; administer stool softeners
         (d) Avoid bending, coughing, sneezing, or vomiting

(e) Avoid isometric energy expenditure (i.e., pushing up in bed)

(f) Maintain quiet, darkened environment

(g) Prohibit television or radio

(h) Encourage bedrest

(i) Limit visitors

(j) Prohibit rectal medications or temperatures

(2) Assess for increases in intracranial pressure

(a) Decreasing level of consciousness (LOC)

(b) Headache

(c) Projectile vomiting

(d) Elevated systolic BP with a stable diastolic pressure—results in a widened pulse pressure

(e) Bradycardia

(f) Pupils, unequal and become fixed and dilated

(g) Hyperthermia

(h) Slow, deep irregular respiratory pattern

(3) Prevent complications of immobility

(a) ROM to prevent contractures and frozen joints

(b) Turning to unaffected side and back q 2 hours to prevent skin breakdown

(c) Pad siderails to prevent injury due to seizures etc.

(d) Monitor bowel and bladder elimination

(e) Administer tube feedings safely

(i) High fowlers position or HOB up at least 30 degrees

(ii) Evaluate tube position in stomach

(iii) Feed slowly; feedings should be at room temperature with blue coloring added

(iv) Check residual q 4 hours to evaluate for full stomach and potential for regurgitation

(4) Maintain communication with client

(a) Use touch and gestures to assist communication

(b) Ask "yes" and "no" questions

(c) Use communication aids such as pictures or word cards

(d) Maintain an accepting environment

(e) Assist with initiation of speech therapy when client is stable

(f) Be patient

      b. Home care regarding client and family education
- (1) Many clients will start their rehabilitative phase in a rehabilitation center, preparing for home care from that level
- (2) Goals of rehabilitation
  - (a) Motor improvement
  - (b) Speech improvement
  - (c) Cognitive improvement
  - (d) Social and mental readjustment to new limitations
  - (e) Return of autonomy especially in activities of daily living (ADLs)
  - (f) Restoration of social activity and interpersonal relationships

10. Evaluation protocol
- a. How do I know that my interventions were effective?
  - (1) No assessment findings associated with increased intracranial pressure
  - (2) No complications of immobility
  - (3) Nutritional needs met safely
  - (4) Communication needs met with minimal frustration for the client
- b. What criteria will I use to change my interventions?
  - (1) Client exhibits assessment findings associated with increased intracranial pressure
  - (2) Client exhibits one or more complication of immobility (pressure sores, contractures, etc.)
  - (3) Client is losing weight indicating nutrition is not adequate or client is not tolerating feedings; complications of tube feedings are apparent
  - (4) Client is unable to make needs known and is becoming frustrated
- c. How will I know that my client teaching has been effective?
  - (1) Mobility is improved
  - (2) Speech is improved
  - (3) Client is gaining independence related to feeding and hygiene
  - (4) Client is performing one or more ADL per week
  - (5) Client is renewing interpersonal relationship with significant other

11. Older adult alert
- a. Because the older client is at higher risk for the complications of immobility, the nurse must be more vigilant in the prevention and early identification of problems

  b. The older adult population is most affected by CVAs

  c. When caring for an older client following a CVA, the nurse must consider other medical problems the client may have when planning care

B. **Brain tumors**

 1. Definition—abnormal growth in the cranial cavity; may be benign or malignant; may be a primary tumor or a metastatic lesion

 2. Pathophysiology—all brain tumors have the potential for being life threatening; early diagnosis gives a more promising outcome if the tumor is benign or malignant; the tumor is space occupying and creates pressure on brain tissue; edema will follow and eventually herniation of the brain down into the foramen magnum will cause death

 3. Etiology—many metastatic lesions originate from the lung or the breast; no known cause for primary brain tumors that do not metastasize to other areas of the body

 4. Incidence—equal incidence among males and females; metastatic lesions are more common than primary lesions

 5. Assessment

  a. Ask the following questions

   (1) Have you noticed any weakness in one area of your body?

   (2) Do you ever feel pins and needles or numbness in any area of your body?

   (3) Do you ever have difficulty speaking?

   (4) Do you ever have difficulty walking?

   (5) Do you experience headaches, dizziness, or seizures?

  b. Clinical manifestations

   (1) Weakness of an area of the body or half of the body (right or left)

   (2) Paresthesia

   (3) Difficulty speaking

   (4) Gait, personality, or vision changes

   (5) Headaches

   (6) Dizziness

   (7) Seizures

  c. Abnormal diagnostic tests

   (1) Skull x-rays—identifies lesion

   (2) Chest x-rays—may identify primary site

   (3) CT scan—identifies tumors, ventricular changes, shifts in brain mass

   (4) MRI—same as CT scan

        (5)   EEG—identifies slowing in areas of the brain that are affected by the tumor

        (6)   Cerebral angiogram—identifies tumor vascularity

6. Expected medical interventions
   a. Depends on type and location of the tumor
   b. Chemotherapy—intrathecal, in CSF
   c. Radiation therapy
   d. Intracranial surgery to remove or debulk tumor
7. Nursing diagnoses
   a. Anxiety related to unknown outcome of illness
   b. Pain related to pressure exerted on surrounding structures by tumor
   c. Risk for injury related to weakness or seizure activity secondary to cerebral edema
   d. Self-care deficit, bathing, and hygiene related to impaired mobility
8. Client goals
   a. Client will state that anxiety is decreased
   b. Client will state that pain is relieved or improved on a scale of 0 to 10; is 0 to 2
   c. Client will not be injured during hospitalization
   d. Client will begin to bathe self, each day bathing one more body area
9. Nursing interventions
   a. Acute care—postoperative care
      (1) Measures to decrease intracranial pressure (see CVA Acute Care)
      (2) Monitoring intracranial pressure—always compare postoperative vital signs and neurologic signs to preoperative signs (see CVA, Acute Care)
      (3) Assess I & O carefully; clients are usually kept slightly dehydrated to prevent cerebral edema
      (4) Assess head dressing for drainage and bleeding
      (5) Assess for any drainage from the nose or ears; if drainage identified, dipstick for glucose which if positive indicates cerebral spinal fluid
      (6) Do not pack ears or nose if drainage identified—may increase intracranial pressure
      (7) Use scrupulous aseptic technique when caring for incision and changing dressing (if ordered by physician) because risk for infection or meningitis is very great

        (8) Pad siderails to prevent injury as a result of seizure activity

    b. Home care regarding client and family education

        (1) Note changes in infection

        (2) Note changes if tumor increases in size or reestablishes

        (3) Increasing mobility in the home

        (4) Increasing independence in the home

10. Evaluation protocol

    a. How do I know that my interventions were effective?

        (1) Client exhibits no findings associated with increased intracranial pressure

        (2) Vital signs are within 10% of baseline for the client

        (3) Intake is approximately 10% less than output, keeping the client in a minimally dehydrated state

        (4) No bleeding from incision noted

        (5) No evidence of CSF leak

        (6) No evidence of infection

        (7) No seizure activity or injury

    b. What criteria will I use to change my interventions?

        (1) Increased ICP

        (2) Vital signs are not within 10% of baseline for the client

        (3) Intake is greater than output indicating fluid overload

        (4) Bleeding noted from incision

        (5) CSF leak noted

        (6) Increased temperature, increased WBC—indicative of postoperative infection

        (7) Seizure activity noted

    c. How will I know that my client teaching has been effective?

        (1) Client-family able to state signs and symptoms of infection

        (2) Able to state signs and symptoms of increasing tumor size

        (3) Mobility increases each day

        (4) Client becomes more independent each day

11. Older adult alert—as a normal course of aging the elderly client may exhibit slower reflexes. Careful preoperative evaluation must be done to establish a baseline for the client before surgery. Comparison of the postoperative status to the baseline will alert the nurse to appropriate changes in the postoperative period.

C. **Head injury**
   1. Definition—trauma or injury to the skull and/or brain as a result of impact to the head
   2. Pathophysiology
      a. Concussion—no changes in brain tissue; brain shaken causing a brief change in neurologic status
      b. Contusion—bruise of brain itself; caused by blow to the head
      c. Skull fracture—break in the skull; may be a linear fracture, nondisplaced fracture, or displaced fracture
      d. Hematomas (Figure 2-1)
         (1) Epidural—injury resulting in damage to an artery with rapid formation of a blood collection above the dura; death will occur if not treated very quickly
         (2) Subdural—injury resulting in damage to a vein with formation of a collection of blood below the dura; may be slow forming and assessment factors may not appear for weeks; classified as acute, subacute, or chronic differentiated by the length of time of hematoma formation
         (3) Intracerebral—associated with a cerebral laceration and edema of surrounding tissue; may be seen following a contusion
   3. Etiology—trauma from motor vehicle accidents, falls, and assaults
   4. Incidence—teenagers and young adults most frequently affected age group; over 2 million injuries occur per year

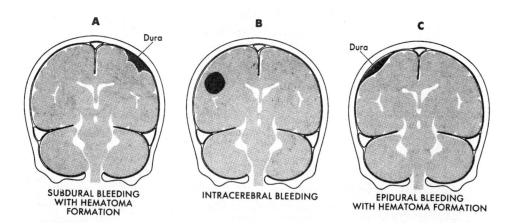

Figure 2-1. Types of hematomas. **A,** Subdural bleeding with hematoma formation. **B,** Intracerebral bleeding. **C,** Epidural bleeding with hematoma formation. (From Beare PG and Myers JL: *Principles and practice of adult health nursing,* ed 2, St Louis, 1994, Mosby.)

5. Assessment
   a. Ask the following questions
      (1) Do you have a headache?
      (2) Did you lose consciousness after your injury?
      (3) Tell me who you are? Where you are? What the date is?
      (4) Do you feel sick to your stomach?
   b. Clinical manifestations may include any or all of these
      (1) Decreased LOC
      (2) Posturing—usually in response to stimulation (usually bilateral but can be unilateral) (Figure 2-2)
          (a) Decorticate—indicates cortical damage
          (b) Decerebrate—indicates severe hemispheric damage
      (3) Headache
      (4) Pupil changes—size, equality, reaction
      (5) Nausea, vomiting
      (6) Elevated systolic BP with widened pulse pressure
      (7) Bradycardia
      (8) Slow, irregular respiratory pattern

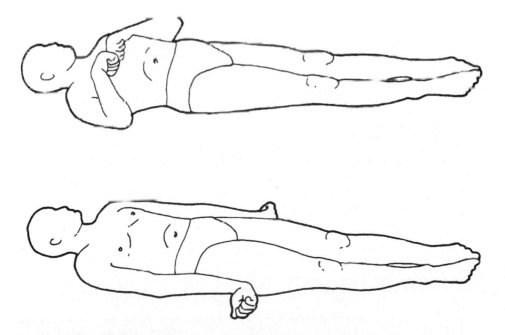

Figure 2-2. **A,** Decorticate posturing. **B,** Decerebrate posturing. (From AJN/Mosby *Nursing Board Review*, ed 9, St Louis, 1994, Mosby.)

    c. Abnormal laboratory findings
       (1) Electrolytes—hypernatremia or hyponatremia related to pressure on the hypothalamus and inappropriate antidiuretic hormone (ADH)
       (2) Serum alcohol elevated—high degree of injuries are alcohol related
    d. Abnormal diagnostic tests
       (1) Skull x-ray—fractures
       (2) Cervical x-ray—fracture or displacement; high incidence of cervical injury associated with cranial injury
       (3) CT scan—hematoma, shift of brain contents
       (4) MRI—same as CT scan
       (5) EEG—abnormal waves; used to help identify brain death
       (6) PET scan—brain tissue normal but metabolically hypoactive

6. Expected medical interventions
    a. Surgery—suture lacerations, drain hematomas and repair vascular injuries, debride wounds, repair skull abnormalities
    b. Drug therapy
       (1) Mannitol—to decrease cerebral edema
       (2) Anticonvulsants—to prevent seizure activity
       (3) Corticosteroids—to prevent or decrease cerebral edema
       (4) Antibiotics—prevent meningitis
    c. Mechanical ventilation if respiratory effort impaired; maintain slight respiratory ALKALOSIS, pCO_2 25 to 30, to help decrease cerebral edema for a maximum of 48 hours or if ICP is rising; refer to physician protocol
    d. ICP monitoring—to identify and treat increases in intracranial pressure >20
    e. Nutritional support—tube feeding or TPN until client is able to eat

7. Nursing diagnoses
    a. Ineffective airway clearance related to decreased neurologic status
    b. Pain related to injured cerebral tissue
    c. Impaired verbal communication related to decreased neurologic status
    d. Fluid volume excess or deficit related to altered ADH production and release

8. Client goals
   a. Client will maintain patent airway as evidenced by clear upper airway sounds
   b. Client will state head pain is decreased or relieved
   c. Client will verbally communicate with staff appropriately or write notes indicating needs
   d. I & O will be balanced; daily weight is stable within 1 kg of client baseline
9. Nursing interventions—identical to the care required of the client with a brain tumor or CVA
10. Evaluation protocol—identical to the evaluation protocol for the client with a brain tumor or CVA
11. Older adult alert
   a. If an older client is suffering from a head injury, it is usually related to a fall. The fall may be associated with another neurologic impairment such as a CVA. The client must be evaluated carefully for all possible injuries.
   b. Older client will also be at higher risk for all complications associated with a head injury
   c. Rehabilitation of older adult clients may be more difficult with the presence of other illnesses or of decreased endurance

D. Spinal cord injury (SCI)
   1. Definition—damage to the spinal cord as a result of fractured or displaced vertebrae, resulting in a loss of sensation and motor function below the level of the cord damage
   2. Pathophysiology—any movement in the vertebrae can cause compression, tearing, or transection of the cord; common areas affected are the cervical or lumbar vertebrae
   3. Etiology—trauma, such as motor vehicular accidents (MVA), falls, diving accidents, tumors, congenital defects, infectious or degenerative diseases
   4. Incidence—over 10,000 per year; usually seen in the young adult
   5. Assessment
      a. Ask the following questions
         (1) Are you having any difficultly breathing?
         (2) Can you feel me touching you here? Touch several areas below the level of injury.
         (3) Can you wiggle your toes? your fingers?
      b. Clinical manifestations
         (1) Loss of movement below the level of injury
         (2) Loss of sensation below the level of injury
         (3) Decreased or absent bowel and bladder function

         (4) Loss of perspiration below the level of injury

         (5) All autonomic functions are uncertain below the level of injury

         (6) Pain

         (7) Fever

         (8) Spinal shock

             (a) Total loss of sensory, motor, and autonomic function below the level of injury. Example: urine retention

             (b) Hypotension

             (c) Bradycardia

             (d) Lasts several days to several months

   c. Abnormal laboratory findings

         (1) Serum chemistry—hypoglycemia or hyperglycemia, electrolyte imbalance

         (2) CBC—decreased H&H

   d. Abnormal diagnostic tests

         (1) Spinal x-rays—vertebral fractures or displacement

         (2) CT scan—spinal cord edema and injury

         (3) MRI—same as CT scan

6. Expected medical interventions

   a. Immobilization of entire spine requires use of Gardner tongs or Halo traction and a specialized bed, such as a Stryker frame or rotational bed for turning and care (Figure 2-3)

   b. Surgery to remove bone fragments and, in some instances, to place bone graft to bring stability to vertebral column

   c. Corticosteroids—high dose is now recommended

   d. Support of respiratory function with use of mechanical ventilation if necessary

   e. Support fluid volume as necessary

7. Nursing diagnoses

   a. Altered cardiac output related to loss of vascular tone secondary to spinal cord injury

   b. Ineffective breathing pattern related to interrupted spinal cord impulses

   c. Impaired physical mobility related to loss of muscle control below the level of spinal cord injury

8. Client goals

   a. Client will demonstrate an appropriate cardiac output as evidenced by BP within 10% of baseline

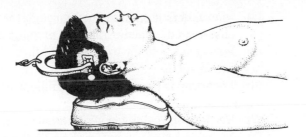

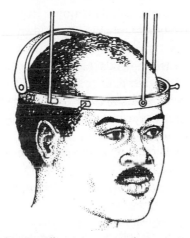

Figure 2-3. **A,** Gardner-Wells tongs. **B,** Halo ring. (From Beare PG and Myers JL: *Principles and practice of adult health nursing,* ed 2, St Louis, 1994, Mosby.)

    b. Client will demonstrate an effective breathing pattern as evidenced by respiratory rate and depth within 10% of baseline

    c. Client will demonstrate appropriate muscle tone in all appropriate muscle groups

9. Nursing interventions

    a. Acute care

      (1) Respiratory function is maintained either through the use of mechanical ventilation or through coughing and deep breathing q 2 hours

      (2) Cardiovascular status is assessed and maintained with the use of fluid and vasopressor therapy per physician order

      (3) Vertebral immobility and skeletal traction with appropriate alignment is maintained per physician orders

(4) Joint mobility is maintained through the advent of passive and/or active range of motion exercises

(5) Wrist contractures are prevented through the use of splints

(6) Foot-drop is prevented through the use of high-top sneakers or splints

(7) Evaluate for pulmonary infections

(8) Maintain bladder function through the use of continuous or intermittent bladder drainage

(9) Monitor for urinary tract infection

(10) Begin bowel training program once bowel function has resumed; daily timed Bisacodyl suppository

(11) Prevention of skin breakdown through use of turning regime and meticulous hygiene

(12) Nutrition needs met per physician orders via tube feed, enteral, or parenteral nutrition

(13) Assist with psychologic impact of injury

b. Home care regarding client and family education—rehabilitative phase

(1) Autonomic dysreflexia—any client with lesion above T6 is at risk

(a) Result of noxious stimuli below the level of the injury causing organ reflex activity

(b) Bowel or bladder distention is common cause

(c) Distention causes exaggerated stimulation of sympathetic nervous system

(d) Rapid increase in BP

(e) Bradycardia

(f) Severe headache

(g) Flushing

(h) Profuse sweating

(i) Treatment

(i) Remove cause

(ii) Decrease BP with short acting antihypertensive agent

(iii) Elevate head of bed to help decrease BP

(2) Self-intermittent catheterization if client is able

(3) Monitoring respiratory status for findings associated with infection

(4) Monitoring urinary tract for findings associated with infections

(5) Skin care, a long-standing need

        (6) Maintaining mobility

        (7) Maintaining joint function and contracture prevention with active-passive range of motion

10. Evaluation protocol

    a. How do I know that my interventions were effective?

        (1) Appropriate respiratory status—rate is 16 to 20 breaths per minute with appropriate depth and ABGs within 10% of client baseline

        (2) BP and pulse within 10% of client baseline

        (3) Appropriate skeletal alignment with no further cord damage

        (4) Appropriate joint functions

        (5) No contractures

        (6) No foot-drop

        (7) No pulmonary or genitourinary infections

        (8) Acceptable attainment of bowel training

        (9) No skin breakdown

        (10) Minimal or no weight loss (less than 5 kg)

        (11) Psychological adjustment to impairment

    b. What criteria will I use to change my interventions?

        (1) BP, HR, RR or depth of respiration are greater than 10% of client baseline

        (2) New neurologic instability

        (3) Joint immobilities

        (4) Foot-drop

        (5) Pulmonary or genitourinary (GU) infection

        (6) Fecal incontinence or constipation

        (7) Skin breakdown

        (8) Weight loss >5 kg

        (9) Emotional liability and inability to discuss body changes

    c. How will I know that my client teaching has been effective?

        (1) Client-family able to state cause, signs, symptoms, and treatment of autonomic dysreflexia

        (2) Able to demonstrate appropriate intermittent catheterization technique

        (3) Able to state findings associated with respiratory and GU infections that should be brought to the attention of the physician

        (4) Able to demonstrate correct skin care

        (5) Able to demonstrate correct range of motion exercises and methods to maintain joint function

11. Older adult alert
   a. The nurse must be very aware of the complications associated with the spinal cord injured client and remember the older adult client is a higher risk for these complications
   b. The older adult client suffering from congestive heart failure or chronic lung disease may not be able to lay flat
   c. The older adult client is easily disoriented. One method to hinder this is to prevent sensory deprivation by ensuring that the older adult client is wearing glasses and hearing aids to maintain appropriate sensory input.

E. **Chronic degenerative neurologic diseases—Parkinson's syndrome, multiple sclerosis, amyotrophic lateral sclerosis, and myasthenia gravis. For the definition, etiology, incidence, pathophysiology, assessment, and expected medical intervention, see Table 2-2.**
   1. Nursing diagnoses
      a. Self-care deficit, bathing, and hygiene related to physical mobility impairment and weakness
      b. Body image disturbance related to changes in body function and inability to perform functions independently
      c. Impaired home maintenance management related to weakness and immobility
      d. Ineffective individual-family coping related to deteriorating health status
   2. Client goals
      a. Client will continue to perform several aspects of the ADL as long as possible and assist when possible
      b. Client will state comfort with changes occurring in the body
      c. Client will indicate that home maintenance is managed by other family members or resources as necessary
      d. Client will attain acceptable coping skills
   3. Nursing interventions
      a. Maintain independence
         (1) Help client identify optimal activity level
         (2) Teach client to balance rest and activity
         (3) Encourage use of assistive devices

Table 2-2. Comparison of Chronic Degenerative Neurological Diseases

	Parkinsonism	Multiple Sclerosis	Amyotrophic Lateral Sclerosis	Myasthenia Gravis
Onset age	50-60 years	20-40 years	40-70 years	20-50 years
Sex	Male > female	Female > male	Male > female	Female > male
Etiology	Unknown	Unknown; virus/autoimmune origin suspected	Unknown; virus/autoimmune origin suspected	Unknown; autoimmune origin suspected; occurs in cool climates
Area affected	Substantia nigra cells in basal ganglia	Disseminated demyelinated plaques in white matter of brain and spinal cord	Motor neurons in brain and spinal cord	Myoneural junction of voluntary muscle
Pathophysiology	Impaired coordinated muscle movement and autonomic dysfunction because of deficiency of dopamine	Impaired nerve impulse conduction because of destruction of myelin	Impaired nerve impulse conduction because of degeneration of motor neurons	Impaired transmission of nerve impulse to skeletal muscle possibly because of acetylcholine deficiency
Findings	Rigidity Slow movements Nonintentional tremor Autonomic dysfunction	Depends on site of plaque: ▶ Visual problems ▶ Spastic weakness/paralysis ▶ Poor coordination ▶ Paresthesias	Twitching Muscle weakness, progressing to atrophy and paralysis of upper and lower extremities	Profound muscle weakness and fatigue Can progress to respiratory failure (myasthenic crisis)

Continued.

43

Table 2-2. Comparison of Chronic Degenerative Neurological Diseases—cont'd

	Parkinsonism	Multiple Sclerosis	Amyotrophic Lateral Sclerosis	Myasthenia Gravis
		▶ Speech defects ▶ Intentional tremor ▶ Bowel/bladder dysfunction ▶ Emotional disorders ▶ Exacerbations and remissions	Usually fatal 2-15 years after onset	
Treatment	Supportive Medication	Symptomatic	Symptomatic	Supportive Medication Surgery sometimes: thymectomy
Medication	Levodopa Carbidopa/levodopa (Sinemet)	Muscle relaxants Antiinflammatories (steroids) during exacerbation	Antibiotics for respiratory and urinary tract infections	Anticholinesterase: Diagnosis—Edrophonium chloride (Tensilon) Maintenance—Pyridostigmine bromide (Mestinon) Antiinflammatories (steroids) during acute phase

From *AJN/Mosby: AJN/Mosby Nursing Boards Review*, ed 9, St Louis, 1994, Mosby.

      b. Prevent complications
- (1) Assist client in diet selections-planning that will prevent constipation and maintain nutritional status
- (2) Help client and family be alert to skin care needs, risk of breakdown, and prevention of breakdown
- (3) Encourage ROM exercises and deep breathing exercises for the prevention of joint and muscle disuse and pulmonary infections
- (4) Implement the use of self-catheterization if necessary to prevent GU infection

      c. Provide appropriate care and guidelines in all settings
- (1) When hospitalization is necessary and when a long-term care facility may be necessary
- (2) How to obtain help in the home with care and instruction
- (3) How to obtain physical therapy and vocational therapy as needed

      d. Provide education and emotional support for client and family—assist them in making contact with appropriate support groups and agencies that offer resources for education or care assistance

  4. Evaluation protocol

      a. How will I know that my interventions and teaching were effective?
- (1) Client-family able to demonstrate independence and ability to cope with new situations
- (2) Able to identify those situations that require physician intervention or hospitalization
- (3) Able to indicate how to obtain help from community agencies or other resources
- (4) Able to state how to prevent some of the more common complications of the disease process

  5. Older adult alert

      a. The older adult client will develop complications of the disorders more often than the younger adult and must be evaluated aggressively for these difficulties

F. **Glaucoma**

  1. Definition—disorder characterized by an increase in intraocular pressure, resulting in blindness if untreated. Primary open-angle glaucoma (POAG), the most common form, has slow onset with few symptoms; closed-angle glaucoma has acute onset with severe eye pain.

2. Pathophysiology
   a. Open-angle—resistance to flow of aqueous humor out of posterior chamber as a result of thickened collecting channels or canal of Schlemm (normal drainage canal)
   b. Closed-angle—iris is abnormally situated and prevents drainage through the normal drainage canal
3. Etiology
   a. Heredity
   b. Eye trauma
   c. Diabetes
   d. Eye surgery
4. Incidence—leading cause of blindness; higher incidence in the African American population
5. Assessment
   a. Ask the following questions
      (1) Have you noticed that you have been losing the ability to see objects to your sides?
      (2) Have you noticed you have been bumping into objects lately?
      (3) Have you experienced halos around lights or blurring of vision?
      (4) Have you experienced eye pain?
   b. Clinical manifestations
      (1) Chronic open-angle
         (a) Loss of peripheral vision
         (b) Eventual loss of central vision
      (2) Acute closed-angle
         (a) Early stage findings suggest it often occurs in the evening and is intermittent
            (i) Blurred vision
            (ii) Halos around lights
            (iii) Frontal headache
            (iv) Eye pain
         (b) Acute stage findings
            (i) Severe eye pain
            (ii) Photophobia
            (iii) Increased lacrimation
   c. Abnormal diagnostic tests—intraocular pressure measured and higher than 20 mm Hg
6. Expected medical interventions
   a. Miotic ophthalmic drops to constrict the pupil and/or decrease formation of the aqueous humor by the ciliary body

    b. Surgery (iridectomy) or laser (iridotomy) therapy are indicated when medical treatments are not effective; however, the severity of blindness may guide the treatment and outcomes

7. Nursing diagnoses

    a. Anxiety related to vision changes and possible loss of vision

    b. Pain related to increased intraocular pressure

    c. Sensory-perceptual alteration—loss of peripheral vision related to damage to intraocular structures

8. Client goals

    a. Client will state anxiety is decreased

    b. Client will state pain or other findings is decreased or relieved

    c. Client will indicate accommodations made for loss of peripheral vision

9. Nursing interventions

    a. Acute care

        (1) Bedrest to help relieve pain

        (2) Quiet environment, dimmed lighting

        (3) Analgesics and antiemetics as needed

        (4) Allow sleeping on back and on unoperative side

        (5) Avoid straining at stool

        (6) If eyesight impaired

            (a) Direct all speaking to client

            (b) Avoid nonverbal communication

    b. Home care regarding client education

        (1) How to instill eye drops correctly

        (2) How to prevent further eye damage; damage already done to the eye cannot be reversed

        (3) Need for lifelong medical treatment

        (4) Need for routine eye exams

        (5) Need for avoiding upper body strength activities to prevent increased intraocular pressure

        (6) How to alter diet to decrease sodium intake

10. Evaluation protocol

    a. How will I know that my interventions were effective?

        (1) Pain is relieved

        (2) Communication with client is acceptable

    b. What criteria will I use to change my interventions?

        (1) Pain is unrelieved

        (2) Communication is frustrating for the client

      c. How will I know that my client teaching has been effective?
- (1) Client able to demonstrate correct eye drop administration
- (2) Able to state instillation of eye drops is a must for remainder of life
- (3) Able to state that routine exams must be done at least yearly
- (4) Able to indicate which activities should not be performed to prevent increased IOP
- (5) Able to state change after eliminating salt from diet

11. Older adult alert
- a. Glaucoma must be considered when assessing an older adult client with visual disturbances

G. Cataracts

1. Definition—opacity of the crystalline lens of the eye
2. Pathophysiology—the thickness and the denseness of the lens increases with age as a result of the formation of new fiber cells in the lens; also a result of molecule deterioration caused by the absorption of ultraviolet radiation
3. Etiology—breakdown of the metabolic process of the lens, or trauma
4. Incidence—found commonly in population >55 years of age
5. Assessment
   - a. Ask the following questions
     - (1) Do you have difficulty seeing?
     - (2) Have you just recently noticed difficulty seeing or has this been a gradual change?
     - (3) Do you have any pain in your eye?
   - b. Clinical manifestations
     - (1) Blurred vision
     - (2) Gradual loss of vision
     - (3) Painless changes in vision
   - c. Abnormal diagnostic test—ophthalmoscopic exam indicating presence of cataracts
6. Expected medical interventions
   - a. Surgical removal of the lens, usually on an outpatient basis
   - b. Intraocular lens placement following surgery
   - c. Contact lenses may be prescribed following surgery, or glasses to replace natural lens
7. Nursing diagnoses
   - a. Sensory-perceptual alterations related to changes in visual acuity
   - b. Risk for injury related to change in visual acuity

8. Client goals
   a. Client will indicate having made acceptable adjustments for decreased vision
   b. Client will be free of injury
9. Nursing interventions
   a. Acute care—postoperative in recovery area for 2 to 3 hours before discharge to home
      (1) Deep breaths, no coughing
      (2) Keep head of bed elevated 30 to 45 degrees
      (3) Turn client only to unaffected side to prevent an increase in intraocular pressure in affected eye
      (4) Check under the eye shield and dressing for bleeding
      (5) Treat nausea immediately to prevent vomiting which causes increased intraocular pressure
      (6) Report severe eye pain immediately to physician; could be acute glaucoma
   b. Home care regarding client education
      (1) Do not remove eye shield or dressing until instructed to by physician; afterwards the eye is protected with glasses or a shaded lens during the day with an eye shield at night
      (2) Instill eye medications as ordered
      (3) Visits to physician may be daily for 4 to 5 days if outpatient surgery done
      (4) Avoid activities that would cause straining, bending, or lifting until the initial postoperative physician visit
      (5) Prevent coughing or sneezing until seen by the physician postoperatively
      (6) Do not squeeze the eyelids shut, rub or place pressure on eyes until seen by the physician postoperatively
      (7) Cataract glasses
         (a) Magnify objects by one third
         (b) Vision clear only in the center of the lens
      (8) Contact lenses will be more clear than cataract glasses but more expensive
10. Evaluation protocol
    a. How will I know that my interventions were effective?
       (1) Client is deep breathing but not coughing
       (2) Client is turning only to the unaffected side
       (3) No bleeding noted
       (4) Nausea was treated and vomiting averted
       (5) No severe pain noted

        b.   What criteria will I use to change my interventions?
- (1) Client is coughing or vomiting
- (2) Client is turning to affected side
- (3) Bleeding noted on dressing
- (4) Client admits to pain, becoming more severe

        c.   How will I know that my client teaching has been effective?
- (1) Client able to state activities to be avoided
- (2) Able to state appropriate home care for dressings, physician visits
- (3) Able to state how the cataract glasses or contact lenses will affect vision
- (4) Able to demonstrate installation of ordered eye medication

11. Older adult alert
    a.   As a common disorder of the older adult, cataracts must be considered when assessing an older adult client with visual disturbances
    b.   The older adult client may not be able to provide self-care postsurgery due to eye shield and impaired vision; may require assistance for a period of time

H. **Retinal detachment**
1. Definition—fluid collecting between the neural and pigment layers of the retina
2. Pathophysiology—vitreous humor seeps through an opening in the retina and separates the retina from the pigment epithelium and choroid
3. Etiology—recent or previous trauma, retinal degeneration, and recent cataract surgery
4. Incidence—more common after the age of 50 but can occur as a result of trauma at any age
5. Assessment
    a.   Ask the following questions
- (1) Did you notice a flash of light or sparks in front of your eyes?
- (2) Do you ever see small specks, spots, or clumps floating in front of your eyes?
- (3) Did you experience the loss of part of your vision?

    b.   Clinical manifestations
- (1) Flashes—described as flashes of light, or sparks in front of eyes; more common when entering a dark room
- (2) Floaters—described as specks, spots, or clumps before the eyes

        (3)   Curtain effect—described as a shade being pulled over part of the visual field

        (4)   Blurred vision that becomes worse

        (5)   Loss of visual field

        (6)   On ophthalmoscopic exam the retina hangs like a torn curtain

6. Expected medical interventions
   a. Cryotherapy or laser photocoagulation to seal any breaks in the retina
   b. Scleral buckling—suturing a compatible material on the sclera at the site of the break
7. Nursing diagnoses—same as for the client with cataracts
8. Client goals—same as for the client with cataracts
9. Nursing interventions
   a. Acute care
      (1) Preoperative
         (a) Bilateral patching may be ordered to decrease eye movement
         (b) Mydriatics and antibiotic eye medications may be used
      (2) Postoperative—care identical to the care of the client having cataract surgery
   b. Home care—same as the client having cataract surgery
10. Older adult alert—same as the client having cataract surgery

I. Deafness
1. Definition— complete or partial loss of hearing
2. Pathophysiology
   a. Conductive hearing loss—sounds cannot be conducted through the outer and middle ear; can be improved by hearing aid because the inner ear structures are intact
   b. Sensorineural hearing loss—impaired sensory or neural components of hearing in the inner ear; will not benefit from a hearing aid
3. Etiology—infection, ototoxic substances, trauma, noise, aging process
4. Incidence—most common disability in the United States; over 25 million Americans suffer from this disorder
5. Assessment
   a. Ask the following questions
      (1) Do you have difficulty understanding words?
      (2) Do you have a ringing in your ears?

      b. Clinical manifestations
         (1) Progressive loss of hearing
         (2) Eventual loss of the ability to understand the spoken word
         (3) Tinnitus
         (4) Distorted or abnormal sounds
      c. Abnormal diagnostic tests—audiometric test—decreased hearing acuity

6. Expected medical interventions
      a. Hearing aid if found to be effective
      b. Cochlear implants

7. Nursing diagnoses
      a. Sensory—perceptual alterations—auditory related to trauma, infection, ototoxic substances, noise, aging process
      b. Risk for injury related to decreased auditory acuity

8. Client goals
      a. Client will state adjustments in lifestyle made to accommodate for changes in hearing
      b. Client will be injury free

9. Nursing interventions regarding client education
      a. How to care for and clean hearing aid device
      b. Keep device free of ear wax
      c. Prevent device from getting wet
      d. How to check the battery
      e. Keep device out of extreme heat

10. Evaluation protocol
      a. How will I know that my client teaching has been effective?
         (1) Client shows correct method for placing device
         (2) Client demonstrates how to test battery
         (3) Client demonstrates correct cleaning
         (4) Client states in what type of environment device should be stored

11. Older adult alert
      a. Being a more common disorder of the older adult, hearing assessment is important to include as part of routine assessment

REVIEW QUESTIONS

1. The client who experienced neurologic changes in relation to a transient ischemic attack will typically have had evidence of these changes for
   a. Several hours
   b. Several days
   c. Longer than 24 hours
   d. Over 2 to 3 months

2. In reading a client's plan of care the nurse has identified interventions which relate to the client's hemiparesis. The nurse would expect to see
   a. Padded siderails
   b. Full active range of motion
   c. Full active and passive range of motion
   d. The use of picture aids for communication

3. When assessing a client for an increase in intracranial pressure, the nurse would prioritize the assessment in which manner?
   a. Level of consciousness, respiratory rate, blood pressure, pupillary reaction
   b. Pupillary reaction, level of consciousness, respiratory rate, blood pressure
   c. Blood pressure, level of consciousness, respiratory rate, pupillary reaction
   d. Respiratory rate, blood pressure, level of consciousness, pupillary reaction

4. When caring for the client with head trauma, a priority of care would be to prevent transient increases in intracranial pressure. A nursing intervention aimed at preventing this would be to
   a. Administer antiemetics as soon as nausea occurs
   b. Maintain the client in a flat position with proper head and neck alignment
   c. Encourage television and radio for sound diversion
   d. Perform only rectal temperatures for accuracy

5. A classic finding associated with an increase in intracranial pressure is
   a. Tachycardia
   b. Hypotension
   c. Projectile vomiting
   d. A slow deep regular respiratory pattern

6. The client who has suffered a spinal cord injury is at great risk for foot-drop. This is best prevented through the use of
   a. Traction
   b. Physical therapy
   c. High-top sneakers
   d. Range of motion exercises

7. A complication of spinal cord injury, during the rehabilitative stage, is autonomic dysreflexia and manifested by
   a. Increased BP, decreased HR, severe headache
   b. Decreased BP, increased HR, severe headache
   c. Increased/decreased BP, increased HR, decreased level of consciousness
   d. Increased/decreased BP, increased/decreased HR, dry, hot skin

8. In the client who has undergone cataract surgery, an activity that would be discouraged due to the risk of increased intraocular pressure is
   a. Reading
   b. Sewing
   c. Gardening
   d. Driving

9. Client teaching has been effective if when instilling eye drops the client
   a. Drops the drop onto closed eyes
   b. Holds the upper lid open and allows the drop to drop onto the eye
   c. Pulls down on the lower lid and drops the drop onto the eye
   d. Pulls down the lower lid and drops the drop into the lower lid

10. Client teaching, preoperatively, for clients with a retinal detachment must include
    a. How to instill eye drops
    b. That both eyes will be patched to prevent any eye movement in the affected eye
    c. That they will wear dark glasses before surgery due to photophobia
    d. What activities clients can engage in postoperatively

ANSWERS, RATIONALES, AND TEST-TAKING TIPS

Rationale	Test-Taking Tips

1. **Correct answer: a**

   The client experiencing a TIA should have resolution of symptoms within several minutes or within 24 hours; longer time would be characterized as RIND, an evolving stroke or CVA.

   The key word in the question is "transient." This is a clue to look for a response that is less than 24 hours. Note that responses *b* and *c* are similar—days being the common element; therefore these two responses can be eliminated with *a* and *d* left. Common sense plus the word "transient" in the question eliminates response *d*.

2. **Correct answer: c**

   The client with hemiparesis, or weakness on one side of the body will require active range of motion for the side not affected, and passive range of motion for the side affected with hemiparesis.

   To select the correct response one must focus on the client's strengths and weaknesses. If you only focused on "hemiparesis" the approach was too narrow.

3. **Correct answer: d**

   The client with increasing intracranial pressure must be first assessed for Airway, Breathing and Circulation followed by the first criteria to change—level of consciousness then pupillary reaction.

   ABC's have the priority. Then the major dysfunction becomes the next focus.

4. **Correct answer: a**

   Following head trauma, the client's head must be elevated at least 30 degrees at all times; the client should not be allowed to be stimulated by the television

   The key word is "prevent." The only action that prevents is the response in *a*. Do not assume that a head trauma client cannot respond; if you assumed this then the other choices would have been chosen.

or the radio, and and should
not have rectal stimulation.
Immediately treat nausea to
prevent vomiting.

5. **Correct answer: c**

Manifestations of increased
intracranial pressure are:
hypertension with widened
pulse pressure, slow deep
irregular respiratory pattern,
bradycardia, and projectile
vomiting.

The key words are "classic finding"
of increased ICP. The approach
here is to ask as you read each
option, "Is this a true or false
statement?"

6. **Correct answer: c**

High-top sneakers provide the
best prevention of foot-drop
for clients at risk. All other
responses are too general,
not specific enough, to best
answer the question.

Clustering responses *b* and *d* under
the theme of intermittent therapy
eliminates them. Sneakers are
more of a continuous therapy.
Traction doesn't have anything to
do with foot-drop prevention.

7. **Correct answer: a**

Manifestations of autonomic
dysreflexia are: severe rapid
onset of hypertension,
bradycardia, flushing,
profuse sweating, and severe
headache.

Associate that an autonomic or
sympathetic dysreflexia is a hyper
situation. Narrow the responses to
b or *c* that has hypertension—
match the hyper themes. A
change in LOC has nothing to do
with spinal cord injury especially
in the rehab phase. Think of days
of high stress or sympathetic
stimulation when most people end
up with headaches.

8. **Correct answer: c**

Gardening would require upper
body straining activities,
which are contraindicated in
the client at risk for
increased intraocular

Associate that strain will increase
pressures. The given activity that
will strain the most is response *c*.

pressure; driving would be
contraindicated but not due
to the risk of increasing
intraocular pressure.

9. **Correct answer: d**
   Correct method for a client to
   use to instill eye drops is to
   pull down on the lower lid,
   evert the lid, and place the
   drop on the cup formed by
   the lower lid.

   Recall that the eye is very sensitive
   and this eliminates responses *b*
   and *c*. Common sense eliminates
   response *a*.

10. **Correct answer: b**
    Clients must be taught
    preoperatively the rationale
    for bilateral patching—when
    one eye moves, the other
    will move as well, so to
    restrict movements both
    eyes must be patched;
    postoperative teaching
    would not take priority over
    the education required about
    patching; dark glasses are
    not worn preoperatively.

    Look—retinal detachment—two
    words for the condition means two
    patches on the eyes. Cataracts is
    one word thus use only one patch.

The Cardiac System

CHAPTER

3

STUDY OUTCOMES

After completing this chapter, the reader will be able to do
the following:

▼ Identify major anatomic components and functions of the cardiac
system.
▼ Assess a cardiac client using the appropriate technique and
sequence.
▼ Choose the appropriate nursing diagnoses for the client with a
cardiac disorder.
▼ Implement the appropriate nursing interventions for the client with
a cardiac disorder.
▼ Evaluate the progress of the client with a cardiac disorder for
establishment of new nursing interventions based on evaluation
findings.

KEY TERMS

Cardiac output (CO)	The amount of blood ejected from the ventricles; CO = heart rate × stroke volume.
Conduction	The movement of formed electrical impulses through the heart; these stimulate the chambers of the heart to contract.
Contractility	The force of myocardial contraction.
Diastole	Relaxation of the chambers of the heart; results in filling of the chambers; desired diastolic BP <90 mm Hg.
Systole	Contraction of the chambers of the heart; results in the emptying of the chambers; desired systolic BP <140 mm Hg.

CONTENT REVIEW

I. **The cardiac system is the system in the body responsible for pumping (1) oxygenated blood (arterial) to the cells so that cellular nutrition and oxygenation can be accomplished, and (2) deoxygenated blood (venous) back to the pulmonary system for the purpose of replenishing oxygen**

II. **Structure and function**
   A. The heart is a muscular organ, approximately the size of an adult fist; positioned directly on the diaphragm, between the lungs
      1. Layers of the heart and coverings
         a. The heart is covered with a double thickness membrane— the pericardium
         b. Epicardium—outermost covering
         c. Myocardium—muscle layer itself
         d. Endocardium—innermost covering
      2. Heart chambers
         a. Right atrium—receives venous blood from systemic circulation
         b. Left atrium—receives arterial blood from the lungs
         c. Right ventricle—receives blood from the right atrium; pumps to the pulmonic circulation

      d. Left ventricle—receives blood from the left atrium; pumps out to the systemic circulation

  3. Valves—maintain a forward flow of blood through the heart

      a. Tricuspid—between the right atrium and ventricle and attached to papillary muscle

      b. Pulmonic—between the right ventricle and the lungs; base of pulmonary artery

      c. Mitral—between the left atrium and ventricle and attached to papillary muscle

      d. Aortic—between the left ventricle and aorta

  4. Conduction system

      a. Specialized cells initiate an electrical impulse

      b. Transmits impulse throughout the heart

      c. Stimulates chambers of the heart to contract in a coordinated pattern

      d. Impulse sequence

         (1) Sinoatrial node (SA)—impulse origination

         (2) Impulse fans out across both atria; followed by atrial contraction

         (3) Recollects at the atrioventricular node (AV)

         (4) Travels through the Bundle of His—top of septum

         (5) Moves into the Purkinje fibers in the ventricles; followed by ventricular contraction

      e. Depolarization—ion exchange in conduction cells

         (1) Potassium leaves cell

         (2) Sodium enters cell

         (3) Calcium enters cell through slow calcium channels; calcium is released in large quantities

      f. Repolarization—ions return to normal balance

         (1) Potassium returns to cell

         (2) Sodium leaves cell

III. Targeted concerns

  A. Pharmacology—priority drug classifications

    1. Cardiac glycosides—increase the force of myocardial contraction

      a. Expected effects—increase in cardiac output with increase in urine output in some cases; slows the rate of impulse initiation from the SA node and movement through the AV node in order to decrease in heart rate

      b. Commonly given drugs

         (1) Digoxin (Lanoxin)

         (2) Digitoxin

   c. Nursing considerations
- (1) Hold drug for HR <60 or >120; notify physician within 2 to 3 hours
- (2) Assess for hypokalemia; most common finding is lower leg cramps; low potassium potentiates action of digitalis drugs
- (3) Digoxin toxicity, >2.5 ng/ml digoxin level; most common initial findings are anorexia, nausea, vomiting; later findings may be yellow vision, green halos around objects, dysrhythmias

2. Beta-adrenergic blocking agents—block sympathetic stimulation (epinephrine) to beta receptor sites in the body
   a. Expected effects
- (1) Decreased myocardial contractility; decreased oxygen need of the myocardium, which prevents angina pectoris
- (2) Decreased HR
- (3) Decreased BP
- (4) Mild antianxiety effects

   b. Commonly given drugs
- (1) Propanolol*** (Inderal)
- (2) Metoprolol*** (Lopressor)

   c. Nursing considerations
- (1) Hold drug for heart rate <50; notify the physician
- (2) Caution against abrupt withdrawal—result may be severe angina pectoris
- (3) Assess for orthostatic hypotension—drop in systolic BP >20 mm Hg when changing from lying or sitting to a standing position
- (4) Assess for symptoms of right- and left-sided heart failure

3. Calcium channel blocking agents—block influx of calcium into cells via the slow channels
   a. Expected effects
- (1) Decreased heart rate; slows tachycardic dysrhythmias
- (2) Decreased myocardial contractility; prevents angina pectoris
- (3) Arteriolar vasodilation; lowered BP
- (4) Prevents coronary artery spasm

*** Beta blockers generic names all end in *lol*. Think of the word lull—makes the heart sleepy and slow.

    b. Commonly given drugs
      (1) Nifedipine (Procardia)
      (2) Verapamil (Calan, Isoptin)
      (3) Diltiazem (Cardizem)
    c. Nursing considerations
      (1) Hold for HR <50; notify physician
      (2) Assess for orthostatic hypotension
      (3) Assess for symptoms of right- and left-sided heart failure
      (4) Potentiated action when used with beta blockers

4. Nitrates—dilate vascular smooth muscle
    a. Expected effects
      (1) Peripheral vasodilation, especially venous capacitence and arterial resistance vessels, leads to pooling of blood in the peripheral circulation; this decreases the amount of blood returned to the right side of the heart, preload, and heart workload is decreased
      (2) Collateral circulation of the heart is dilated; increased oxygen is delivered to the myocardium
    b. Commonly given drugs
      (1) Nitroglycerin (Tridil)—IV drip preparation given for acute anginal attacks; clients need to be cardiac monitored
      (2) Nitroglycerin (Nitrostat)—sublingual preparation given for acute anginal attacks
      (3) Nitroglycerin (Nitrobid)—oral preparation given to prevent anginal attacks
      (4) Nitroglycerin (Transderm-Nitro)—transdermal preparation given to prevent anginal attacks
    c. Nursing considerations
      (1) Hold medication and contact physician with a BP <90/60 mm Hg
      (2) Assess for orthostatic hypotension
      (3) Remove old patches, wiping site to remove all medication
      (4) Rotate sites of transdermal preparations
      (5) IV preparation must be mixed in a glass IV bottle and only polyethylene tubing can be used to prevent absorption of the drug into the tubing

5. Antidysrhythmic drugs—suppress or obliterate impulses originating in the conduction pathway and competing with the SA node; in the subclassifications of these drugs, different mechanisms occur to suppress or obliterate dysrythmias
   a. Expected effects—decreased heart rate, regulated heart rhythm
   b. Commonly given drugs
      (1) Lidocaine (Xylocaine) IV only; first sign of toxicity is confusion; severe toxicity will bring on seizures
      (2) Quinidine—major side effect: diarrhea
      (3) Procainamide (Pronestyl)—major concerns: hypotension with IV; rash, arthralgia with p.o.
      (4) Bretylium (Bretylol)—major concerns: hypotension; nausea and vomiting after rapid IV
   c. Nursing considerations
      (1) Monitor for bradycardia and heart block
      (2) Assess for central nervous system abnormalities
6. Lipoprotein lowering drugs—lower the serum lipoprotein levels by a decrease in its production or by a removal of lipoproteins from the body
   a. Expected effect—decrease the risk of developing arteriosclerosis
   b. Commonly given drugs
      (1) Gemfibrozil (Lopid) inhibits synthesis of lipoproteins
      (2) Lovastatin (Mevacor) inhibits synthesis of lipoproteins
   c. Nursing considerations
      (1) May elevate CPK levels
      (2) Administer with food to decrease gastric irritation
      (3) Liver function studies should be monitored periodically for an increase in ALT, AST
      (4) Teach client that cholesterol will be eliminated via the bowel and may cause increased flatus or change in stool consistency

B. Procedures
   1. Electrocardiogram (EKG, ECG)—a record of the electrical activity of the heart; six limb leads and six precordial leads depict the transmission of impulses down through the conduction system. Abnormal electrical activity may indicate

impaired impulse transmission through the heart, which could be caused by ischemic, injured, or infarcted cardiac tissue.

2. Stress test—an ECG tracing done while the client exercises, either on a stationary bike or on a treadmill; evaluates the myocardial response to an increase in oxygen demand; helps diagnose preinfarction angina

3. Echocardiography—ultrasound technique that evaluates the internal structure and function of the heart muscle and valves; evaluates cardiac chamber size, wall action, ejection fraction, and presence of cardiac effusions

4. Cardiac catheterization/coronary angiography—Left: invasive procedure, usually via the femoral artery to the aorta for evaluation of the left chambers of the heart, the coronary arteries, and ejection and filling pressures; patency of the coronary arteries is evaluated through the use of fluoroscopy during dye injection. Remember, dye injection results in diuresis; postprocedure monitor and replace fluids.

5. Cardiac enzymes—released following injury to cells
   a. Creatine phosphokinase (CPK)
   b. Lactate dehydrogenase (LDH)
   c. SGOT, now known as aspartate aminotransferase (AST)
   d. Isoenzymes—more specific to cardiac cell injury
      (1) CK-MB elevated
      (2) $LDH_1 > LDH_2$
   e. Elevation of enzyme levels indicates myocardial infarction
   f. Note: Alphabetically C comes before L; thus it is easy to remember that CK-MB peaks first, within 24 hours, before LDH peaks

C. Psychosocial
   1. Denial—the most common and earliest response to chest pain; clients frequently will attribute chest pain to indigestion or stress; this response may contribute to a delay in treatment
   2. Anxiety—an uncomfortable feeling associated with an unknown direct cause; many clients are unable to discuss the feeling of anxiety, but do, however, feel uneasy about what may happen
   3. Fear—an uncomfortable feeling associated with real danger
   4. Anger—normal sequence of feelings in the cardiac client when lifestyle changes occur; the anger sometimes aimed at caregivers is usually a reaction to required lifestyle changes as a result of client's illness

     5. Lifestyle changes—directly related to the degree of incapacitation the client experiences; changes mainly revolve around the diet, activity, work type, and environment

  D. **Health history—question sequence**
     1. What symptoms are you having that made it necessary for you to seek assistance?
     2. Are you currently being treated by a physician for any other problems?
     3. Have you ever had any injuries or illnesses that you were treated for in the past?
     4. Is there a family history of cardiac disease?
     5. Are you presently taking any prescription or over-the-counter drugs? What are they?
     6. Are you following a diet prescribed by a physician?
     7. Do you follow a specific diet?
     8. Do you smoke or have you ever smoked? If yes, how much?
     9. Do you drink alcohol, coffee, or tea? If yes, how much?
   10. What is your usual activity level? Do you exercise and how much?
   11. Do you live a stressful lifestyle, either in the home or at work?

  E. **Physical exam—appropriate sequence**
     1. Airway, breathing, circulation—vital signs
     2. Chest pain evaluation—scale of 0 to 10
     3. Skin color, temperature, moisture, turgor—compare central vs. peripheral
     4. Arterial pulses
     5. Jugular vein distention—evaluate with client positioned with the head of the bed elevated to at least a 35 degree angle
     6. Inspection of the chest for chest wall movement and pulsations
     7. Palpation of the chest for point of maximal impulse and chest wall pain (Figure 3-1)
     8. Auscultation of heart sounds—use stethoscope
       a. Diaphragm—S1 and S2, high-pitched murmurs
       b. Bell—S3 and S4, low-pitched murmurs
     9. Auscultation of lung sounds—use stethoscope diaphragm

IV. Pathophysiologic disorders

  A. **Coronary artery disease**
     1. Definition—a disorder of diminished blood flow to the coronary arteries; the heart is starved of blood flow, oxygen, and nutrients
     2. Pathophysiology—atherosclerotic plaque lines the walls of the coronary arteries; the plaque continues to grow over the years

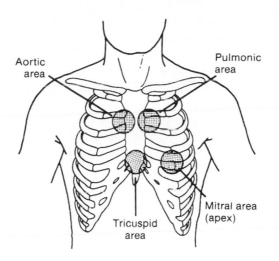

Figure 3-1. Areas of auscultation of heart valves. (From *AJN/Mosby Nursing Board Review*, ed 9, St Louis, 1994, Mosby.)

and results in a decrease in the lumen size of the affected artery. Overall effect: imbalance between the amount of oxygen supplied to the myocardium and the amount of oxygen demanded by the myocardium.

3. Etiology—contributing factors
   a. Heredity
   b. Age
   c. Sex
   d. Hypertension
   e. Hyperlipidemia
   f. Obesity
   g. Diabetes
   h. Smoking
   i. Sedentary lifestyle
   j. Coronary artery spasm
4. Incidence—leading cause of death in the United States, approximately 500,000 deaths a year; it is estimated that close to 5 million people have coronary artery disease
5. Assessment
   a. Ask the following questions
      (1) Where is the pain? Can you point to the pain with one finger?
      (2) How long have you had the pain?

   (3) On a scale of 0 to 10 what number would you assign to your pain? (1 is slight pain, 10 is most severe)

   (4) Does it radiate? If so, where?

   (5) How would you describe your pain?

   (6) What were you doing just before the pain started?

   (7) Did you do anything that made the pain better or worse?

 b. Clinical manifestations

   (1) Angina pectoris—myocardial ischemia

    (a) Chest pain, tightness, or heaviness

    (b) Relieved quickly: 3 minutes to a maximum of 15 minutes by rest or by sublingual nitroglycerin

    (c) Initiated by physical exertion or stress

    (d) Radiation of pain may or may not be present

   (2) Printzmetal's angina, caused by coronary artery spasm: chest pain that occurs during rest or sleep

   (3) Myocardial infarction—myocardial necrosis

    (a) Severe crushing, stabbing chest pain—more severe than client's angina

    (b) Not relieved by rest or medication

    (c) Pain lasts much longer than angina: >20 minutes

    (d) Frequently associated with shortness of breath, nausea, diaphoresis

    (e) May or may not have radiation of pain

 c. Abnormal laboratory findings

   (1) Angina pectoris

    (a) Lipid levels—may be elevated indicating atherosclerotic involvement

   (2) Prinzmetal's angina

    (a) Lipid levels—may be elevated indicating some associated atherosclerosis

   (3) Myocardial infarction

    (a) Enzymes—CK-MB, LDH_1, LDH_2 elevation indicate myocardial necrosis

    (b) CBC—elevated WBC

 d. Abnormal diagnostic tests

   (1) Angina pectoris

    (a) ECG—ST segment elevation and T wave inversion more common in unstable angina; most often during pain-free periods ST segment and T wares are normal

    (b) Exercise stress test—during test exhibits chest pain, ST segment elevation, bradycardia, or exaggerated tachycardia

    (c) Echocardiography—may show abnormal wall motion, decreased ejection fraction <50%

    (d) Cardiac catheterization—shows impaired blood flow, partial obstruction or narrowing of coronary arteries

   (2) Prinzmetal's angina

    (a) ECG—ST segment elevation before or during pain, then returning to normal when pain relieved; dysrhythmias not uncommon during pain

    (b) Exercise stress test—helps to distinguish between Prinzmetal's angina and angina pectoris; results would be normal with Prinzmetal's angina

    (c) Cardiac catheterization—coronary artery spasm can be induced during test to differentiate between types of angina

   (3) Myocardial infarction

    (a) ECG in specific leads ST segment elevation—injured cardiac tissue; T wave inversion—ischemia, seen in the acute stages, Q waves larger or wider than normal in specific leads—indicative of myocardial necrosis

    (b) CXR—may show various degrees of left ventricular failure or pulmonary congestion

    (c) Echocardiography— identifies abnormal wall motion of ventricles, abnormal chamber size, septal abnormalities, valvular dysfunction, reduced ejection fraction <50%

    (d) Radionuclide blood pool imaging with technetium 99m—pinpoints myocardial damage; size of infarct; degree of ventricular dysfunction

6. Expected medical interventions

  a. Angina pectoris

   (1) Nitrate therapy

   (2) Beta blocker and calcium channel blocker therapy to decrease oxygen consumption by the heart

   (3) Low fat, low cholesterol, calorie controlled diet

   (4) Diagnostic studies to determine extent of coronary artery impairment

   (5) Percutaneous transluminal coronary angioplasty (PTCA) to dilate coronary arteries if indicated

   (6) Cornary artery bypass graft (CABG) to occluded or partially occluded coronary arteries

      b. Printzmetal's angina
- (1) Procardia to prevent coronary artery spasm
- (2) Change in lifestyle as deemed necessary

      c. Myocardial infarction
- (1) Admission to the hospital in a monitored unit, either telemetry or coronary care
- (2) Pain medication for chest pain relief
- (3) Maintenance of BP as needed
- (4) Thrombolytic therapy if chest pain <6 hours, and client has not had recent surgery, trauma, pregnancy, or a bleeding disorder or has not recently taken anticoagulants
- (5) Emergency heart catheterization followed by PTCA or CABG surgery if indicated
- (6) Antidysrhythmic therapy as needed
- (7) Bedrest, sedatives if necessary

7. Nursing diagnoses
- a. Chest pain related to imbalance between oxygen supply and demand of myocardium
- b. Anxiety related to threat of physical well-being
- c. Decreased cardiac output related to cardiac rhythm disturbances
- d. Decreased cardiac output related to decreased ventricular contractility
- e. Activity intolerance related to decreased cardiac contractility

8. Client goals
- a. Client will state chest pain is relieved
- b Client will state feeling more relaxed and calm
- c. Client will exhibit vital signs that are within 10% of baseline
- d. Client will increase activity without associated symptoms by 5% each day (10 more feet walked, and so on)

9. Nursing interventions
- a. Acute care
  - (1) Top priority—pain relief, once airway, breathing, and circulation have been stabilized
  - (2) Administer oxygen and other medications as directed
  - (3) Monitor at least every hour for indications of decreased cardiac output—sustained HR >20 BPM over baseline; lowered BP, decreased urine output
  - (4) Monitor cardiac rhythm for premature ventricular contractions (PVCs), the most common dysrhythmia, treat with Lidocaine

        (5)   Monitor lung sounds for crackles, wheezes, consolidation

        (6)   Maintain a patent IV line

        (7)   Maintain a restful environment

        (8)   Give brief explanations for all procedures, tests, and equipment

        (9)   Encourage verbalization of feelings

  b. Home care regarding client education

        (1)   Short and long-acting nitrates, how to administer and store them

            (a)   Sublingual nitrates

                (i)   Take sublingual nitroglycerin at pain onset, then × 2 at five-minute intervals; if pain persists, call for assistance and transport to an emergency department

                (ii)   Store in dry, dark bottle

                (iii)   Obtain new bottle every 6 months, shelf life is 3 to 6 months once bottle is opened; a tingling under the tongue indicates potency of medication

            (b)   Transdermal nitrates

                (i)   Rotate sites in nonhairy areas above the knees or elbows

                (ii)   Wash site after patch removed

        (2)   Interventions for evaluation of medication effectiveness

            (a)   How to take radial pulse daily; best before getting out of bed

            (b)   What adverse reactions would require medical assistance, such as persistent anorexia, nausea, vomiting, or change in vision

        (3)   How to increase activity level slowly

        (4)   How to weigh daily, before breakfast, wearing the same amount of clothing; report losses or gains of >2 lb per week

        (5)   Diet changes, usually a low fat, low cholesterol, moderate to low salt diet

        (6)   When sexual activity can resume; usually when client can climb a flight of stairs without SOB or chest pain

  c. Evaluate home environment

        (1)   Location of bedrooms, bathrooms, kitchen

        (2)   Need to walk steps

        (3) Roles of family members

        (4) Need for job counseling

10. Evaluation protocol

    a. How do I know that my interventions were effective?

        (1) Has client chest pain improved?

        (2) Does client feel any shortness of breath or dizziness?

        (3) Does client feel anxious right now?

    b. What criteria will I use to change my interventions?

        (1) Chest pain is not relieved or is not reduced to a comfortable level for the client

        (2) Shortness of breath is not relieved or is exacerbated

        (3) Client unable to tolerate even simple activities, such as turning in bed or ambulating in room, without SOB or diaphoresis

    c. How will I know that my client teaching has been effective?

        (1) Client demonstrates correct technique for evaluating own pulse

        (2) Client will walk 10 feet further each day, without chest pain or SOB

        (3) Client will take one nitroglycerin when in pain and then only two more, 5 minutes apart

11. Older adult alert—older adult clients as a normal course of aging exhibit some similar characteristics

    a. Decrease in renal excretion with an increased risk for digitalis toxicity

    b. Decreased skin turgor and dry mucous membranes; inspection of the tongue best indicates dehydration or decreased fluid volume

    c. Decreased cardiac output

B. **Cardiac dysrhythmias**

  1. Definition—a disorder of the electrical system of the heart, causing abnormal HR and/or rhythm

    a. Most common effect—decreased cardiac output

    b. Most severe effect—sudden cardiac death

    c. Most dangerous—ventricular dysrhythmias

    d. Least dangerous—atrial dysrhythmias

    e. Tachycardias more dangerous than bradycardias as a result of the decreased coronary artery filling time associated with tachycardias; clients are more likely to experience chest pain and shortness of breath with tachycardias

  2. Pathophysiology—three mechanisms may trigger cardiac dysrhythmias

    a. Reentry mechanism—the conducted impulse is permitted to enter into a rapid circle-like motion through conduction pathways that result in tachycardia

    b. Increased automaticity—the electricity that is required to stimulate a cell to depolarize is reduced and the cell is easily stimulated, allowing for abnormal impulse formation that result in premature beats

    c. Impaired conduction—impulse is either slowed or blocked in conduction pathways, usually resulting in bradycardia or A-V heart block—1st, 2nd, or 3rd degree; most common site for impaired conduction is the AV node

3. Etiology—most commonly arise from the following

    a. Myocardial cellular hypoxia, from a cardiac, hematologic (anemia) or respiratory disorder

    b. Electrolyte imbalance

    c. Drug toxicity

4. Incidence—major cause of death in the client suffering from an acute myocardial infarction

5. Assessment

    a. Ask the following questions

        (1) Have you felt any palpitations or a feeling as if your heart is flipping over in your chest?

        (2) Have you felt dizzy or light-headed?

        (3) Have you had blurred vision?

        (4) Have you had any chest pain or SOB?

    b. Clinical manifestations

        (1) Irregular heart rhythm with a rate >100 or <60 beats per minute

        (2) Pale skin color, diaphoresis

        (3) Feeling of increased anxiety, nervousness leading to confusion, lethargy, comatose state

        (4) Hypotension, BP <90/60

    c. Abnormal laboratory findings

        (1) Arterial blood gases—hypoxemia: P_aO_2 <80 mm Hg; acidosis with pH <7.35

        (2) Electrolytes—severe high or low levels, especially potassium, magnesium, or calcium

        (3) Toxicology studies—elevated levels

    d. Abnormal diagnostic tests

        (1) ECG—conclusive evidence of the type of dysrhythmia; should be obtained when client is symptomatic

        (2)   Holter monitor, 24-hour ambulatory ECG—gives information regarding dysrhythmia, in relation to client activity, especially if dysrhythmia is intermittent. Note: Important for client to maintain activity log during monitoring.

        (3)   Electophysiologic studies (EPS)—in hospital, medically induced dysrhythmias for accurate diagnosis of the site of origin and effectiveness of selected drugs

6.   Expected medical interventions

   a.   Cardioversion or defibrillation for life-threatening dysrhythmias as indicated

   b.   Antidysrhythmic drugs

   c.   Pacemaker insertion, temporary and/or permanent as indicated

7.   Nursing diagnoses

   a.   Decreased cardiac output related to ineffective cardiac rhythm

   b.   Activity intolerance related to ineffective cardiac output

   c.   Anxiety related to change in health status

8.   Client goals

   a.   Client will have appropriate cardiac output as evidenced by HR within 10 to 20 beats per minute of baseline and rhythm without ectopy; BP systolic within 20 mm Hg of baseline

   b.   Client will increase activity without associated symptoms by 5% each day (10 more feet walked, and so on)

   c.   Client will state the feeling of being more relaxed and calm

9.   Nursing interventions

   a.   Acute care

        (1)   Cardiac monitoring in a critical care or telemetry unit

        (2)   Initiate prompt treatment for life-threatening dysrhythmias—Lidocaine for PVCs, ventricular tachycardia; pacemaker for third-degree heart block

        (3)   Monitor lung sounds, evaluate for left ventricular failure

        (4)   Administer antidysrhythmic drug therapy and evaluate for adverse reactions

   b.   Home care regarding client education

        (1)   Medication therapy—adverse reactions, desired effects, symptoms to report

        (2)   Encourage client to cease any activity if dysrhythmic symptoms occur and take peripheral pulse for one minute at that time—note rate, regularity

   (3) Explain dietary restrictions ordered due to their stimulant effect, such as coffee, tea, and chocolate products

   (4) Discourage smoking

 10. Evaluation protocol

  a. How do I know that my interventions were effective?

   (1) Has client felt any symptoms of heart rhythm problem?

   (2) Has client felt any shortness of breath?

  b. What criteria will I use to change my interventions?

   (1) Increased or sustained symptoms associated with dysrhythmia

   (2) Blood pressure decreases with a change in level of consciousness

   (3) Evidence of shortness of breath at rest

  c. How will I know that my client teaching has been effective?

   (1) Client uses decaffeinated coffee and tea, is not eating chocolate

   (2) Client reports no difficulties taking scheduled medication and has noted no side effects

   (3) Client states that if palpitations or dizziness occur, a rest period of at least 15 to 30 minutes is required with the radial pulse taken at beginning and end of rest period

 11. Older adult alert

  a. Older adult clients have a decreased cardiac output as a normal course of aging, so it is imperative to have baseline vital signs to determine changes after medication is begun

  b. Since renal excretion in older adult clients is decreased, these clients are more vulnerable to drug toxicity from the antidysrhythmic drugs

  c. Quinidine, a common antidysrhythmic drug, is known to cause severe watery diarrhea. In older adult clients, this could quickly lead to metabolic acidosis, electrolyte imbalance, and water dehydration from the loss of potassium and buffers.

C. Congestive heart failure (CHF)

 1. Definition—heart is unable to produce a cardiac output that is sufficient to meet the metabolic demands of the body

 2. Pathophysiology—many causes of CHF; most causes fit into two categories of etiologies

  a. The etiologies that cause a decrease in contractility of the myocardium

  b. The etiologies that cause the myocardium to work harder

    c. Cardiac compensatory mechanisms—to improve cardiac output
      (1) Tachycardia
      (2) Ventricular dilation
      (3) Ventricular hypertrophy
    d. Left ventricular failure is manifested first in most clients
      (1) Left ventricle is unable to propel blood in a forward motion into the arterial circulation
      (2) Blood that cannot be propelled forward will back up into the left atrium and then into the pulmonary vessels and lung fields
      (3) Pulmonary vessels become engorged with blood, and plasma begins to leak out of the vessels into the interstitial and alveolar spaces
      (4) Life-threatening form is referred to as acute pulmonary edema and exhibits frothy pink sputum, gas exchange abnormalities
    e. Right ventricular failure is commonly caused by overwork of the right ventricle attempting to pump blood into greatly engorged pulmonary vessels. Since blood cannot be propelled forward, it backs up into the systemic circulation (not considered a life-threatening situation).
3. Etiology—many conditions can cause CHF, including MI, systemic and pulmonary hypertension (increased afterload), valvular abnormalities, myocarditis
4. Assessment
    a. Ask the following questions
      (1) Are you having difficulty breathing?
      (2) Does minimal activity make it even more difficult to breathe?
      (3) When you sleep, how many pillows do you place under your head?
      (4) Do you ever wake up feeling as if you are smothering?
      (5) Do you have difficulty with your ankles or feet swelling? What time of day does this occur?
      (6) Do you feel fatigued or tired on a daily basis?
    b. Clinical manifestations
      (1) Left-sided failure—think **L**eft = **L**ung
        (a) Dry cough, eventually productive
        (b) Fatigue
        (c) Dyspnea on exertion, then at rest

(d) Crackles or rales in lung fields, usually bilaterally at the bases

(e) Orthopnea—unable to sleep flat

(f) Paroxysmal nocturnal dyspnea (PND): awakens from sleep with a smothering feeling

(g) S3 heard over left ventricle

(2) Acute pulmonary edema

(a) Profound dyspnea, progressing to respiratory failure and arrest

(b) Pink, frothy sputum production

(c) Crackles in all the lung fields

(d) Respiratory acidosis, hypoxemia

(e) Metabolic acidosis

(3) Right-sided failure

(a) Jugular venous distention

(b) Easy fatigability

(c) Hepatomegaly—enlarged liver

(d) Dependant, pitting edema—if bedrest: sacral edema; if ambulatory: ankles and feet edematous

(e) S3 heard over right ventricle

c. Abnormal laboratory findings

(1) ABGs—hypoxemia = PaO_2 <80, hypercapnia = $PaCo_2$ >45

(2) Electrolytes—low sodium, from vascular fluid overload, low potassium and magnesium from diuretic therapy

(3) Liver function studies—slight elevation AST, bilirubin, alkaline phosphatase from hepatomegaly

d. Abnormal diagnostic tests

(1) CXR—left-sided failure only: pulmonary congestion and interstitial edema

(2) ECG—changes indicative of hypertrophy of the left or right ventricle; would also be diagnostic for dysrhythmias

(3) Echocardiogram—left-sided failure: abnormal wall movement, may be hypokinetic, diminished ejection fraction of <50%

5. Expected medical interventions

a. Digitalis preparations—to increase pumping capability of the myocardium

b. Diuretics to decrease fluid load in the interstitial spaces

c. Oxygen as SOB and fatigue become more of a problem

6. Nursing diagnoses
   a. Decreased cardiac output related to poor left or right ventricular pumping capability
   b. Fluid volume excess: interstitial spaces related to increased vascular pressures and shifting of fluid into interstitial spaces
   c. Impaired gas exchange related to fluid layer in the alveoli and small airways
   d. Activity intolerance related to decreased oxygenation of body tissues from decreased cardiac output
   e. Anxiety related to SOB and fatigue, secondary to decreased oxygenation of the body tissues
7. Client goals
   a. Client will exhibit vital signs that are within 10% of baseline
   b. Client will exhibit decreased crackles in the lung field by 10% within 2 hours
   c. Client will exhibit a decrease in edematous extremities circumference by 1 inch within 2 days of initial therapy
   d. Client will maintain a PO_2 of 80 to 100 mm Hg and a PCO_2 of 35 to 45 mm Hg; if COPD client PO_2 and PCO_2 at 60 mm Hg +/– 5 mm Hg
   e. Client will increase activity without associated symptoms by 5% each day; 10 feet or more walked, increase number of steps climbed by 5
   f. Client will state feeling less anxious, facial features will exhibit a relaxed look
8. Nursing interventions
   a. Acute care
      (1) Left-sided failure
         (a) Give medications by IV route
         (b) Evaluate heart and lung sounds initially and then every 30 minutes after initial therapy; when clear, at least every 2 to 4 hours
         (c) Administer oxygen as ordered or during periods of SOB or during activity
         (d) Maintain head of bed with elevation at least 40 to 60 degrees, mid to high fowlers when in bed
         (e) Balance rest and activity to meet client needs
      (2) Right-sided failure
         (a) Weigh client daily, before breakfast—same time, same scale, same amount of clothing; expect a loss; report any daily weight changes when client is on diuretic therapy

            (b)   Elevate edematous extremities above the level of the heart when in bed; in chair, elevate to prevent dependency of lower legs below knee level; monitor edema for a decrease

            (c)   Turn and reposition at least every 2 hours; use skin protective devices (heel protectors); consider use of air pressure beds or mattresses

            (d)   Ambulate client or move from bed to chair at least three times a day; promotes circulation and prevents venous stasis

    b.   Home care regarding client education

        (1)   Proper weight monitoring; instruct client to weigh self daily, write on calendar, report a 2 lb or greater weight gain per week

        (2)   Limit salt in diet by cooking with no salt; add salt at table only to maintain a sodium restricted diet; caution the use of salt substitutes since some contain high potassium

        (3)   Pulse monitoring done daily, either prior to getting out of bed or at rest if taking digitalis preparations; if experiencing extreme dyspnea or frothy sputum, take pulse; notify physician

        (4)   Potassium replacement in diet if taking nonpotassium sparing diuretics as furosemide (Lasix) and bumetanide (Bumex); increase foods such as oranges, prunes, bananas, watermelon, potatoes, and beans

9. Evaluation protocol

    a.   How do I know that my interventions were effective?

        (1)   Is client fatigue improving?

        (2)   Does client feel any dizziness?

        (3)   Has client's shortness of breath improved?

        (4)   Has client swelling decreased in client's ankles and feet?

    b.   What criteria will I use to change my interventions?

        (1)   Sustained or increased fatigue and intolerance to activity with therapy

        (2)   A client visibly short of breath, or a client who states an increase in shortness of breath, especially at rest

        (3)   Reports of dizziness and a systolic BP having dropped >10% of client baseline

        (4)   Reports that swelling in client's ankles and feet has increased with or without a weight gain

     c. How will I know that my client teaching has been effective?

        (1) Client takes a 20 minute rest after any activity that increases the respiratory rate or effort in breathing

        (2) Client maintains daily weight at +/− 1 1b every day to average no more than a 2 lb gain per week

        (3) Client sustains HR between 60 to 100 beats per minute each day, either before getting out of bed or at rest

        (4) Client adds no salt to food except at the table

10. Older adult alert

     a. The older adult clients with a susceptibility to orthostatic hypotension have increased risk for falls when taking diuretics and/or antidysrhythmic drug therapy

     b. Hypotension may be a dysfunction even more profound in older adult clients. Normal expectation in the aging process is an increased BP.

     c. Older adult clients are at even greater risk for skin breakdown since their skin tends to be thinner and more fragile. This risk is severely increased in clients with peripheral edema, poor circulation, and poor nutritional status.

D. Valvular heart disease

1. Definition—a dysfunction of one or more of the cardiac valves

     a. Stenosis—restriction of blood flow in a forward motion through the heart

     b. Regurgitation—unpredictable blood flow through the heart; some moving forward, some regurgitating backward into the previous chamber

2. Pathophysiology—two fundamental irregularities

     a. Stenosis

        (1) The valve's lumen decreases significantly from thickened or calcified leaflets

        (2) Restricted blood flow through the lumen

        (3) Reduced blood output from the chamber attempting to push blood through the stenosed lumen

        (4) Hypertrophy eventually occurs from a rise in chamber pressure

        (5) End result: right- or left-sided failure, depending on the valves affected

     b. Regurgitation or insufficiency

        (1) Leaflets of valve are unable to close completely from scarring, calcium deposits, or papillary muscle dysfunction

(2) Result in a reduced blood output from the chamber attempting to empty blood; some blood is ejected forward; some is ejected backward

(3) Eventually the volume of regurgitated blood is added to blood already present in the chamber, which then increases the pressure and workload

(4) Walls of the affected chambers will hypertrophy

(5) Eventually symptoms of right- or left-sided failure occur, depending on the valve affected

3. Etiology—valvular heart disease is most commonly acquired from rheumatic heart fever, bacterial endocarditis, myocardial infarction, and congenital disorders

4. Incidence—the incidence of the illnesses is different for each valvular condition

   a. Mitral abnormalities

      (1) Stenosis is more common in females

      (2) More common in the population younger than 45

   b. Aortic abnormalities

      (1) More common in males

      (2) Aortic stenosis is most common valvular abnormality in the older adult population

5. Assessment

   a. Ask the following questions

      (1) Are you having any chest pain? If yes, where?

      (2) Do you have any shortness of breath?

      (3) Do you have shortness of breath only with exercise or all the time?

      (4) Do you feel very tired? If yes, describe pattern.

   b. General clinical manifestations with any valve dysfunction

      (1) Fatigue

      (2) Dyspnea on exertion

      (3) Chest pain on exertion

      (4) Orthopnea

      (5) Palpitations

      (6) Heart murmur (different with each valve abnormality)

   c. Abnormal laboratory findings—there are no specific laboratory studies utilized in the diagnosis of valvular heart disease

   d. Abnormal diagnostic tests

      (1) Echocardiogram—most diagnostic; valve movement and impairment, such as poor ejection fraction are visualized

(2) ECG—most changes are associated with chamber enlargement; atrial dysrhythmias are common, as are AV blocks
(3) CXR—chamber enlargement, pulmonary congestion
(4) Cardiac catheterization
  (a) Pressure increased in the affected chambers
  (b) Percentage of blood ejected from the chambers can be calculated; called ejection fraction; usually >50%
  (c) Regurgitation amount with dye injection
6. Expected medical interventions
  a. Treat findings as they occur
   (1) Digitalis preparations, diuretics for findings associated with CHF
   (2) Antidysrhythmic drugs for atrial dysrhythmias
  b. Valvuloplasty to repair leaflets
  c. Valvular commissurotomy to free fused leaflets
  d. Valvular replacement
  e. Oral anticoagulants for life following valvular replacement surgery
7. Nursing diagnoses
  a. Fatigue related to poor tissue perfusion
  b. Ineffective breathing pattern related to fluid in airways
  c. Activity intolerance related to poor tissue perfusion and oxygenation
8. Client goals
  a. Client will state fatigue has decreased
  b. Client will demonstrate a respiratory rate of 18 to 22 breaths per minute and of normal depth at rest
  c. Client will increase daily activity without associated symptoms by 5% each day (10 more feet walked, 5 more steps climbed)
9. Nursing interventions
  a. Acute care
   (1) Assess lung sounds for crackles and heart sounds for murmurs or increased intensity of murmur at least every 2 hours
   (2) Administer oxygen during acute episode of shortness of breath or cardiac dysrhythmias
   (3) Balance rest and activity—45 minute to 1 hour rest period after meals or a bath; no activity longer than 15 to 20 minutes

    b. Home care: regarding client education
- (1) Antibiotic prophylaxis required before any invasive procedure or dental work, to prevent bacterial endocarditis
- (2) Daily weights in the morning upon rising to evaluate fluid status; same time of day, same scale, same amount of clothing—report weight gain of more than 2 lb per week to physician
- (3) Expected effects and side effects of medication therapy
- (4) Low-salt diet; minimal caffeine

10. Evaluation protocol
    a. How do I know that my interventions were effective?
- (1) Does client feel more energetic?
- (2) How many pillows is client sleeping on?
- (3) Does client feel breathing is comfortable?
- (4) Was client able to ambulate further today before becoming short of breath?

    b. What criteria will I use to change my interventions?
- (1) Client indicates that fatigue is no better or worse
- (2) Client's respiratory rate is rapid and labored at rest or with minimal activity
- (3) Client is unable to increase activity level by any amount before becoming short of breath
- (4) Client sleeps on three or more pillows or with head of bed >60 degrees

    c. How will I know that my client teaching has been effective?
- (1) Client will obtain a prescription for antibiotics before dental work, and so on
- (2) Client weighs self every morning before breakfast, at the same time and with the same amount of clothing
- (3) Client is not putting any salt on food until after it is prepared
- (4) Client takes diuretic in the morning or afternoon rather than at night

11. Older adult alert
    a. Many of the drug therapies older adults will experience may cause orthostatic hypotension. Older adult clients, as a result of the aging process, are more prone to orthostatic hypotension.
    b. Elderly clients sent home on anticoagulants must be reminded to be evaluated for prothrombin time frequently through the physician office, usually every week or month

      c. The vascular tone in older adult clients is not as responsive to cardiovascular stress, so clients may not respond appropriately to fluids or medications in the face of hypotension

E. **Inflammatory heart disorders**

  1. Definition—a group of cardiac disorders involving an inflammatory process of the layers of the heart

      a. Endocarditis—an inflammation of the endocardium; the innermost layer of the heart; may include the cardiac valves and papillary muscles

      b. Myocarditis—an inflammation of the myocardium, the actual heart muscle

      c. Pericarditis—an inflammation of the visceral and parietal pericardium, the outermost layer of the heart

  2. Pathophysiology

      a. Endocarditis

         (1) Acute—develops on normal valves, progresses rapidly, causes severe destruction; may be fatal without treatment

         (2) Subacute—occurs on damaged heart valves, progresses slowly, survival possible without treatment

         (3) In both of the above, bacteria in the circulation are attracted to the sluggish blood in the atrial floor or to the damaged areas of the heart, most frequently on the valves

         (4) Vegetations result from clumped bacteria

         (5) Vegetations erode and destroy cardiac and valvular tissue; leads to impaired pumping efficiency, intractable heart failure

         (6) Vegetation growth produces fragile cardiac lesions that can break off, embolize, cause ischemia, and/or infarct organs; most common in the brain

      b. Myocarditis

         (1) Insidious process that does not resemble a myocardial infarction; may be diffuse or local damage from a pathogen or toxin

         (2) May take one of three paths

            (a) No signs of heart failure

            (b) Latent period of approximately 1 year, then findings of heart failure

            (c) Rapid onset of heart failure

   c. Pericarditis
      (1) Acute—the two layers of the pericardium are inflamed and roughened; friction between the layers may result in increased fluid production in the space between the two layers; a dry form, fibrinous pericarditis, lasts less than 6 weeks; adhesions form between the sac layers with restriction of heart filling and pumping
         (a) Cardiac tamponade—complication with a fluid build-up, pericardial effusion will occur of either serous, purulent, or hemorrhagic type; a point of increased pressure on the heart results in ineffective pumping
            (i) Treatment immediately required: pericardiocentesis leads to withdrawal of fluid from the pericardial sac
            (ii) Pericardiotomy—incision or window in the pericardium, will prevent further occurrences of cardiac tamponade
      (2) Chronic—constrictive pericarditis; from the reoccurrence of a preexisting condition, the two layers of pericardium eventually become thickened, fused, and scarred together; the pericardium then will act as a large band surrounding the heart, actually constricting the pumping action of the heart and leading to minimal cardiac filling and output; treatment involves imperative removal of the pericardium to restore appropriate cardiac pumping

3. Etiology
   a. Endocarditis—entry of pathogens during dental work, IV drug use, or any invasive procedures; bacteria is the most common pathogen
   b. Myocarditis—most common infecting agent is a virus; bacteria, protozoal, or rickettsial diseases less common
   c. Pericarditis—causes
      (1) Infectious—most common source is viral or idiopathic (unknown)
      (2) Noninfectious—after acute myocardial infarction, trauma, uremia: Dressler's syndrome: 1 to 4 weeks post-myocardial infarction
      (3) Autoimmune—rheumatic disease, systemic lupus erythematosus

4. Incidence
   a. Endocarditis—5 of every 1000 clients admitted to the hospital have infective endocarditis; mean age is 50; ratio of men to women 2:1; decrease in the number caused by streptococci, but an increase in the number caused by atypical organisms such as yeasts and fungi
   b. Myocarditis—impossible to evaluate because the incidence changes within the age groups and within groups that are affected by different etiologies
   c. Pericarditis—far more common in the male population
5. Assessment
   a. Ask the following questions
      (1) Do you have chest pain? Where is it?
      (2) Have you been running a fever? How high has your fever gone?
      (3) Have you been experiencing flu-like symptoms?
      (4) Do you have a prosthetic valve?
      (5) Have you had any prior infections, dental work, or procedures?
   b. Clinical manifestations (Table 3-1)
   c. Abnormal laboratory findings (Table 3-2)
   d. Abnormal diagnostic tests (Table 3-3)
6. Expected medical interventions
   a. Endocarditis
      (1) Parenteral antibiotic therapy, 4 to 6 weeks
      (2) Antipyretics, analgesics
      (3) Valvular surgery if needed, usually at a later date
   b. Myocarditis
      (1) Supportive treatment
      (2) Treat dysrhythmias as they occur
      (3) Antibiotics: organism can be identified
   c. Pericarditis
      (1) Antiinflammatory agents; nonsteroidal antiinflammatory agents are drugs of choice
      (2) Analgesics, antipyretics—aspirin is drug of choice
      (3) Pericardiocentesis for cardiac tamponade—removal of pericardial fluid via needle insertion into the epigastric area
      (4) Pericardial window—open chest drainage of pericardial fluid, pericardium left open to prevent future episodes of cardiac tamponade

Table 3-1. Clinical Manifestations of Inflammatory Heart Disorders

Assessments	Endocarditis	Myocarditis	Pericarditis
Unique Findings	Splinter hemorrhages of nail beds Petechiae— common around conjunctiva, mucous membranes	History of a viral syndrome within weeks, common in spring and fall Sudden unexplained heart failure	Pericardial friction rub
Pain	Not common	Chest pain: pericardial	Chest pain: pleuritic,↑ when lying flat,↓ when upright and leaning forward; may radiate to neck, shoulder back and arms— common between the shoulder and base of their neck; exaggerated with inspiration and body movements
Heart Sounds	Heart murmur— present or intensified	None specific	Distant muffled heart sounds
Pertinent Findings	Fever acute: high >101°F subacute: low grade of 99-100°F Fatigue, malaise	Malaise, easy fatigability Exertional dyspnea	Fever Malaise, fatigue Anxiety Nonproductive cough, orthopnea

Table 3-2. Abnormal Laboratory Findings of Inflammatory Heart Disorders

Laboratory Studies	Endocarditis	Myocarditis	Pericarditis
CBC—WBC	↑	↑	↑
ESR	↑	↑	↑
Blood culture	Positive for infecting organism	Not done	Not done
Rheumatoid factor	+ In 50% of cases	Negative	Negative
Cardiac enzymes	May be ↑	↑	May be ↑

Table 3-3. Abnormal Diagnostic Tests of Inflammatory Heart Disorders

Diagnostic Tests	Endocarditis	Myocarditis	Pericarditis
ECG	Normal initially, later conduction abnormalities, cardiac dysrhythmias	ST segment and T wave abnormalities, Q wave appearance	Elevated ST segment in all leads
Echocardiogram	Identify vegetation on cardiac structures and valvular abnormalities	Dilated ventricles, poor wall contraction	Presence of pericardial fluid, decreased wall motion during systole, abnormal septal movement
Other tests	CXR—cardiomegaly	Endomyocardial biopsy—inflammatory process in myocardial cells, myocardial necrosis, CXR—cardiomegaly	CXR—enlarged cardiac silhouette

         (5)   Pericardiectomy—removal of both layers of pericardium for fibrous pericarditis or constrictive pericarditis

7. Nursing diagnoses
    a. Chest pain related to cardiac inflammatory process
    b. Decreased cardiac output related to poor contractile state of the myocardium
    c. Altered body temperature related to cardiac inflammatory process
8. Client goals
    a. Client will state that chest pain is decreased or relieved
    b. Client will exhibit BP and HR within 20% of baseline
    c. Client will exhibit body temperature of 37° C or 98.6° F or baseline for the client
9. Nursing interventions
    a. Acute care
        (1) Endocarditis
            (a) Evaluate for congestive heart failure changes and evidence of embolization
            (b) Administer antipyretics as needed for temperature elevation; administer antibiotics as ordered
            (c) Evaluate for improvement of murmurs and activity intolerance
        (2) Myocarditis
            (a) Monitor for congestive heart failure changes
            (b) Offer pain relief for chest discomfort
            (c) Evaluate for less fatigability and exertional dyspnea
        (3) Pericarditis
            (a) Offer pain relief for chest pain
            (b) Administer fever-reducing agents for temperature elevation
            (c) Evaluate client frequently for complications
                (i) Cardiac tamponade—distended neck veins that remain distended during inspiration (Kussmaul's sign), shortness of breath
                (ii) Pericardial effusion—increased anxiety and restlessness, dyspnea, hypotension, muffled heart sounds
    b. Home care regarding client education
        (1) Endocarditis

      (a)   Home administration of IV antibiotics
           (i)   Importance of evaluating IV access before each administration
          (ii) Findings associated with infection in IV access
        (iii) Importance of giving medications on time and not missing a dose
      (b)   Gradual increase of activity
           (i)   Balance rest and activity
          (ii) Frequent rest periods
        (iii) No activity lasting longer than 15 to 20 minutes
         (iv) Increase activity by 5 minutes per day
          (v) Stop activity when fatigued or short of breath
      (c)   Avoidance of people with upper respiratory infections
      (d)   Careful adherence to antibiotic prophylaxis for any dental or invasive procedure
  (2) Myocarditis
      (a)   Monitoring techniques for any changes, especially in HR or rhythm, flu-like symptoms, report to physician immediately
      (b)   How to monitor for findings associated with heart failure
      (c)   Need for family members to learn CPR techniques in case of life-threatening dysrhythmia
  (3) Pericarditis
      (a)   Seek help immediately
           (i)   Chest pain, eased by an upright, leaning forward position
          (ii) Sudden shortness of breath
      (b)   Wear a medical alert bracelet or necklace with indicated condition
      (c)   Avoid fatigue
10.   Evaluation protocol
    a.   How do I know that my interventions were effective?
      (1) Has client's chest pain gone away or improved?
      (2) Does client feel warm? If yes, check temperature.
      (3) Does client feel less short of breath or have less or no swelling in ankles or feet?

     b.   What criteria will I use to change my interventions?
- (1)   Client indicates chest pain has become worse or has not decreased in intensity
- (2)   Client states a feeling of being warm with a temperature elevation
- (3)   Client exhibits sudden sustained shortness of breath, audible crackles in the lungs, increased anxiety and restlessness, jugular venous distension at 35 degree or higher angle, or has developed edema of the ankles and/or feet

     c.   How will I know that my client teaching has been effective?
- (1)   Client-family able to demonstrate correct technique for taking a pulse and identify correct criteria for calling physician
- (2)   Able to demonstrate correct technique for home IV antibiotic administration
- (3)   Able to correctly identify circumstances that require prophylactic antibiotic administration

11.   Older adult alert
     a.   Older adult clients' inelastic vascular systems will not respond as quickly or as effectively to the situations of inflammatory heart disorders. Little compensation will occur for a sudden drop in cardiac output, thus clinical findings may be more acute.
     b.   Older adult clients with prior angina may attempt to treat pain associated with inflammatory heart disorders as if it were angina pectoris

REVIEW QUESTIONS

1. During client assessment the nurse identifies jugular venous distention. The evaluation of this finding is that the client may be manifesting
   a. Left-sided heart failure
   b. Right-sided heart failure
   c. Dehydration
   d. Pulmonary congestion

2. When assessing a client's chest pain, she indicates that it has a sharp character; she points to her sternum when asked where her pain is located; and she indicates that it radiates up into her neck. What other information is needed to distinguish this pain from a possible myocardial infarction? The client
   a. Took two nitroglycerin at home without relief of pain
   b. States the pain is accompanied by nausea
   c. Has a family history of coronary artery disease in women
   d. Took a third nitroglycerin on arrival at the hospital, which relieved her pain

3. The priority assessment in the client experiencing an acute myocardial infarction would be
   a. Peripheral pulses
   b. Heart rate
   c. Airway
   d. Chest pain

4. Appropriate intervention for a client hospitalized for cardiac dysrhythmias and for complaints of difficulty breathing would be
   a. Give the ordered morphine
   b. Place oxygen on the client
   c. Start an IV
   d. Call the physician

5. The client describes a nightly ritual of going to bed, laying flat in bed, and waking up around 2:00 A.M. and feeling as if he is smothering. This would be documented as
   a. Orthopnea
   b. Dyspnea
   c. Paroxysmal nocturnal dyspnea
   d. Nocturnal dyspnea

6. The most appropriate nursing intervention for the client with complaints of exertional dyspnea would include
   a. Frequent rest periods
   b. Ordered oxygen available for periods of exertion
   c. Nitroglycerin available for periods of exertion
   d. Ambulating the client close to the bed so the client can rest while ambulating as needed

7. A client is in pulmonary edema. Which one of the following STAT physician orders is most appropriate to question?
   a. Arterial blood gas evaluation
   b. Digoxin 0.25 mg IV
   c. Lasix 40 mg IM
   d. Oxygen at 4 liters per minute

8. A client with mitral valve disease requires more teaching when the client tells you
   a. "I take my penicillin only when the dentist has to drill a tooth"
   b. "I take my penicillin before every dentist visit"
   c. "I weigh myself every morning at 7:00 with my pajamas on, before I eat breakfast"
   d. "I have removed the salt shaker from the stove so I can't add salt as I cook"

9. A priority for client teaching for the client returning home following a brief hospitalization for bacterial endocarditis is
   a. Monitor daily weight
   b. Balance rest and activity
   c. Avoid people with upper respiratory infections
   d. IV antibiotic administration technique

10. An assessment finding the pericarditis client should be alerted to is
    a. Sudden palpitations
    b. Sudden sustained SOB
    c. Lethargy
    d. Sleeplessness

ANSWERS, RATIONALES, AND TEST-TAKING TIPS

Rationale	Test-Taking Tips

1. Correct answer: b

Jugular venous distention is a result of back flow of blood from a failing right ventricle. Assess the *L*ungs for *L*eft heart failure. Dehydration results in a dry client and neck veins would be down, not distended.

Eliminate *a* and *d* since both deal with the lung. Use common sense: if dehydrated, the neck veins would be flat, sometime even when the client is supine.

2. Correct answer: d

The third nitroglycerin, relieving her pain gives valuable information—she is within the criteria of three NTG tablets allowed for angina before further interventions; nausea is not necessarily associated with an acute MI. Family history of coronary artery disease, male or female, contributes only to high risk, not to differentiation between angina and MI.

The key words are "distinguish the pain." THE ONLY way to differentiate angina from MI pain is by evaluation of the effects of three nitroglycerine 5 minutes apart. If pain is not relieved, MI is suspected.

3. Correct answer: c

Airway is always a priority of assessment in any client. Responses *b* and *d* are appropriate but not the priority. They would be done secondly. Response *a* would be done last in this given list.

ABC's guide priority assessment no matter what the given situation is. Remember to select the answer that supports what you KNOW— not what you don't know. Cluster options *a, b,* and *d* with the theme cardiac—select *c,* if you have no idea of the correct answer.

4. **Correct answer: b**

Placing oxygen on a client who is short of breath is the correct intervention; that would take priority over starting an IV, giving morphine, or calling the physician.

The most common error on this question is to read into the words of "cardiac dysrhythmias" to mean ventricular dysrhythmia. As written these terms could mean atrial dysrhythmias which are not as life threatening as ventricular. Thus, difficulty breathing is the major focus of the question.

5. **Correct answer: c**

Going to bed in a flat position but waking up in the middle of the night feeling as if you are smothering is referred to as paroxysmal nocturnal dyspnea (PND). Orthopena is difficulty breathing lying down. Dyspnea is difficulty breathing. Nocturnal dyspnea is difficulty breathing at night without definition of how it happens.

Responses *a, b,* and *d* do describe the situation. However, they are too general of a description. Use common sense to narrow the selections to *c* or *d* since the event happens at night. Then, narrow it down further with the use of common sense; the situation happens suddenly and the word paroxysmal means sudden or outburst.

6. **Correct answer: b**

The best response here is to have oxygen available for any periods of exertion; the options a and d may be appropriate but not the best option or most realistic.

Option *a* is too general of a selection. Frequent rest periods WHEN? It doesn't give enough information. Common sense: option *c* is appropriate for pain *not* dyspnea. And option *d* sounds good yet contradicts itself to say ambulate close to the bed yet rest "while ambulating as needed"; if ambulating as needed then the client could go wherever desired.

7. **Correct answer: c**

Lasix IM must be questioned; a client in pulmonary edema must have Lasix IV to bring about quick diuresis and decreased lung water; all other responses are appropriate orders.

The key words "pulmonary edema" guides one to determine that the left heart has acutely failed and can't get blood out through the systemic circulation; thus circulation will be poor and the injection is inappropriate.

8. **Correct answer: a**

The client must be taught to take prophylactic antibiotics before any dental procedure; all other statements are correct.

The word "only" in option *a* makes the client response too narrow. This alerts the reader to use common sense to suspect that there are many other precautions this client type would need to follow.

9. **Correct answer: d**

The priority teaching need for a client going home following hospitalization for bacterial endocarditis is how to administer the IV antibiotics at home, required for 4 to 6 weeks.

The key word "brief" alerts the reader that longer treatment for an infection, endocarditis, at home would be needed. Recall that in general most infections commonly require 10 to 14 days of therapy.

10. **Correct answer: b**

Sudden sustained shortness of breath is the best response indicative of cardiac tamponade, a life-threatening complication of pericarditis. Responses *c* and *d* are indicative of increased P_aCo_2 >45 or intracranial pressure. Response *a* is most indicative of mitral valve dysfunction.

Of the given options, use the concept of the ABC's—airway, breathing, circulation takes priority to guide assessments and interventions. Thus, *b* is the correct response.

The Vascular System

STUDY OUTCOMES

After completing this chapter, the reader will be able to do
the following:

▼ Identify major anatomic components and functions of the vascular
  system.
▼ Identify assessment findings of clients with alterations of the
  vascular system.
▼ Choose appropriate nursing diagnoses for the vascular disorders
  discussed.
▼ Implement appropriate nursing interventions for the client with
  a vascular disorder.
▼ Evaluate progress of the client with a vascular disorder for
  establishment of new nursing interventions based on evaluation
  findings.

KEY TERMS

Peripheral vascular resistance (PVR)	Also called *afterload*. An impedance to blood flow, involves three factors: 1. Aortic pressure 2. Vessel size 3. Blood viscosity
Vasoconstriction	Contraction or squeezing of the walls of the blood vessels causing a decrease in diameter of the vessel lumen.
Vasoconstrictor	Any agent that will cause contraction of the walls of the blood vessels.
Vasodilatation	Expansion of the size of a blood vessel, causing an increase in the diameter of the lumen of the vessel.
Vasodilator	Any agent that will cause an increase in the size of a blood vessel.

CONTENT REVIEW

I. The vascular system has many functions

A. System responsibilities
1. Carry oxygenated blood and nutrients to tissues and cells
2. Carry deoxygenated blood back to lungs for reoxygenation
3. Carry waste material away from tissues and cells, back to organs of excretion

B. The lymph system—part of the vascular system
1. System responsibilities
   a. Remove fluid and proteins from interstitial space
   b. Return them to the circulating fluid volume
   c. Similarly transport immune components back into the circulatory system via the lymph system

II. Structure and function

A. Arteries
1. Carry blood rich in oxygen and nutrients away from the heart to tissues and cells via the aorta

    2. Have a very muscular, thick wall structure, composed of three layers
       a. Outer layer—tunica adventitia
       b. Middle layer—tunica media
       c. Inner layer (contacts with blood flow)—tunica intima
    3. Arterioles—smallest branches of arteries, connecting to capillaries
    4. Exception: Pulmonary artery—carries unoxygenated blood away from right side of heart to lungs

B. **Veins**
    1. Carry unoxygenated blood back to right side of heart for reoxygenation and waste removal
    2. Have thinner walls; this allows for easier contraction and expansion
    3. Walls contain the same three layers as arteries; wall thickness is greatly reduced
    4. Uniqueness
       a. Contain valves at various intervals to ensure blood flow will continue in a forward motion toward the heart
       b. Flow driven by pumping of skeletal muscle and suction generated by respiratory movements, especially inspiration
    5. Venules—smallest branches of veins, connected from capillaries
    6. Exception: Pulmonary vein carries oxygenated blood back to left side of heart away from lungs

C. **Capillaries or capillary bed**
    1. Microscopically small vessels connecting arterioles and venules
    2. Site of transfer of nutrition, fluids, and gases into the tissues
    3. Collect waste from excretory organs

D. **Lymph vessels**
    1. Component of the capillary bed
    2. Similar to veins in structure and flow, with the same three layers and intermittent valves to propel lymph fluid forward
    3. Collect fluid and proteins from the interstitial space and return them to the circulating blood volume via the thoracic ducts to the subclavian veins
    4. Introduce important elements of the immune system such as antibodies and lymphocytes into the circulating blood volume
    5. Lymphatic structures—tonsils, spleen, thymus

E. **Sequence of flow—blood and lymph**

Outlet of the left ventricle

Aorta, 100 mm Hg
Highest pressure in the vascular system

Arteries

Arterioles

Capillaries ► Small lymphatics

Venules   Larger lymphatics

Veins   Thoracic ducts

Inferior vena cava   Subclavian veins at the
                            junction of the subclavian
Superior vena cava ◄   ◄   and internal jugular veins

Right atria 0 to 5 mm Hg
Lowest pressure in vascular system

Right ventricle

Pulmonary artery

Lungs

Left atria

III. Targeted concerns

A. **Pharmacology—priority drug classifications**

   1. Antihypertensive drugs

      a. Beta adrenergic blockers (discussed in Chapter 3, p. 62)

      b. Calcium channel blockers (discussed in Chapter 3, pp. 62-63)

      c. Angiotensin converting enzyme (ACE) inhibitors—interrupts the renin–angiotensin-aldosterone system; prevents the formation of angiotensin II, a potent vasoconstrictor from angiotensin I, also inhibits aldosterone release

(1) Expected effects—decreases the production of aldosterone, and thus decreases sodium and water retention with decreased circulating blood volume; a decrease in vascular tone results in vasodilation

(2) Commonly given drugs
   (a) Captopril**** (Capoten)
   (b) Enalapril**** (Vasotec)

(3) Nursing considerations
   (a) Administer 1 hour before meals, at the same time each day
   (b) Monitor labs—electrolytes; for elevated levels of creatinine, AST, ALT, slight elevation of potassium; for diminished counts of WBC
   (c) Monitor BP carefully with initiation or change of therapy
   (d) Volume-depleted clients may exhibit a profound decrease in BP or sustained orthostatic hypotension
   (e) Orthostatic hypotension common with first dose
   (f) Major side effects—proteinuria, renal failure, agranulocytosis, neutropenia
   (g) Rebound hypertension if suddenly stopped

d. Alpha–adrenergic receptor blockers—inhibit the action of the sympathetic nervous system at some point along the system

(1) Expected effects—venous and arteriolar vasodilation, lowered BP or sustained orthostatic hypotension

(2) Commonly given drugs
   (a) Clonidine (Catapres)
   (b) Methyldopa (Aldomet)
   (c) Prazosin (Minipress)

(3) Nursing considerations
   (a) Since any sympathetic inhibitor can cause orthostatic hypotension, lying and standing BP are imperative; check at least daily or, if changes in dosage, check prior to medication administration
   (b) Renal monitoring is imperative, such as creatinine and BUN monitoring and strict I&O; all of these drugs may cause a decrease in renal blood flow
   (c) Monitor BP carefully and frequently if client has findings associated with dehydration

**** ACE inhibitors end in *pril.*

            (d)   More common side effects
                (i)   CNS depression
                (ii) Impotence
               (iii) Psychotic disturbances such as nightmares, depression, delirium
            (e)   Major side effects
                (i)   Aldomet: thrombocytopenia, leukopenia
                (ii) Catapres: CHF

e.   Direct smooth muscle relaxants—directly dilate the arterioles

    (1)   Expected effects—decreased peripheral resistance, afterload, decreased BP

    (2)   Commonly given drugs
        (a)   Hydralazine (Apresoline)
        (b)   Minoxidil (Loniten)

    (3)   Nursing considerations
        (a)   Laboratory tests before starting—CBC, creatinine, LE prep, ANA titer, electrolytes
        (b)   Severe rebound hypertension if stopped; warn client not to stop without physician's orders
        (c)   Teach client to rise slowly from chair or bed because of high risk of orthostatic hypotension
        (d)   Monitor BP carefully, especially after first dose and with any changes in dosage; for Minoxidil check HR prior to dose for reflex tachycardia
        (e)   Minoxidil used topically for alopecia

f.   Diuretic agents—induce excretion of water, sodium, and/or potassium from the body

    (1)   Expected effects—reduction in circulating blood volume, preload, decreased BP

    (2)   Commonly given drugs
        (a)   Hydrochlorothiazide (Hydrodiuril)—potassium lost, thiazide diuretic
        (b)   Furosemide (Lasix)—potassium lost, loop diuretic
        (c)   Bumetanide (Bumex)—potassium lost, loop diuretic
        (d)   Spironolactone (Aldactone)—potassium saved

    (3)   Nursing considerations
        (a)   Monitor sodium, potassium, magnesium, and chloride levels; check baseline levels before initial dose is given

  (b) Teach client to evaluate
    (i) Daily weight, report sharp loss or gain—
        >2 lb/day
    (ii) Postural hypotension from loss of fluid
    (iii) Electrolyte replacement if needed
  (c) Monitor for metabolic alkalosis from loss of
      chloride—circumoral and extremity numbness
      and tingling, feeling of lightheadedness,
      apprehension, irritability, disorientation,
      confusion, or more severe findings of
      hypocalcemia such as seizures or tetany
g. Drugs used for hypertensive crisis—given only
   intravenously; cause potent, rapid vasodilation of arteriolar
   bed
  (1) Expected effect—rapid drop of BP, within
      minutes
  (2) Commonly given drugs
    (a) Nitroprusside (Nipride)—IV drip only
    (b) Diazoxide (Hyperstat)—IV bolus only
  (3) Nursing considerations
    (a) Monitor BP continuously, every 1 to 10 minutes
        if using a noninvasive BP
    (b) Use arterial pressure line—best evaluation for
        continuous monitoring
2. Anticoagulant agents—interferes with coagulation pathway at
   some point
  a. Expected effect—prevent blood clotting
  b. Commonly given drugs
    (1) Oral anticoagulant—most common
      (a) Warfarin sodium (Coumadin)—fully therapeutic
          in 2 to 3 days; lasts about 7 to 10 days after final
          dose
      (b) Antidote—vitamin K (Aquamephyton), given IM,
          IV slowly
    (2) Parenteral anticoagulant—most common
      (a) Heparin sodium—effects immediately; lasts
          about 4 hours after final dose
      (b) Antidote—Protamine sulfate, given IV slowly
  c. Nursing considerations
    (1) Monitor activated partial thromboplastin time
        (APTT) for heparin administration; on the average,
        normal level is 30 seconds for APTT

       (2) Monitor prothrombin time (PT) for warfarin administration; on the average, normal level is 15 seconds

       (3) Do not administer aspirin to clients taking oral anticoagulants

       (4) Evaluate all urine, stools, and vomitus for blood

       (5) Institute bleeding precautions—soft toothbrush, avoid IM injections, evaluate venipunctures for bleeding

       (6) Therapeutic level for both oral and parenteral drugs is 1.5 to 2 times the normal control levels

       (7) Side effects

          (a) Coumadin—nausea, vomiting, anorexia

          (b) Heparin—alopecia with long term use

       (8) Major toxic effect of both preparations is bleeding

3. Antiplatelet agents—prevent aggregation of platelets

   a. Expected effect—decreased thrombus formation

   b. Commonly given drugs

       (1) Aspirin

       (2) Dipyridamole (Persantine)

       (3) Ticlopidine (Ticlid)

   c. Nursing considerations

       (1) Caution clients against taking aspirin to treat fever and chills for more than 24 hours; it may mask a serious infection or blood dyscrasia

       (2) Instruct client not to take aspirin with coumadin; results would enhance coumadin effect with increased bleeding risk; coumadin may be given with dipyridamole post valve replacement

4. Thrombolytic agents—dissolve a thrombus or embolus

   a. Expected effects—return of blood flow to vessel obstructed by a thrombus; stops showering of emboli

   b. Commonly given drugs

       (1) Streptokinase (Streptase)

       (2) Alteplase (Activase)

   c. Nursing considerations

       (1) Clients must be started on heparin drip concurrently with thrombolytic agent to prevent more thrombus formation

       (2) Monitor client for excessive bleeding; monitor all body excrement for blood

       (3) Institute bleeding precautions; soft toothbrush, no IM injections, evaluate all venipunctures for bleeding

        (4)   Assess client carefully for severe allergic reaction or anaphylaxis; most commonly seen with streptokinase

5. Sympathomimetic agents—mimics the effect of stimulation of organs and blood vessels by the sympathetic nervous system; vasopressor
   a. Expected effect—elevated BP
   b. Commonly given drugs
      (1) Dopamine (Intropin)
      (2) Dobutamine (Dobutrex)
      (3) Ephedrine
   c. Nursing considerations
      (1) For best results, blood volume must be adequate prior to starting IV drip; minimal or no effective response in the dehydrated client
      (2) Continuous BP monitoring is imperative—every 2 to 5 minutes
      (3) Best evaluation of BP—arterial line
      (4) Must titrate drug carefully to prevent hypertension
      (5) Monitor IV sites carefully for infiltration, may cause sloughing of tissue
      (6) Best administration method—central line

B. **Procedures**
   1. Doppler ultrasonography—noninvasive test; identifies presence of a decrease in arterial blood flow by evaluating audible arterial signals; arterial flow: intermittent solid sounds; venous flow: more continuous swish sound
   2. Computerized tomography (CT scan)—permits visualization of arterial walls and adjacent structures; helpful in diagnosis of aortic aneurysms
   3. Angiography (arteries) and venography (veins)—invasive tests; contrast medium is injected into artery or vein; x–ray studies completed of the area injected; actual obstructions can be visualized

C. **Psychosocial**
   1. Noncompliance—a major concern in hypertensive clients; a major factor: lack of symptoms associated with hypertension; symptoms tend to remind clients to take their medication
   2. Fear—a major concern in many clients with vascular disease; directly related to danger of death or loss of limb
   3. Lifestyle changes—a major issue in clients with arterial occlusive disease, which may eventually end in limb amputation; other issues considered: need for change of diet, exercise, cessation of smoking or of caffeine use

D. **Health history—question sequence**
 1. What symptoms are you having that made it necessary for you to seek assistance?
 2. Are you being treated for other disorders?
 3. Is there a family history of vascular disease?
 4. Are you presently taking any prescription or over-the-counter drugs?
 5. Have you noticed a change in your weight? Either a loss or gain? How much and over what period of time?
 6. Do you smoke? How much and for how long?
 7. Do you use alcohol? How much and for how long?
 8. Are you presently following a special diet? What kind?
 9. Do you have a history of high cholesterol or triglycerides?
 10. Do you exercise? How much and how often?
 11. Do you have pain in your legs when walking? How far must you walk before the pain begins?
 12. Do you live or work in a stressful environment? How do you cope with this stress?
 13. Do you have headaches? How often? How do you relieve these?
E. **Physical exam—appropriate sequence**
 1. Airway, breathing, circulation—vital signs
 2. Level of consciousness—awake, alert, and oriented; pupillary response
 3. Skin color, temperature, moisture, and turgor; mucous membranes
 4. Examine neck for distended neck veins
 5. Inspection of the chest, bilateral chest movements, abnormal chest movements
 6. Palpation of the chest for tenderness, growths
 7. Auscultation of heart sounds
 8. Inspection of abdomen for pulsations, asymmetry
 9. Auscultation of abdomen for abnormal sounds, bruit
 10. Palpation of abdomen
 11. Examination of peripheral pulses, especially feet

IV. Pathophysiologic disorders
A. **Shock**
 1. Definition—insufficient tissue perfusion; if untreated or resistant to treatment, result is inadequate tissue oxygenation and cellular death
 2. Pathophysiology—shock is the state in which clients have lost one of the three important functions of the circulatory system: circulating blood volume, a balance between vasoconstriction

and vasodilation, or a competent pumping action of the heart. Clients pass through several stages of shock, regardless of the cause of the syndrome.

   a. Stage I, compensated—body uses compensatory mechanisms: increased heart rate, vasoconstriction of peripheral and gastrointestinal vessels to maintain near normal cardiac output and BP

   b. Stage II, decompensated—beginning drop in cardiac output and BP

      (1) Massive vasoconstriction, which causes vasodilation of the microcirculatory system (capillary circulation)

      (2) Extensive pooling of blood in capillaries of the microcirculatory system

      (3) Transfer of fluid from blood into the interstitial space and edema

      (4) Drastic reduction in venous return with a significant drop in BP

      (5) Lack of cellular oxygenation occurs because of the decrease in capillary blood flow

      (6) Lactic acidosis production begins because cells are functioning in anaerobic metabolism

   c. Stage III, progressive

      (1) Occurs if tissue perfusion is not improved

      (2) Shock becomes more profound with cell necrosis

      (3) Eventually organ death and client demise

  3. Etiology

   a. Hypovolemic shock—lack of adequate circulating blood volume; frequently from blood loss with trauma; plasma loss as with burns; dehydration syndrome with fluid loss, such as with gastrointestinal losses

   b. Cardiogenic shock—severely decreased cardiac output from poor pumping capability of the heart; more common after an extensive myocardial infarction or with chronic cardiomyopathy

   c. Distributive shock—blood vessels dilate throughout the vascular bed causing a redistribution and pooling of blood; also termed vasogenic

      (1) Three types

         (a) Anaphylactic shock—allergic or hypersensitive reaction to an allergen; clients also manifest bronchial constriction with acute respiratory distress or arrest

        (b) Neurogenic shock—inability of the nervous system to control dilation of the blood vessels; most common after spinal cord injury, spinal anesthesia, and severe vagal stimulation induced by pain, trauma, or stress

        (c) Septic shock—pathogenic organisms present in the blood lead to a release of vasoactive materials, such as histamine, prostaglandins, bradykinins, and leukotrienes, causing massive vasodilation

4. Assessment
   a. Ask the following questions
      (1) What is your name? Where are you? What day or year is it?
      (2) Do you feel weak or nauseated?
      (3) Do you feel short of breath?
      (4) Clinical manifestations (Table 4-1)
   b. Abnormal laboratory findings (Table 4-2)
   c. Abnormal diagnostic studies
      (1) ECG—tachycardia, also may show ischemia and dysrhythmias
      (2) CXR—pulmonary congestion in later stages of shock, especially cardiogenic
5. Expected medical interventions
   a. Fluid replacement as necessary with crystalloids, normal saline, or lactated ringers; colloids, hetastarch (hespan) or human albumins or other plasma expanders; and blood; packed cells may be given more than whole blood
   b. Fluid volume monitoring with central venous pressure (CVP) line, or pulmonary artery line; keep CVP >8 cm H_2O, systolic pressure >90, mean arterial pressure (MAP) between 70 and 90
   c. Oxygen to improve tissue oxygenation
   d. Mechanical ventilation as necessary to maintain respiratory status
   e. Vasopressor agents to maintain BP
   f. Laboratory test monitoring for evaluation of the treatment of abnormalities
   g. Nutritional support via enteral or parenteral routes
6. Nursing Diagnoses
   a. Impaired gas exchange related to diminished circulation
   b. Altered tissue perfusion (gastrointestinal, cerebral, cardiac, pulmonary, renal) related to impaired circulation

Table 4-1. Clinical Manifestations of Shock

Assessment Findings	Hypovolemic	Cardiogenic	Distributive
Respiratory	Rapid, shallow	Same	Same
Cardiovascular	Rapid, weak, thready pulse, hypotension	Same	*Anaphylactic—* same *Neurogenic—* bradycardia hypotension *Septic—same*
Integumentary	Cool, clammy, pale skin	Cool, clammy, pale skin	*Anaphylactic and Neurogenic—*dry, cool, pale skin *Septic—*early: warm, dry flushed skin late: same as hypovolemic
Neurologic	Anxiety, irritability nervousness, restlessness, leading to confusion, and loss of consciousness	Same	*Anaphylactic—*same, *Neurogenic—*same *Septic—*drowsiness leading to stupor then coma
Gastrointestinal and Genitourinary	Decreased bowel sounds, oliguria	Same	Same

    c. Decreased cardiac output related to poor cardiac pumping capability, inadequate blood volume, vascular pooling

    d. Fluid volume deficit related to blood loss, fluid shift into the interstitial spaces and tissues

  7. Client goals

    a. Client will maintain a P_aO_2 >80 mm Hg, pH between 7.35 and 7.45, and a P_aCO_2 between 35 and 45 mm Hg

    b. Client will maintain adequate tissue perfusion of all organs as evidenced by minimal adequate functioning of those organs i.e., clients can state name, location, and correct date or year; urine output at least 30 ml/hr, bowel sounds present without diarrhea

    c. Client will keep BP and HR within 20% of baseline

Table 4-2. Abnormal Laboratory Findings of Shock

Laboratory Findings	Hypovolemic	Cardiogenic	Distributive
Hemoglobin/ hematocrit	↓	–	–
WBC	↑	↑	↑
ESR	↑	↑	↑
Blood cultures	–	–	+ growth of causative agent, most common gram + or gram –
Electrolytes	K↑ from cellular death	Same	Same
BUN	↑ from dehydration, blood loss, breakdown of old blood in gut, decreased renal perfusion	↑ from decreased renal perfusion	↑ from decreased renal perfusion
Creatinine	↑ related to decreased renal perfusion	Same	Same
Blood glucose	↑ in response to stress	Same	Same
PT, PTT	↑	↑	↑
Platelets	↓	↓	↓
Arterial blood gases	Hypoxemia, metabolic acidosis, respiratory alkalosis	Same	Same

      d. Client will maintain adequate fluid volume as evidenced by urine output of at least 30 ml/hr

  8. Nursing interventions

      a. Acute care

          (1) Maintain patent airway while monitoring breathing patterns for tiring and increased respiratory effort

          (2) Monitor circulatory parameters every 10 to 15 minutes until stable

          (3) Maintain at least one large bore IV, 16 or 18 gauge, for fluid and blood products administration

(4) Be prepared to utilize a modified Trendelenburg (body flat, legs elevated) position to maintain organ perfusion when therapy is ineffective or when therapy is being started

(5) Give all medications intravenously

b. Home care regarding client education

(1) If shock has been induced by an allergen, clients must be instructed to wear a medical-alert bracelet to alert health care personnel to allergy; facilitate clients obtaining and learning how to use epinephrine kit; must carry with them at all times

(2) Clients who have experienced a critically ill situation such as shock, may leave the hospital confused and somewhat disoriented or forgetful. They will need help at home to reorganize their thinking processes and bring this aspect of their illness to completion.

9. Evaluation protocol

a. How do I know that my interventions were effective?

(1) Does client know own name? location? date or year?

(2) Does client feel dizzy or weak?

(3) Does client feel short of breath?

b. What criteria will I use to change my interventions?

(1) Client confused as to person, place, and time

(2) Client indicates dizzy and weak feelings, even in a flat or modified Trendelenburg position; assessment findings indicate vital signs are not stabilizing

(3) Client indicates shortness of breath with assessment findings that indicate increased respiratory effort, shallow respirations, and no energy to deep breathe

c. How will I know that my client teaching has been effective?

(1) Client describes the situation that would require the use of an epinephrine kit, and demonstrates use of the kit

(2) Client orders a medical-alert bracelet

(3) Client states feeling less anxious, with fewer periods of confusion or forgetfulness at home, and progressing to a state of normalcy experienced before the illness

10. Older adult alert

a. Older adult clients, have increased peripheral vascular resistance as a normal change of aging. Thus, little compensation is available for those in shock. Vital signs will change more rapidly than in younger adults.

    b. Older adults have decreased elasticity of the blood vessels. This results in a decrease in the normal compensatory mechanism for vasoconstriction seen in younger adults.

    c. Older adult clients may have a higher BP as a result of increased vascular resistance. Therefore, in evaluation of vital signs keep in mind the clients' baseline. Older adults may tend to have a higher baseline BP. Be aware that a drop in BP >20 mm Hg may have significant effects especially on renal glomerular filtration rate; don't wait for a drop to 100/60 to seek intervention.

    d. If on cardiac medication, older adult clients will have inhibition of the normal compensatory action, i.e., increased HR of >100. Look for a sustained increase in HR of >20 beats per minute over client baseline HR. Consider this increase as a possible sign of shock.

B. **Atherosclerosis**

  1. Definition—one type of arteriosclerosis that represents a broad class of arterial wall changes associated with decreased elasticity; occlusive arterial disease, affects mainly the coronary, cerebral, and femoral arteries as well as the aorta

  2. Pathophysiology—involves the accumulation of cholesterol and lipids, called lesions, in the wall of affected arteries

    a. Layer of the wall most commonly affected is the intima rather than the medis or adventia

    b. Progression of lesions

      (1) Start with a fatty streak

      (2) Progress to a fibrous plaque

      (3) Proceed to a lesion made up of the fibrous plaque, calcium, and a thrombus

      (4) Lesions progress over many years; eventually occlude the affected artery to as high as 100% of the lumen

  3. Etiology—many factors characterized as modifiable factors and nonmodifiable factors are believed to precipitate the onset of atherosclerosis

    a. Nonmodifiable factors

      (1) Heredity

      (2) Age

      (3) Gender

      (4) Race

    b. Modifiable factors

      (1) Environment, including dietary factors

      (2) Smoking

      (3) Hypercholesteremia

        (4) Hypertension

        (5) Diabetes

        (6) Obesity

        (7) Stress

        (8) Sedentary lifestyle

  4. Incidence—underlying cause of most cardiac and vascular diseases

  5. Assessment—widely variable depending on the vessels affected. The various disorders that can occur will be discussed in detail within the chapters in which the disorders belong, i.e., coronary artery disease—the cardiac system.

C. **Hypertension**

  1. Definition

    a. A consistent elevation of BP on three or more checks

    b. Systolic >140 and/or diastolic >90

    c. Hypertensive crisis is an acute rise in BP to a life-threatening level, >200 mm Hg systolic and >110 mm Hg diastolic

  2. Pathophysiology—some factors increase BP

    a. Change in hormones that regulate BP, such as aldosterone, renin, ADH

    b. Increase in circulating blood volume

    c. Increase in HR

    d. Circumstances that cause vasoconstriction

    e. Circumstances that stimulate the sympathetic nervous system

  3. Etiology

    a. Classified as having primary or essential hypertension—meaning the cause is unknown; 90% of clients

    b. Or, secondary hypertension—meaning hypertension is from a known cause, i.e., renal disease, pregnancy; 10% of clients

  4. Incidence—estimated that over 85 million Americans have hypertension, but nearly half of that population is unaware of their problem

  5. Assessment

    a. Ask the following questions

    Remember—Hypertension is asymptomatic in the majority of clients. These questions are leading toward clients who are *beginning* to have symptoms.

        (1) Do you have trouble remembering?

        (2) Do you ever have dizzy spells or a feeling of light-headedness?

        (3) Do you feel tired quite often?

(4) Do you suffer from headaches? If yes, when do they occur most often? Is there a pattern to the headaches?

(5) Do you ever have nose bleeds?

(6) Do you feel as if you have a lot of stress in your life, and if so how do you handle it?

b. Clinical manifestations

(1) Usually none in the client with mild to moderate hypertension

(2) Moderate to severe

(a) Difficulty remembering

(b) Headaches, common upon waking

(c) Palpitations

(d) Epistaxis—very common in hypertensive crisis or very high undiagnosed hypertension

(3) BP >140/90 on three separate occasions

c. Abnormal laboratory findings—with renal involvement

(1) Urinalysis—proteinuria, hematuria

(2) Creatinine elevated

(3) BUN elevated

(4) Cholesterol and lipid levels elevated

d. Abnormal diagnostic tests

(1) ECG—left ventricular hypertrophy

(2) CXR—left ventricular enlargement

6. Expected medical interventions

a. Weight reduction as necessary

b. Encourage cessation of smoking

c. Low-salt diet

d. Restriction of caffeine and alcohol in diet

e. Encourage increased exercise

f. Antihypertensive medication if lifestyle alterations are ineffective after implementation at least 6 months

7. Nursing diagnoses

a. Knowledge deficit regarding medical regime related to incomplete client teaching

b. Risk for noncompliance to medical regime related to asymptomatic illness and side effects from medication regime

8. Client goals

a. Client will explain individualized medical regime

b. Client will follow medical regime as evidenced by controlled BP and loss of weight

9. Nursing interventions
   a. Acute care—hypertensive crisis
      (1) BP every 5 to 15 minutes until stable and controlled
      (2) Maintain cardiac monitoring for dysrhythmias
      (3) Evaluate neurologic status every 30 min to every hour for changes
      (4) Maintain IV access for antihypertensive drug therapy
      (5) Monitor laboratory values—creatinine, electrolytes, H&H, for hydration status and renal function
   b. Home care regarding client education
      (1) Low-sodium, low-fat, limited-caffeine, and possibly reduced-calorie diet
      (2) Expected effectiveness of medications ordered with possible side effects; client side effects should be reported to physician
      (3) Follow-up exams with physician and frequent BP monitoring
      (4) Discuss the relationship between exercise, diet, medications, weight loss, and BP control
      (5) Caution use of over-the-counter substances such as cold medications and their ability to raise BP
10. Evaluation protocol
    a. How do I know that my interventions were effective? Note: Acute care interventions will be best evaluated by objective data.
       (1) BP is maintained at a level compatible with organs not being compromised
       (2) Neurologic status is stable and minimal or no deficit is noted
       (3) Cardiac dysrhythmias are not apparent
    b. What criteria will I use to change my interventions?
       (1) Unstable BP
       (2) Neurologic deficit or deterioration noted in assessment
       (3) Significant cardiac dysrhythmias present
    c. How will I know that my client teaching has been effective?
       (1) Client uses small amounts of salt at the table only
       (2) Client reads labels before buying and prepares low-fat foods
       (3) Client maintains appropriate weight as directed by physician

          (4) Client can describe method of taking medication, side effects necessary to alert physician, and BP pattern

          (5) Client knows frequency of physician visits and time of next appointment

    11. Older adult alert

      a. Due to decreased vascular elasticity seen normally in older adult clients, it is likely that BP readings will be labile

      b. It would not be uncommon for these clients to suffer adverse hypotension from antihypertensive medications, especially if they are volume depleted

D. Peripheral arterial occlusive disorders

    1. Definition—a group of disorders that causes a decrease in lumen diameter and/or damage to the wall of the lumen; includes three common disorders

      a. Arteriosclerosis obliterans

      b. Raynaud's disease

      c. Thromboangiitis obliterans (Buerger's disease)

    2. Pathophysiology

      a. Arteriosclerosis obliterans (partial obstruction) caused by atherosclerotic plaque—vessel diameter becomes progressively smaller; skin color of extremity usually pale

          (1) Collateral circulation does increase blood flow to the area that may be affected

          (2) Collateral vessels will, with time, not be sufficient to feed affected area with oxygen and nutrients

          (3) Ischemic tissue will eventually turn into necrotic tissue if no medical intervention

          (4) Process can take many years before client begins to have symptoms

          (5) Formation of a fresh thrombus in an affected vessel may lead to acute necrosis of the affected area

          (6) Arteries most commonly affected—carotid, iliac, and femoral

      b. Raynaud's disease—vasospasm of the small arteries or arterioles; skin color changes of digits—whiteness to cyanosis; with spasm as artery relaxes color changes to rubor or redness with throbbing or burning pain from reactive hyperemia, which indicates greater artery relaxation

          (1) Often aggravated from a response to cold, stress, or use of vibrating tools

          (2) Tobacco is thought to be a major precipitating factor

    c. Buerger's disease—thromboangiitis obliterans, significant inflammatory occlusive changes in the peripheral arteries and veins of hands and feet; skin color of extremity usually reddened, rubor

       (1) Possibly related to an autoimmune response

       (2) Untreated can lead to necrosis and loss of extremities

       (3) Tobacco is thought to be a major contributing factor

3. Etiology
    a. Atherosclerosis
    b. Autoimmunity
    c. Inflammation
    d. Thrombus
    e. Trauma
    f. Vasospasm

4. Assessment
    a. Ask the following questions

       (1) Do you have pain in your calf when you walk? This is intermittent claudication.

       (2) Does your leg pain stop when you stop walking?

       (3) Do you have pain in your legs or hands when you are resting?

       (4) Do your feet or hands feel cold to you?

       (5) Do you ever have changes in your eyesight or hearing for a brief period of time?

       (6) Do you ever have a time when you feel like you cannot think clearly? Does this occur when you are stressed?

    b. Clinical manifestations (Figure 4-1, Table 4-3)

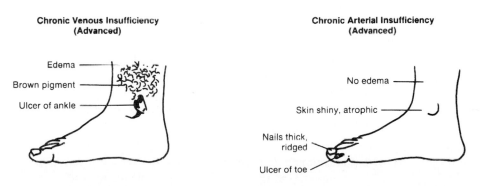

Figure 4-1. Common manifestations of chronic arterial and venous peripheral vascular problems. (From *AJN/Mosby Nursing Board Review,* ed 9, St Louis, 1994, Mosby.)

Table 4-3. Clinical Manifestations of Peripheral Arterial Occlusive Disorders

Disorders	Primary Manifestations	Secondary Manifestations
Carotid occlusion	Visual or auditory disturbances, headache	Slowed mental processes, seizures
Femoral—Iliac occlusion	Intermittant Claudication—pain upon walking in calf of legs, pain at rest in the extremities	Cool extremities, poor peripheral pulses, hypertrophied toe nails, capillary refill >3 seconds
Raynaud's disease	Paleness of the digits, then cyanosis, cold, numbness (which is the vasospastic period)	Previous symptoms are followed by an extreme rubor in the extremity with throbbing or burning pain (blood reenters the extremity)
Buerger's disease	Intermittent claudication first felt in the arch of the foot then the calf, pain at rest in extremity, hair distribution sparse	Ischemic digits, parathesias, dependant rubor in the extremity, capillary filling >3 seconds

    c. Abnormal laboratory findings—none specific
    d. Abnormal diagnostic tests
       (1) Noninvasive
         (a) Doppler ultrasonography—demonstrates degree of ischemia experienced by client
         (b) Plethysmography—indicates decline in peripheral circulation
       (2) Invasive—angiography—with a contrast dye, circulation with occlusions are visualized
  5. Expected medical interventions
    a. Nitrate or calcium channel blocker drugs to dilate collateral circulation
    b. Weight reduction
    c. Smoking cessation—"cutting down" is ineffective
    d. Anticoagulants, antiplatelet drugs
    e. Peripheral angioplasty
    f. Thrombolytic therapy
    g. Bypass grafting
    h. Endarterectomy, surgical or laser
    i. Extraanatomic bypass grafting
    j. Amputation as necessary

6. Nursing diagnoses
   a. Altered peripheral tissue perfusion related to impedance of flow in the vessels
   b. Pain related to decline in oxygenation secondary to decreased blood flow to the affected area
   c. Risk for impaired skin integrity related to poor tissue oxygenation, secondary to a decline in peripheral circulation
7. Client goals
   a. Client will exhibit an increase in peripheral tissue perfusion as evidenced by warmth in the affected area
   b. Client will state pain is minimal or relieved in affected area
   c. Client will not lose skin integrity to the affected area
8. Nursing interventions
   a. Acute care—may be a postsurgical period
      (1) Follow guidelines for care of the postsurgical client
      (2) Avoid strain over incision to prevent graft dislodgement or incisional disruption
      (3) Monitor for hemorrhage—arterial bleeding; check underneath client's extremity
      (4) Administer ordered anticoagulants
      (5) Place client in reverse Trendelenburg if ordered by the physician to increase blood flow to lower extremities; avoid extremity elevation
      (6) Evaluate neurovascular status of affected extremity with each check of vital signs
         (a) Pulses distal to site
         (b) Skin temperature, color as compared to nonaffected extremity
         (c) Sensation
         (d) Movement
   b. Home care regarding client education
      (1) Need to eliminate nicotine and caffeine
      (2) Discourage use of any heat products to area; encourage a warm living environment
      (3) Instruct client to seek physician's advice for any skin breakdown of lower extremities
      (4) Encourage a mild exercise program—walking, interspersed with adequate rest and relaxation exercises
         (a) Lie flat in bed with legs elevated above heart for 2 to 3 minutes
         (b) Dangle on side of bed with legs relaxed for 2 to 3 minutes

(c) Exercise feet—flex, extend, invert, and evert; hold each position for 30 seconds

(d) Afterwards, lie flat in bed, legs at heart level and covered with blanket for 5 minutes

(5) Need to wear warm socks and gloves when entering a cold weather environment

(6) Technique for capillary refill checks, skin and foot care

9. Evaluation protocol

a. How will I know that my interventions were effective? The acute care interventions are best evaluated by objective data.

(1) Vital signs are stable

(2) No bleeding noted from incision

(3) Neurovascular status is intact and unchanged from baseline after surgery

(4) Pain is controlled

b. What criteria will I use to change my interventions?

(1) Bleeding noted at the dressing site, sustained elevated HR >20 BPM over baseline, drop in BP >20 mm Hg from baseline

(2) Loss of peripheral pulses distal to the surgical site

(3) Loss of sensation, warmth, movement, or change in color of extremity distal to the surgical site

(4) Change in neurologic status

c. How will I know that my client teaching has been effective?

(1) Clients state they have stopped smoking cigarettes and drinking caffeinated beverages

(2) Clients state they keep their homes at 72 degrees in the winter and always wear warm clothing on hands and feet when outside

(3) Clients indicate they have been walking a half a block more each day without pain, followed with 30 minutes of rest and a relaxation exercise

(4) Clients will have minimal or no break in skin integrity on lower extremities

10. Older adult alert

a. Realize that tissue perfusion in older adult clients may be even more compromised from poor vascular elasticity

b. A positive note: since older adult clients have had many years to develop their obstructive disorder, reliable collateral circulation may be present

c. The older adult clients' perceptions of pain may be altered by decreased nerve ending functioning and also concurrent disorders such as arthritis; pain assessment of these clients may be more difficult

E. **Peripheral venous disorders**
1. Definition—disorders that decrease normal venous return from the peripheral circulation to the heart
    a. Chronic venous insufficiency—poor venous return, with venous stasis and eventual venous status ulcer
    b. Deep vein thrombosis—inflamed deep vein of leg or pelvis with a thrombus in area of inflammation
2. Pathophysiology
    a. Chronic venous insufficiency
        (1) Valves in the veins have become incompetent
        (2) Blood pools in the vessels of the lower extremities
        (3) Venous pressure in these areas increases
        (4) Blood pooling hinders efficient oxygen and nutrient exchange in the capillary area
        (5) Area becomes edematous, brown in pigmentation, and stasis ulceration is inevitable
        (6) Stasis ulcers are difficult to heal as a result of poor oxygenation and nutrition to the tissue areas involved
    b. Deep vein thrombosis
        (1) Common in clients likely to have venous stasis, such as those on strict bedrest or with sedentary jobs
        (2) Stasis of blood facilitates thrombus formation
        (3) States of hypercoagulability: either increased clotting factors or increased viscosity of the blood, i.e., high hemoglobin and hematocrit levels or severe dehydration; allows for clumping of red blood cells and platelets, with thrombus formation beginning
        (4) Any injury to a vessel wall causes platelets and blood debris to be attracted to the area and clots to easily form
3. Etiology
    a. Chronic venous insufficiency—caused by nonfunctioning valves in veins of lower extremities; gravity allows blood to pool in lower vasculature
    b. Deep vein thrombosis—occurs in response to hypercoagulabity, venous stasis, or actual injury to a vessel wall
4. Incidence
    a. Chronic venous insufficiency
        (1) Follows an episode of deep vein thrombosis
        (2) May take many years to manifest

    b. Deep vein thrombosis
       (1) More common in the female population
       (2) Found in one-third of all clients who have had major surgery or a major illness

5. Assessment
    a. Ask the following questions
       (1) Do you have any pain in either of your legs? in a relaxed position? with your toes pointed toward your head?
       (2) Is there any swelling in either of your legs?
       (3) Do you feel any warm areas in your legs?
    b. Clinical manifestations
       (1) Chronic venous insufficiency (see Figure 4-1)
         (a) Chronically edematous limbs—usually around the ankles; commonly bilateral
         (b) Thick, rough, brownish colored skin around the ankles
         (c) Venous stasis ulcers—more common by ankles
       (2) Deep vein thrombosis
         (a) Pain at site of thrombus
         (b) Swelling at site of thrombus, usually in one leg only
         (c) Redness and warmth at site of thrombus
         (d) CLINICAL EMERGENCY—assessment findings of pulmonary embolism
    c. Abnormal laboratory findings—none specific
    d. Abnormal diagnostic tests
       (1) Doppler ultrasonography—documents diminished circulation to area and impedance to venous blood flow
       (2) Plethysmography—documents diminished circulation to the area

6. Expected medical interventions
    a. Chronic venous insufficiency
       (1) Elevate leg as much as possible
       (2) Wear knee length support hose
       (3) Use wet saline dressings for stasis ulcers
    b. Deep vein thrombosis
       (1) Bedrest, elevate affected limb at least 4 to 6 inches in acute phase
       (2) Heparin drip approximately seven days
       (3) Coumadin for 3 to 6 months
       (4) Thrombolytic drug therapy

7. Nursing diagnoses
   a. Impaired skin integrity related to poor venous return and venous pooling
   b. Impaired tissue integrity related to poor venous return and venous pooling
   c. Pain related to inflammation in area of thrombus or ulceration
8. Client goals
   a. Client will exhibit that skin impairment will not increase in size and begin granulation healing
   b. Client will exhibit that tissue integrity improves as evidenced by decreased ankle edema by ¼" per week
   c. Client will state pain has been relieved by measures instituted
9. Nursing interventions
   a. Acute care—deep vein thrombosis
      (1) Monitor vital signs at least every 2 to 4 hours until stable
      (2) Monitor for sudden changes in respiratory effort or lung sounds which may be indicative of pulmonary embolism
      (3) Maintain patent IV for heparin drip
      (4) Monitor activated partial thromboplastin times (APTT) to be 1.5 to 2 times normal
      (5) Maintain bedrest for 5 to 7 days
      (6) Elevate legs above level of heart to enhance venous return while on bedrest
      (7) Maintain warm, moist compresses to affected legs
   b. Home care regarding client education
      (1) How to take oral anticoagulant drugs, how often to have APTT studies drawn, and how to institute bleeding precautions
      (2) Need to eliminate tobacco and caffeine substances
      (3) Not to wear restrictive clothing around lower extremities; not to cross legs at the knee
      (4) Use birth control medication with gynecologist follow-up if relevant; these medications often are associated with venous thrombosis
      (5) Avoid standing or sitting for periods longer than 1 hour
      (6) Need to elevate legs above level of heart, at least eight hours each day
10. Evaluation protocol
    a. How do I know that my interventions were effective?
       (1) Has client leg pain improved?

          (2) Has swelling in client's leg decreased?

          (3) Is client having any shortness of breath?

    b. What criteria will I use to change my interventions?

          (1) Vital signs changes of more than 20% from baseline for client

          (2) Findings associated with pulmonary embolism

          (3) Pain in client's extremity

          (4) Minimal or no decrease in size of extremity swelling

    c. How will I know that my client teaching has been effective?

          (1) Client has an APTT drawn every week in physician's office

          (2) Client raised foot of bed six inches for sleeping with legs elevated

          (3) Client, if female, no longer wears garters

11. Older adult alert

    a. As a normal course of aging the venous valves in the blood vessels become inefficient; older adult clients are at great risk for venous insufficiency

    b. Older adults are at greater risk for venous occlusion from decreased cardiac output and changes in vein wall integrity, decreased mobility, and a tendency to dehydrate from lack of sufficient fluid intake

F. **Aortic aneurysm**

1. Definition—a dilation of the aorta

2. Etiology—most common pathology

    a. Atherosclerosis

    b. Hypertension plays a key role in the development

3. Incidence—more common in the male population, usually after 50 years of age

4. Pathophysiology

    a. Abdominal aortic aneurysms

          (1) More common than thoracic aortic aneurysm

          (2) Walls of aorta are under high pressure due to pressure directly exerted on them with each ventricular ejection

          (3) For this reason, and as a result of changes associated with atherosclerosis, the media of the aorta wall begin to weaken and bulge outward

          (4) Pressure continues on the walls and eventually the intima will tear

          (5) The tear will allow blood to be diverted into the wall of the aorta → this is referred to as a false aneurysm

        (6)   The wall fills with blood which then clots

        (7)   The wall now bulges outward and into the lumen; this increases peripheral vascular resistance and increases BP

        (8)   Over a period of time the outer wall may tear allowing for rupture of the aneurysm which is a medical emergency and requires immediate surgery

5. Assessment

  a. Ask the following questions

        (1)   Have you experienced any pain in your groin or along your sides?

        (2)   Have you been experiencing light-headedness?

  b. Clinical manifestations

        (1)   MOST ARE ASYMPTOMATIC UNTIL THEY DISSECT OR RUPTURE

        (2)   Pain is SEVERE with a dissection and acute rupture

        (3)   Thoracic aneurysms—pain between the shoulder blades

        (4)   Abdominal aneurysms—flank or groin pain

           (a)   Pulsatile mass in mid-abdominal area

           (b)   Decreased peripheral pulses—unilaterally or bilaterally

           (c)   Bilateral pale, lower extremities

  c. Abnormal laboratory findings: CBC—in an acute rupture may indicate decreased hemoglobin and hematocrit, several hours after incident

  d. Abnormal diagnostic tests

        (1)   CXR, abdominal x-ray—may show calcification of aneurysm and highlight its outline

        (2)   CT scan—documents size of the aneurysm

        (3)   Aortography—with contrast medium can delineate aneurysm and determine if there are other arteries compromised

6. Expected medical interventions

  a. Medications to decrease BP to lowest point tolerable for client

  b. Surgical repair with graft if aneurysm is larger than 6 cm

7. Nursing diagnoses

  a. Decreased cardiac output related to alternate flow of blood into the wall of the aorta

  b. Alteration in peripheral tissue perfusion related to blood pooling in arterial wall

    c. Severe anxiety related to fear of death

    d. Pain related to effects of aortic changes

8. Client goals

    a. Client will maintain BP and HR within 20% of baseline

    b. Client will exhibit palpable peripheral pulses and warm extremities

    c. Client will show a decrease in anxiety as evidenced by relaxed facial features

    d. Client will state that measures used to relieve pain have done so

9. Nursing interventions

    a. Acute care

      (1) Take vital signs every 5 to 15 minutes

      (2) Monitor neurologic signs at least every 30 minutes

      (3) Monitor lung and heart sounds at least every hour

      (4) Prepare client physically and mentally for surgery

      (5) Medicate for pain as vital signs permit

      (6) Monitor lower extremities for changes in neurovascular status

      (7) Measure abdominal girth every hour, before and after surgery; do not palpate site of aneurysm

    b. Home care regarding client education

      (1) If clients have aneurysms that must be evaluated every 6 months by ultrasound, they must be taught the importance of those follow-up visits

      (2) Postoperative home care

        (a) Get return demonstration for incision care

        (b) Inform about activity restrictions

        (c) Teach that lifting is usually not permitted for at least 6 weeks; afterwards only 2 lb can be lifted, with a gradual increase

        (d) Teach how to avoid a pulling or straining situation

        (e) Inform that driving usually is restricted until at least the first postoperative visit with the physician

10. Evaluation protocol

    a. How do I know that my interventions were effective?

      (1) Has client pain improved with pain medication? Rate on a scale of 0 to 10

      (2) Does client know own name? location? date or year?

      (3) Are client's vital signs within 20% of baseline?

    (4) Are peripheral pulses present? Are extremities warm and of normal color for client?

  b. What criteria will I use to change my interventions?

    (1) Unstable vital signs

    (2) Rapidly changing neurologic signs

    (3) Neurovascular status in lower extremities has changed to indicate impairment

    (4) Abdominal girth is increasing

    (5) Pain is unrelieved or becoming more severe

  c. How will I know that my client teaching has been effective?

    (1) Client demonstrates correct technique for incisional care

    (2) Client plans for a friend to drive to physician's office for follow-up visit

    (3) Client identifies how to avoid exertion while at home, and to rest at least 3 times a day

11. Older adult alert

  a. Due to the decreased cardiovascular status of older adult clients, decreased cardiac output and decreased vascular elasticity, these clients are usually unable to withstand the trauma of aortic rupture. Periodic checkups should be encouraged to identify aortic aneurysms in their intact state so a surgical repair can be offered.

  b. The sudden illness and life-threatening nature of the illness make it imperative that clients and significant others have time together before surgery and as much time as possible after surgery. Many times they have been together for >30 years and need that time to adjust and support one another.

REVIEW QUESTIONS

1. The most effective method of monitoring fluid volume in the client suffering from hypovolemic shock is
   a. Blood pressure evaluation
   b. Heart rate evaluation
   c. Central venous pressure monitoring
   d. Arterial line monitoring

2. The client suffering from cardiogenic shock will show evidence of improved tissue perfusion by a/an
   a. Decreased level of consciousness
   b. Increased urine output
   c. Decrease in bowel sounds
   d. SaO_2 of 88%

3. The appropriate body position for a client suffering from hypovolemic shock with compromised vital signs is
   a. Supine
   b. Reverse Trendelenburg position
   c. Modified Trendelenburg position
   d. Trendelenburg position

4. In a health screening fair the nurse has identified a client with a BP of 200/100 mm Hg. The intervention at this point would be to
   a. Begin diet teaching on low-salt diet
   b. Retake the BP to verify the reading
   c. Refer client to their physician for further evaluation
   d. Ask the client to proceed to the emergency department

5. The client is told that he or she has a 100% occlusion of their left femoral artery. The assessment of the left lower extremity reveals a warm, pink foot, with appropriate blanching, sensation, and movement. The nurse is aware that the reason for appropriate neurovascular status is
   a. The client's daily walking periods
   b. The use of warm socks at all times
   c. Venous circulation that has assumed the roles of arteries
   d. The presence of healthy collateral circulation

6. During an initial assessment of a newly admitted client, the client indicates the inability to walk as far as he used to due to pain in the right calf. Another question the nurse would want to ask the client to confirm a suspicion is which of the folllowing?

a. How often do you have your discomfort?
b. How far can you walk before you have pain?
c. Does your pain stop when you stop walking?
d. When does your pain occur?

7. The purpose of a heparin drip in a client with deep vein thrombosis is to
   a. Prevent further clot formation
   b. Dissolve the clot
   c. Decrease inflammation
   d. Decrease interstitial edema

8. A drug that should be available when the client is receiving heparin, in case of bleeding emergency, is
   a. Vitamin C
   b. Protamine sulfate
   c. Aquamephyton
   d. Coumadin

9. An imperative assessment factor of high priority in the client postoperative for thoracic aortic aneurysm repair is
   a. Urine output
   b. Bowel sounds
   c. Neurologic status
   d. Heart sounds

10. When assessing a client with an intact abdominal aortic aneurysm, the nurse identifies that the lower extremities are cool to touch, but pulses are palpable. This is a result of
    a. Poor venous return from the lower extremities
    b. Peripheral edema from the increased interstitial pressure
    c. Poor cardiac output in the lower extremities
    d. Loss of cardiac output in false channels of the aorta

ANSWERS, RATIONALES, AND TEST-TAKING TIPS

Rationale	Test-Taking Tips

1. Correct answer: c

Central venous pressure monitoring will give the best information about fluid balance in your client. If the CVP is low, <5 cmH$_2$O the patient is hypovolemic; if CVP >12 cmH$_2$O the patient is hypervolemic.

BP and arterial line are measurements of arterial function. Cluster these two and eliminate as a possible choice. Heart rate can be dependent on fluid balance—if over or under hydrated the heart rate increases. However, it is not the most effective method for fluid volume evaluation.

2. Correct answer: b

The only criteria listed which shows improvement of body organs is increased urine output.

Cluster options *a, c,* and *d* into the category of deterioration of circulation or into the category of "decreased" vs. *b* stands alone because of the word increased.

3. Correct answer: c

Modified Trendelenburg position increases blood flow to vital organs but does not induce increased cerebral edema.

Use common sense—in shock the brain needs blood, not congestion, and venous return need to be increased. Supine position does neither of these. Trendelenburg congests the brain, so eliminate it as an option even though venous return is increased. Reverse Trendelenburg is the opposite of Trendelenburg—minimal blood to brain and pool blood in veins—eliminate as an option.

4. **Correct answer: c**

The best response here is to refer the client to a physician for further work-up. A repeat BP may be elevated due to anxiety from first reading, so may not be therapeutic or accurate.

If you have no clue to the correct response, try a cluster approach. Cluster options *a, b,* and *d* under the category of specific as compared to option c which is a more general or global response. Select the one that is different.

5. **Correct answer: d**

Collateral circulation is feeding the lower extremities to a point of maintaining a reasonable neurovascular status at this point.

The use of common sense will guide the correct selection. Daily walks improve all circulation not just the left leg. To have "warm" socks "all" the time would be impossible. Note that the absolute word "all" will also eliminate this as an answer. Venous circulation will not assume the role of arterial circulation.

6. **Correct answer: d**

Asking when the pain occurs opens up the conversation to discuss the pain and does not lead the client to answer questions in any certain direction.

Options *a, b,* and *c* are more specific types of questions that can be clustered under that category of too specific.

7. **Correct answer: a**

Heparin drip in a client with deep vein thrombosis is used to prevent further clots from forming.

Cluster options *c* and *d* because of the word "decrease" and eliminate these as possible answers. Recall that to dissolve clots the therapy is several doses of medications rather than a drip.

8. **Correct answer: b**

Protamine sulfate is the antidote for heparin.

Recall that coumadin may result in bleeding; aquamephyton is vitamin K to counteract overdose of coumadin; vitamin C is most important in healing of tissues.

9. **Correct answer: c**

   Neurologic status is imperative following thoracic aortic aneurysm repair due to the fact that cerebral arteries that feed the brain flow off of the thoracic aorta.

   If you have no clue to the correct response, try a cluster approach. Cluster options *a, b,* and *d* under the category of specific as compared to option *c* which is a more general or global response. Select the one that is different.

10. **Correct answer: d**

    Some of the blood flow is trapped in the false channels of the aortic aneurysm, causing a decrease in peripheral vascular status.

    The important words in the stem are "abdominal aneurysm" and then recall that the pathology may result in false channels that defer some of the blood.

The Hematologic System

STUDY OUTCOMES

After completing this chapter, the reader will be able to do
the following:

▼ Identify the major components and functions of the hematologic
system.

▼ Identify assessment findings of clients with alterations of the
hematologic system.

▼ Choose appropriate nursing diagnoses for the client with a disorder
of the hematologic system.

▼ Implement appropriate nursing interventions for the client with a
disorder of the hematologic system.

▼ Evaluate the progress of the client with a disorder of the hematologic
system for the establishment of new nursing interventions based on
evaluation findings.

KEY TERMS

Hemostasis	Termination of bleeding by chemical or mechanical means.
Plasma	Liquid portion of the blood.
Serum	Plasma that has had some substances removed.

CONTENT REVIEW

I. The hematologic system is responsible to
  A. Transport oxygen
  B. Transport nutrients to the body's cells
  C. Transport waste to the kidneys, skin, and lungs
  D. Transport hormones to the body's tissues
  E. Protect from life-threatening microorganisms
  F. Facilitate heat transfer from the body

II. Structure and function
  A. Blood volume is 55% plasma and 45% cells
  B. Blood is comprised of three types of cells—erythrocytes, platelets, and leukocytes
  C. Plasma is a pale yellow liquid comprised of water, blood proteins, and other dissolved solutes
  D. The part of the blood volume that is made up of cells is called the hematocrit and is largely comprised of erythrocytes. The hematocrit is expressed as a percentage.
  E. Erythrocytes house hemoglobin, necessary for carrying oxygen
  F. Platelets become sticky when in contact with a foreign substance or a damaged blood vessel
  G. Leukocytes (WBC) are responsible for fighting disease in the body; several divisions
    1. Granulocytes—have granules in their cytoplasm
      a. Neutrophils
      b. Basophils
      c. Eosinophils
    2. Agranulocytes—no granules in their cytoplasm
      a. Lymphocytes
      b. Monocytes

III. Targeted concerns

A. Pharmacology—priority drug classifications

1. Hemostatic agents—inhibit plasminogen activator; has antifibrinolytic action
   a. Expected effect—controls excessive bleeding
   b. Commonly given drugs
      (1) Aminocaproic acid (Amicar)
      (2) Thrombin (Thrombinar)
   c. Nursing considerations
      (1) Urine will turn reddish brown
      (2) May cause postural hypotension

2. Antihemophilic agents—synthetic factor VIII
   a. Expected effect—treatment of hemophilia A to enhance clotting process
   b. Commonly given drugs
      (1) Human antihemophilic factor (synthetic factor VIII)
      (2) Factor IX complex (Konyne)—increases blood levels of clotting factors II, VII, IX, X
   c. Nursing considerations
      (1) Infuse at prescribed rate
      (2) Monitor for ↑ HR, ↓ BP, ↑ RR—may indicate reaction

3. Vitamins—essential for normal cell reproduction
   a. Expected effect—maturation of RBCs
   b. Commonly given drugs
      (1) Cyanocobalamin (vitamin B_{12})
      (2) Folic acid (vitamin B_9, folvite)
   c. Nursing considerations
      (1) Give with food
      (2) Clients must be educated about the risks of vitamin overdose; more of a problem with fat-soluble vitamins because they accumulate in the tissues; excess water-soluble vitamins are normally excreted through the kidney

4. Plasma/volume expanders—increase the colloidal osmotic pressure
   a. Expected effect—expands volume to maintain cardiac output
   b. Commonly given drugs
      (1) Human albumin (salt poor albumin)
      (2) Dextran 40 (Rheomacrodex)

               (3) Hetastarch (Hespan)

               (4) Plasma protein (Plasmanate)

        c. Nursing considerations

               (1) Monitor for signs of hypervolemia

               (2) Monitor vital signs for increases during administration

    5. Colony stimulating modifiers/factors—stimulates production of several types of hematopoietic precursor cells

        a. Expected effects—increase RBC production; stimulates neutrophil production

        b. Commonly given drugs

               (1) Erythropoietin (Epogen)—for increase in RBCs

               (2) Recombinant human granulocyte colony-stimulating factor (Neupogen)—for increase in neutrophils

        c. Nursing considerations

               (1) Monitor BP every 2 to 4 hours; H&H daily

               (2) Do not shake vial, may cause deactivation of drug

B. Procedures

    1. Complete blood count and differential—provides information about cells in the hematologic system

    2. Hemoglobin electrophoresis—identifies abnormal hemoglobin

    3. Erythrocyte sedimentation rate (ESR)—elevated level indicates inflammatory, neoplastic, and/or necrotic processes

    4. Peripheral blood smear—all three blood cells can be identified

    5. Reticulocyte count—evaluates bone marrow function

    6. Iron level and total iron-binding capacity—detects abnormal levels of iron and iron-binding capacity

    7. Serum ferritin—identifies iron-deficiency anemia

    8. Platelet count—actual count of platelets

    9. Bone marrow examination—evaluates hematopoiesis

   10. Lymphangiography—X-ray examination of the lymph system using radioactive dye

   11. Lymph node biopsy—identifies metastatic involvement

C. Psychosocial

    1. Anxiety—an uncomfortable feeling associated with an unknown cause; common in the client treated for a malignancy

    2. Fear—an uncomfortable feeling associated with a known cause; also common in the client who has been diagnosed with a malignancy; the fear is most often the fear of death

    3. Denial—may be seen in the client with a malignancy as a stage of grieving

    4. Life-style—baseline of activities to evaluate need for change

    5. Activities of daily living (ADL)—ability to perform or not

  D. **Health history—question sequence**

    1. What problem would you like to discuss with the physician?

    2. What symptoms have you been experiencing?

    3. Are you presently being treated for any illnesses?

    4. Have you been treated for other illnesses in the past?

    5. Have you had any surgical procedures?

    6. Have you ever received a blood transfusion? For what reason?

    7. Did you have an adverse reaction to your blood transfusion? If so, what was the reaction?

    8. Are you currently taking any medications either prescriptions and over-the-counter medications?

    9. Do you have any allergies?

    10. Is there a family history of any blood disorders?

    11. What is your occupation?

    12. Are you following any special diet?

    13. Do you use alcohol?

    14. Have you lost any weight lately?

  E. **Physical exam—appropriate sequence**

    1. Airway, breathing, circulation—vital signs

    2. Inspect skin, hair, nails

    3. Inspect and palpate lymph nodes   head to toe approach (Figure 5-1)

    4. Inspect, palpate, and auscultate the cardiovascular system

    5. Inspect, palpate, percuss, and auscultate the respiratory system

    6. Assess neuromuscular function

    7. Assess sensory function

    8. Evaluate pain history

    9. Inspect, auscultate, percuss, and palpate the abdomen

    10. Inspect and palpate the genital system

IV. Pathophysiologic disorders

  A. **Anemia**

    1. Definition—decrease in RBC count, function or structure, with a subsequent decrease in oxygen-carrying capability of the blood

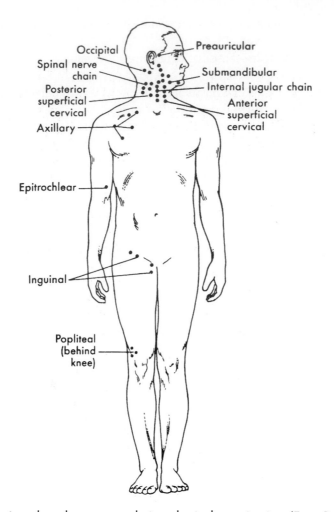

Figure 5-1. Lymph nodes to assess during physical examination. (From Beare PG and Myers JL: *Principles and practice of adult health nursing,* ed 2, St Louis, 1994, Mosby.)

    a. Types
        (1) Pernicious anemia—vitamin B_{12} deficiency from a lack of intrinsic factor in the stomach
        (2) Folic acid deficiency anemia—a lack of folic acid intake or absorption
        (3) Aplastic anemia—low RBCs caused by bone marrow abnormality
        (4) Iron deficiency anemia—low hemoglobin in RBCs
        (5) Hemolytic anemia—caused by breakup of RBCs
        (6) Blood loss anemia—loss of RBCs

(7) Sickle-cell anemia—abnormal hemoglobin; causes RBC to assume a sickled shape

2. Pathophysiology
   a. Bone marrow not producing sufficient number of RBCs
   b. RBCs not synthesized effectively as a result of a lack of essential factor
   c. Folic acid lacking in diet or absorption blocked, such as in the alcoholic client
   d. Too many RBCs destroyed due to hereditary factors or to an acquired disorder
   e. RBC loss due to acute or chronic bleeding
3. Etiology—blood loss, abnormal production of RBCs, or increased destruction of RBCs
4. Incidence—more common in older adult clients, also common in clients whose nutrition is poor
5. Assessment
   a. Ask the following questions
      (1) Do you ever feel short of breath?
      (2) Do you frequently feel tired?
      (3) Do you ever feel your heart beating too fast?
      (4) Does the cold bother you?
      (5) Do you suffer from headaches or dizziness?
   b. Clinical manifestations
      (1) Moderate anemia
         (a) SOB
         (b) Fatigue
         (c) Palpitations
      (2) Severe anemia
         (a) Paleness
         (b) Feeling of exhaustion
         (c) Sensitivity to cold
         (d) Dizziness, headaches
   c. Abnormal laboratory findings
      (1) RBC count decreased
      (2) Hemoglobin decreased
      (3) Hematocrit decreased
   d. Abnormal diagnostic tests—bone marrow aspirate; identifies specific type of anemia
6. Expected medical interventions
   a. Identify cause
   b. Treat cause if possible
   c. Iron preparations, diet management

     d. Folic acid, B_{12} administration

     e. Blood transfusions or fluid resuscitation

     f. Oxygen therapy for severe anemia

7. Nursing diagnoses

     a. Decreased cardiac output related to a decrease in circulating blood volume

     b. Activity intolerance related to reduced oxygen-carrying capacity of the blood

     c. Self-care deficit, bathing, and hygiene related to fatigue secondary to decreased oxygenation

8. Client goals

     a. Cardiac output will be appropriate as evidenced by BP within 10% of baseline

     b. Client will increase tolerance to activity as evidenced by ADL for 15 minutes without SOB

     c. Client will bathe upper body without SOB

9. Nursing interventions

     a. Acute care

         (1) Transfusion therapy

            (a) Proper identification of blood product and recipient must be completed by two licensed nurses FIRST! Most states require the RN to spike the blood bag then start the flow.

            (b) Vital signs must be taken before administration, paying special attention to the temperature; report any elevation to physician

            (c) Blood infusion must have its own IV site with at least a 20 gauge needle

            (d) During administration, monitor carefully for reactions to transfusion; the first 15 minutes is most critical and nurse must be present in the room

               (i) Anaphalytic: wheezing, tachycardia, tachypnea, hypotension, cardiac-respiratory arrest

               (ii) Allergic: hives, itching, chills, fever (febrile reaction)

               (iii) Hemolytic: low back pain, chills, chest pain

            (e) Stop blood immediately in the face of a reaction; hang new fluid, usually normal saline, and tubing; inform physician; return blood to blood bank; get urine sample and send to lab

       b. Home care regarding client education
          (1) How to balance rest and activity effectively—prioritize activities
          (2) What foods to eat to increase RBC production—high in iron, folic acid, and B_{12}

10. Evaluation protocol
       a. How do I know that my interventions were effective?
          (1) Transfusion therapy completed without reaction
          (2) Transfusion reaction managed quickly and effectively
       b. What criteria will I use to change my interventions?
          (1) Transfusion reaction noted
          (2) Transfusion reaction managed in a less then timely manner
       c. How will I know that my client teaching has been effective?
          (1) Client demonstrates methods to balance rest and activity
          (2) Client produces a food diary indicating food choices that are appropriate to increase RBC production

11. Older adult alert
       a Older adult clients are very prone to B_{12} deficiency anemia, from either a lack of B_{12} intake or an intrinsic factor. The nurse must assess for this anemia. It is best to be alert for clients with poor nutritional intake, a history of gastric ulcers or gastric resection, and to monitor hemoglobin and hematocrit values of older adult clients.

B. Acute leukemia
   1. Definition—an overgrowth of immature cells of the bone marrow
       a. Acute nonlymphocytic leukemia (ANLL)—overgrowth of the primitive cells from the myeloid stem cell line
       b. Acute lymphocytic leukemia (ALL)—proliferation of primitive lymphocytes
   2. Pathophysiology
       a. ANLL—malignant cell is an immature myeloblast; the cell generates and infringes on other normal components of the bone marrow
       b. ALL—malignant cell is an immature lymphoblast; as in ANLL, the malignant cell infringes on the other normal components of the bone marrow
   3. Etiology
       a. ANLL
          (1) Genetic abnormalities
          (2) Ionizing radiation

        (3) Viruses
        (4) Immunosuppressive agents
        (5) Chloramphenicol
        (6) Chemotherapeutic agents
    b. ALL
        (1) Radiation exposure
        (2) Genetic abnormalities

4. Incidence
    a. ANLL—adults over the age of 60; over 6000 new cases a year
    b. ALL—a childhood illness; approximately 20% of adult cases; over 5000 new cases a year

5. Assessment
    a. Ask the following questions
        (1) Do you suffer from frequent infections?
        (2) Do you feel fatigued much of the time?
        (3) Do you bruise easily, or bleed at unusual times?
        (4) Do you ever feel a deep pain in your bones?
    b. Clinical manifestations
        (1) Frequent or recurring infections
        (2) Fatigue and lassitude
        (3) Bruising, unusual bleeding
        (4) Pale complexion
        (5) Enlarged lymph nodes
        (6) Enlarged spleen
        (7) Bone pain
        (8) ANLL may be preceded by an anemia
        (9) ALL has a rapid onset
    c. Abnormal laboratory findings
        (1) ALL—WBC >10,000; increased lymphocytes
        (2) ANLL—WBC ↑ blasts
    d. Abnormal diagnostic tests
        (1) Bone marrow aspiration
            (a) ALL— >50% lymphoblasts
            (b) ANLL— >50% myeloblasts

6. Expected medical interventions
    a. Chemotherapy to eliminate the malignant cell
    b. Bone marrow transplant

7. Nursing diagnoses
    a. Pain related to increased production of leukemia cells in bone marrow
    b. Risk for infection related to ineffective, immature WBCs

8. Client goals
   a. Client will state that pain is decreased or relieved
   b. Client will be free of infective processes
9. Nursing interventions
   a. Acute care
      (1) Use of private room to prevent exposure to infection
      (2) Strict Universal Precautions; reverse isolation may be needed
      (3) Immediate evaluation of client for infection if fever, T >99° F becomes apparent, i.e., cultures
   b. Home care regarding client education
      (1) Proper handwashing
      (2) Soft toothbrush with nonabrasive toothpaste
      (3) Use stool softeners for constipation and antidiarrheal agents for diarrhea to prevent skin breaks
      (4) Maintenance of a minimal intake of 2000 to 3000 cc per day to prevent urinary stasis
10. Evaluation protocol
    a. How do I know that my interventions were effective?
       (1) Afebrile client
       (2) No other assessment findings indicative of infection
    b. What criteria will I use to change my interventions?
       (1) Elevated temperature
       (2) Positive cultures
    c. How will I know that my client teaching has been effective?
       (1) Client is using a soft toothbrush and has no gum bleeding
       (2) Client states taking in >2000 ml/day in fluid with no findings of urinary infection
11. Older adult alert
    a. Bone pain may be confused with the pain of arthritis. This must be prevented by complete assessment of the pain older clients report.

C. **Chronic leukemia**
   1. Definition—abnormal proliferation of mature WBCs
      a. Chronic myelogenous leukemia (CML)—increased production of the mature WBCs of the myeloid cell line
      b. Chronic lymphocytic leukemia (CLL)—increased production of poorly functioning mature lymphocytes
   2. Pathophysiology

a. CML—associated with a chromosome aberration, known as the Philadelphia chromosome; a translocation of the genetic material of chromosome 9 and 22
b. CLL—increased production of mature lymphocytes causing an impingement of other cells in the bone marrow
3. Etiology—most common is exposure to ionizing radiation and chemicals
4. Incidence—20% of all leukemias; more common in males >50
5. Assessment
   a. Ask the following questions
      (1) Have you been losing weight?
      (2) Have you been feeling fatigued?
      (3) Do you have pain in your bones?
   b. Clinical manifestations
      (1) May be asymptomatic, symptoms may be vague
      (2) Fatigue
      (3) Weight loss
      (4) Bone pain
      (5) Splenomegaly
      (6) Lymphadenopathy
      (7) Easy bruising
      (8) Skin rashes or lesions
   c. Abnormal laboratory findings
      (1) CLL—in serum: mature WBCs increased, platelets and RBCs decreased
      (2) CML—in serum: mature WBC >50,000
   d. Abnormal diagnostic tests
      (1) CLL—bone marrow, in accelerated phase; large quantities of immature WBCs
      (2) CML—bone marrow, large quantities of immature WBCs
6. Expected medical intervention
   a. Chemotherapy—oral and intravenous
   b. Bone marrow transplant
7. Nursing diagnoses, client goals, nursing interventions, evaluations, and older adult alert—will be identical to the client with acute leukemia

D. **Lymphoma**
   1. Definition—group of malignancies originating from the stem cell in the bone marrow; malignancy occurs in the lymphoreticular system

a. Two types
    (1) Hodgkin's disease
    (2) Non-Hodgkin's lymphoma

2. Pathophysiology
   a. Hodgkin's—malignant cell origin has not been confirmed but theory suggests a B or T lymphocyte
   b. Non-Hodgkin's—the malignant cell is the lymphocyte in any stage of its development; this cell reproduces and then invades the bone marrow

3. Etiology
   a. Hodgkin's—unknown; possible viral, genetic, or environmental factors have been investigated
   b. Non-Hodgkin's—high risk seen in clients with autoimmune illnesses and viruses such as Epstein Barr

4. Incidence
   a. Hodgkin's—over 7000 new cases a year; greater incidence in the male population than in the female; two peak periods of incidence—in the third and sixth decade
   b. Non-Hodgkin's— >35,000 new cases per year; more common in males, after the age of 60

5. Assessment
   a. Ask the following questions
    (1) Do you ever wake up at night soaked in sweat?
    (2) Have you been losing weight?
    (3) Have you noticed that you have been running fevers?
   b. Clinical manifestations—the two lymphomas are similar in manifestations
    (1) Night sweats
    (2) Fevers
    (3) Weight loss
    (4) Enlarged painless lymph nodes
   c. Abnormal laboratory findings
    (1) CBC—mild anemia, increased WBC, decreased lymphocytes, increased ESR
    (2) Chemistries—increased alkaline phosphatase, increased gammaglobulins
   d. Abnormal diagnostic tests
    (1) Lymph node biopsy—malignant
    (2) Lymphangiography—abnormal lymph nodes and possibly lymph vessel impairment
    (3) Bone marrow biopsy—abnormal cells
    (4) Staging laparotomy—lymph node site involvement

6. Expected medical interventions
   a. Staging laparotomy with splenectomy—splenectomy improves effects of chemotherapy
   b. Chemotherapy
   c. External beam radiation therapy
7. Nursing diagnoses
   a. Pain related to progression of disorder to the bones
   b. Risk for infection related to impaired immune system
   c. Altered nutrition—less than body requirements related to increased metabolic demands of the malignant disorder
8. Client goals
   a. Client will state that pain is improved or has been relieved
   b. Client will show no evidence of infection, i.e., fever
   c. Client will lose no more weight, but increase weight by ½ kg per 2 week period
9. Nursing interventions
   a. Acute care
      (1) The client who is postoperative for the staging laparotomy must be cared for with all the routine nursing interventions discussed in Chapter 10, p. 315
      (2) This client is also at high risk for infection, so nursing interventions must be aimed at vigorous prevention of postoperative infection
   b. Home care regarding client education
      (1) Infection prevention
      (2) How to prepare medications at home if client is giving chemotherapy in the home; technique for preparation and administration must be discussed
      (3) How to cope with side effects of chemotherapy and radiation therapy
         (a) How to maintain hydration
         (b) How to administer antiemetics as needed
         (c) How to care for the skin during external radiation therapy
            (i) Not to wash area with soap
            (ii) Not to remove skin markings
            (iii) Not to apply any creams or ointments to the skin unless specifically directed
         (d) How to recognize infection in the early stages
         (e) How to respond to hemorrhage if it occurs

10. Evaluation protocol
    a. How do I know that my interventions were effective?
        (1) Infection has been prevented
        (2) Infection has been identified early and treated appropriately
    b. What criteria will I use to change my interventions?
        (1) Elevated temperature that is not responding to treatment; anything >99° F is of concern in the immunosuppressed client
        (2) Overall status of client is deteriorating
    c. How will I know that my client teaching has been effective?
        (1) Client demonstrates ability to mix and administer chemotherapeutic drugs
        (2) Client demonstrates the ability to treat side effects of chemotherapy and radiation therapy effectively
        (3) Client identifies appropriate skin care during radiation therapy
        (4) Client identifies assessment factors associated with infection that should be reported to the physician
        (5) Client identifies appropriate measure to treat hemorrhage in the home if it occurs
11. Older adult alert
    a. Older adult clients will have greater risk for infection due to the normal decrease in the immune response with age
    b. Evaluate older adult clients carefully for pain which may be bone pain but mistaken for arthritis

E. **Multiple myeloma**
1. Definition—neoplasm of plasma cells
2. Pathophysiology—plasma cells have transformed to a malignant form; an immunoglobulin M-protein is formed by the malignant plasma cells; M-protein is reproduced and prevents appropriate antibody production
3. Etiology—unknown; possible viral; possible inappropriate response to antigenic stimulation
4. Incidence—more than 10,000 new cases per year; more common in the black population; most common after age 60
5. Assessment
    a. Ask the following questions
        (1) Do you ever have a deep pain in your bones?
        (2) Do you ever feel tired?
        (3) Do you suffer from frequent infections?

      b. Clinical manifestations
         (1) Bone pain increases with movement
         (2) Bone demineralization leading to hypercalcemia
         (3) Anemia
         (4) Renal insufficiency leading to renal failure
      c. Abnormal laboratory findings
         (1) Serum calcium elevated
         (2) Urinalysis—increased calcium
         (3) Serum electrophoresis—increased globulin
         (4) Serum creatinine elevated
      d. Abnormal diagnostic tests
         (1) Bone marrow aspiration—increased immature plasma cells
         (2) Skeletal x-rays—demineralization
6. Expected medical interventions
      a. Chemotherapy
      b. Radiation therapy—adjuvant therapy
      c. Bone marrow transplantation
7. Nursing diagnoses
      a. Pain related to bone demineralization and pathologic fractures
      b. Impaired physical mobility related to bone pain and pathologic fractures
      c. Altered nutrition—less than body requirements related to anorexia
8. Client goals
      a. Client will state that pain is relieved or improved on a scale of 0 to 10
      b. Client will demonstrate ability to perform ROM exercises at least BID to prevent muscle atrophy
      c. Client will maintain present weight, no further weight loss, or increase weight by ½ kg per 2 week period if indicated
9. Nursing interventions
      a. Position client for comfort—prevent pathologic fractures
      b. Encourage use of assistive devices
      c. Balance rest and activity
      d. Hydrate >3000 ml/day to treat hypercalcemia for the prevention of renal calculi
      e. Encourage high protein diet with appropriate vitamin intake, but not vitamins A and D—these facilitate absorption of calcium from the gastrointestinal tract

      f. Utilize nursing measures outlined in the client with lymphoma
10. Evaluation protocol
    a. How will I know that my interventions were effective?
      (1) Client states comfort
      (2) No new pathologic fractures
      (3) Appropriate diet intake—high protein and lacking in vitamins A and D
      (4) Urine output of at least 30 ml/hr
    b. What criteria will I use to change my interventions?
      (1) Client has unrelieved pain
      (2) New pathologic fractures noted
      (3) Diet is not tolerated
      (4) Renal function is depressed; complaints of flank pain or other pain related to presence of kidney stones
    c. How will I know that my client teaching has been effective?
      (1) Client demonstrates appropriate fluid and food intake
      (2) Refer to Evaluation Protocol for lymphoma, p. 147
11. Older adult alert—same as for the client with lymphoma

REVIEW QUESTIONS

1. The client who is known to abuse alcohol will also suffer from a low folic acid level caused by
   a. Poor nutrition
   b. Poor dentition
   c. Absorption blocked by alcohol intake
   d. Increased motility in the bowel

2. Assessment findings commonly reported by the client with anemia are
   a. Fatigue, shortness of breath, and palpitations
   b. Fatigue, diarrhea, and shortness of breath
   c. Bone pain, shortness of breath, and headaches
   d. Abdominal pain, shortness of breath, and headaches

3. Before initiating a blood transfusion the nurse must pay special attention to a baseline assessment of
   a. Blood pressure
   b. Heart rate
   c. Temperature
   d. Respiratory rate

4. A priority nursing intervention in the face of a blood transfusion reaction must be
   a. Call the physician
   b. Administer Benadryl intravenously
   c. Increase IV fluid rate
   d. Stop the transfusion

5. An initial manifestation of acute leukemia may be
   a. Alternating diarrhea and constipation
   b. Bruising or unusual bleeding
   c. Dizziness
   d. Bone pain

6. A client with leukemia may be placed in a private room to
   a. Isolate other clients from their infection
   b. Prevent over fatigue from other clients
   c. Allow sleep
   d. Isolate the client from exposure to infection

7. The client receiving external radiation therapy must be taught how to care for the skin in the area of the therapy to prevent skin breakdown. Teaching must include
   a. Cleansing the skin thoroughly after treatments to prevent skin sloughing
   b. Baby oil to the area to prevent the drying effects of the therapy
   c. Caution client not to remove skin markings placed by the physician, to ensure consistent therapy
   d. Suggest that the client expose the radiated area to the sun for at least two 10-minute periods per day

8. An assessment finding most often associated with Hodgkin's disease is
   a. Painful lymph nodes
   b. High fevers
   c. Frequent constipation
   d. Night sweats

9. An important laboratory study done for clients with multiple myeloma is
   a. Urinalysis
   b. Serum potassium
   c. Serum calcium
   d. Arterial blood gases

10. A likely complication associated with multiple melanoma is
    a. Weight loss
    b. Urinary tract infection
    c. Pneumonia
    d. Pathologic fractures

ANSWERS, RATIONALES, AND TEST-TAKING TIPS

Rationale	Test-Taking Tips
1. Correct answer: c Alcohol actually prevents folic acid absorption. Increased motility has nothing to do with the given situation.	Be cautious not to have a bias that abuse of alcohol results in poor nutrition and dentation.
2. Correct answer: a A client who is anemic will typically manifest fatigue, shortness of breath, and palpitations.	Use a vertical technique to read and eliminate. Read down—*a* and *b* fatigue, yes; *c* bone pain, no and *d* abdominal pain, no. So with minimal reading the options have been narrowed to two. SOB is in both. Next identify that the heart is more sensitive to alterations in oxygen than the bowel so *a* is the correct choice.
3. Correct answer: c It is extremely important to obtain a baseline temperature before starting a blood transfusion because a fever is the more common first manifestation of a reaction.	Note the key word in the stem "special attention." A common sense approach is to identify that HR, RR, and BP can vary to a greater degree and still be within normal range. However, temperature variation is more limited and needs special attention.
4. Correct answer: d Stopping the blood immediately in the face of a transfusion reaction may minimize the reaction; this is a priority over giving Benadryl, increasing the IV rate, or calling the physician.	Use common sense here—if you are giving a therapy and a reaction occurs then stop the therapy first.

5. **Correct answer: b**

   Bruising or unusual bleeding is the more common manifestation of acute leukemia and may be the symptom that encourages the client to seek a physician's evaluation.

   The key word "unusual" in option *b* hints that this is the correct response. The other options could be more common manifestations of just being alive. Option *d*, bone pain, is not a common way clients would describe pain.

6. **Correct answer: d**

   A client with leukemia has ineffective WBCs and an inability to fight infection; they must be protected from infections or organisms.

   Cluster options *a* and *b* because of the focus of other clients; eliminate these as a choice. There is insufficient data in the stem to select c, allow sleep.

7. **Correct answer: c**

   The client should be warned not to remove skin markings so that therapy can be consistent; they must not use skin treatments unless instructed to do so by the physician; soap will dry the skin.

   Cluster options *a, b,* and *d* under the theme of "do something to the skin" and eliminate these; note option *c* has a focus of protect.

8. **Correct answer: d**

   With Hodgkin's lymph nodes are painless; there may be low grade fevers; constipation is not common; night sweats are a classic manifestation of Hodgkin's disease.

   Pathology that results in night sweats are limited to: AIDS, TB, Hodgkins, menopause, and hypoglycemia.

9. **Correct answer: c**

   Clients with multiple myeloma have hypercalcemia due to demineralization of the bones.

   Eliminate options *a* and *d* since the systems reflected are different, kidney and lung. Associate that usually potassium is imbalanced except in multiple myeloma it is calcium. Recall tips—myeloma and calcium both have seven letters, so remember they have a relationship.

10. **Correct answer: d**

Pathologic fractures are not uncommon in the client with multiple myeloma due to demineralization of the bones.

Options *b* and *c* are too narrow for a multiple myeloma finding. Weight loss may occur but is not most likely to be a complication.

The Respiratory System

STUDY OUTCOMES

After completing this chapter, the reader will be able to do the following:

▼ Assess a client with a respiratory disorder using the appropriate technique and sequence.

▼ Choose appropriate nursing diagnoses for respiratory disorders.

▼ Identify nursing interventions for the client with a respiratory disorder.

▼ Evaluate the progress of the respiratory client for the maintenance of interventions or for the establishment of new interventions.

KEY TERMS

Exhalation	The second phase of ventilation; air exiting the lungs.
Hypoxemia	PO_2 <80 mm Hg.
Hypoxia	Cellular deprivation of oxygen.
Inspiration	The first phase of ventilation; air entering the lungs.
Perfusion	The flow of blood through blood vessels.
Respiration	The exchange of oxygen and carbon dioxide at the alveolar and cellular level.
Tidal volume	The volume of air inspired and then exhaled during one ventilation; approximately 600 to 800 cc.
Ventilation	Air moving in and out of the lungs.
Work of breathing	The amount of energy expended to accomplish ventilation; the respiratory effort.

CONTENT REVIEW

I. **The respiratory system is responsible for the exchange of oxygen and carbon dioxide in the body which takes place primarily in the alveoli of the lungs**

II. **Structure and function**
   A. Upper airways (nasal passages, pharynx, larynx)—warms, humidifies, and filters air inhaled; transports air to lower airways
   B. Lungs—two cone-shaped organs in the thoracic cavity on each side of the heart; left lung has two lobes and ten smaller partitions known as segments; right lung has three lobes and ten segments
   C. Lower airways (trachea, right and left mainstem bronchus, segmental bronchi, terminal bronchioles)—transport air to the alveoli
   D. Alveoli—found in the lung parenchyma; gas exchange of oxygen and dioxide occurs between alveoli and pulmonary capillaries across the alveolar capillary membrane; millions exist in each lung
   E. Alveoli walls contain type II pneumocytes which secrete surfactant—responsible for decreasing surface tension of alveoli and maintaining alveolar patency

III. Targeted concerns

A. Pharmacology—priority drug classifications

1. Bronchodilators—relax bronchial tree; increase lumen size
   a. Expected effects—decrease rate and effort of breathing
   b. Commonly given drugs
      (1) Theophylline (Theodur), PO
      (2) Albuterol (Ventolin), PO, inhalation
      (3) Aminophylline, IV
   c. Nursing considerations
      (1) Expected side effects—sinus tachycardia, palpitations, feelings of nervousness, dizziness
      (2) Report and evaluate HR >120
      (3) Toxic effects—nausea first sign of toxicity, tremors, theophylline levels >20 ug/ml
      (4) Give with food or milk to prevent gastric distress

2. Mucolytics—cause a breakdown of secretions
   a. Expected effects—make expectoration of sputum easier for client; thin secretions
   b. Commonly given drugs
      (1) Acetylcysteine (Mucomyst)—given by aerosol
      (2) Water or appropriate hydration is felt to be the best to thin secretions
   c. Nursing considerations
      (1) Mucomyst best administered as a nebulizer treatment for a respiratory effect; mucomyst also given orally as an antidote for acetaminophen overdose; multiple doses over a three to four day period
      (2) Evaluate for bronchospasm during treatment especially in clients with asthma

3. Expectorants—add bulk or fluid to sputum
   a. Expected effects—increase effectiveness of cough; soothe mucosa of the bronchial tree
   b. Commonly given drugs
      (1) Guaifenesin (Robitussin)
      (2) Terpin hydrate
      (3) Potassium iodide
   c. Nursing considerations
      (1) Client must have adequate hydration for this drug classification to be effective
      (2) Client must have strong cough effort and energy to cough

      (3)   There may be great controversy over clinical efficacy of this drug classification

4. Antitussives—narcotic and nonnarcotic cough suppressants
    a. Expected effect—relief of cough; used when coughing has become detrimental to client's progress
    b. Commonly given drugs
      (1)   Codeine (narcotic)
      (2)   Dextromethorphan (Benylin DM, a nonnarcotic)
    c. Nursing considerations
      (1)   Evaluate lung sounds frequently to determine if secretions are being appropriately removed now that cough is suppressed
      (2)   With narcotic preparations, monitor client for signs of respiratory depression and tolerance to drug

5. Corticosteroids—decrease inflammatory response in airway and decrease airway edema
    a. Expected effect—increase airway lumen size
    b. Commonly given drugs
      (1)   Prednisone (Deltasone)
      (2)   Methylprednisolone (Medrol)
      (3)   Beclomethasone (Vanceril)
    c. Nursing considerations
      (1)   Drug doses must not be missed and must be tapered off over a four to five day period, not stopped abruptly, to prevent findings of adrenal insufficiency
      (2)   Must be given with food or milk to prevent gastric ulcers
      (3)   Many preparations (such as intranasal) are prophylactic, not for acute attacks

6. Cromolyn sodium—prevents release of histamine from the mast cells of the lungs
    a. Expected effect—prophylactically prevents bronchospasm caused by an allergen or exercise
    b. Nursing considerations
      (1)   Administered by inhalation only
      (2)   Caution client to not discontinue use without physician order
      (3)   Not for use in acute asthma episodes

7. Antimicrobial agents—used to treat respiratory infections; specific agent is chosen based on infecting pathogen
    a. Expected effect—elimination of infection

        b. Commonly given drugs
- (1) Penicillins (Penicillin G, Nafcillin, Ampicillin, Carbenicillin, Ticarcillin)
- (2) Cephalosporins (Cephalexin, Cefazolin, Cefoxitin, Keflex, Kefzol, Mefoxin)
- (3) Aminoglycosides (Gentamicin, Tobramycin, Streptomycin)
- (4) Tetracylines (Doxycycline, Vibramycin)

        c. Nursing considerations
- (1) Monitor for allergic reaction to antibiotic
- (2) Evaluate culture and sensitivity report to determine pathogen sensitivity to drug therapy
- (3) Ascertain specific nursing considerations for each antimicrobial group

8. Tuberculosis chemotherapy—bactericidal action against mycobacterium bacillus

        a. Expected effect—elimination of tuberculosis

        b. Commonly given drugs
- (1) First line drugs
  - (a) Isoniazid (INH)
  - (b) Ethambutol (Myambutol)
  - (c) Rifampin (Rifadin) - orange
  - (d) Streptomycin
- (2) Second line drugs
  - (a) Capreomycin
  - (b) Kanamycin (Kantrex)
  - (c) Ethionamide

        c. Nursing considerations
- (1) Pyridoxine (B_6) must be given with INH to prevent neuritis - infl. of a nerve
- (2) Rifampin may color urine and tears orange
- (3) Therapy may extend from 6 to 18 months; liver function studies must be evaluated monthly for liver impairment

B. Procedures

1. Chest x-ray—reveals abnormalities in lungs and thoracic cavity
2. Computed tomography—gives three-dimensional evaluation of thorax; can see abnormalities in lungs and thorax
3. Bronchoscopy—direct visualization of inside of bronchial tree using a flexible, lighted scope

    4. Thorascopy—direct visualization of the pleura for disorders using a flexible, lighted scope; chest tube required postprocedurally to reexpand lung

    5. Pulmonary angiography—dye injected into the pulmonary vasculature to detect abnormalities such as clots in the vascular system of the lungs

    6. Magnetic resonance imaging (MRI)—use of magnetic fields to create an image of thoracic structures

    7. Thoracentesis—drainage of fluid from the pleural space to decrease respiratory distress; fluid evaluation for abnormalities such as bacteria

    8. Sputum culture—provides evaluation of pathogens responsible for respiratory illness

    9. Pulmonary function testing—provides assessment of changes in lung volumes and capacities to evaluate presence of lung disease and degree of severity

   10. Arterial blood gases—sample of arterial blood evaluated for oxygen and carbon dioxide tensions, pH, bicarbonate level, and oxygen saturation; identifies oxygen and carbon dioxide diffusion abnormalities and bicarbonate abnormalities

   11. Ventilation-perfusion scan—inhalation of radioactive gas; detects ventilation impairment-injection of radioactive dye into blood stream, followed by lung scanning, to detect pulmonary perfusion abnormalities

C. **Psychosocial**

    1. Anxiety—a common finding in clients having difficulty breathing; can exacerbate respiratory distress

    2. Fear—respiratory distress produces great fear in clients; fear of death is quite overwhelming in clients having difficulty breathing

    3. Depression—common in clients with long-term respiratory disease; related to decreased capacity to care for themselves or to complete tasks as they had previously

    4. Denial—may be noted in respiratory clients up to the time when respiratory symptoms are severe and undeniable

    5. Hopelessness—many clients experience this feeling due to the incurable nature of their illness

    6. Social isolation—the physical incapacity of respiratory illnesses, as well as the frequent production of foul-tasting sputum, causes an isolation-type living situation for many clients

D. Health history—question sequence
  1. What symptoms are you experiencing?
  2. What causes your symptoms, or makes them worse?
  3. What makes your symptoms better?
  4. When did you first notice these symptoms?
  5. Are you able to complete your own hygiene?
  6. Are you able to go to work, or do work around the house?
  7. Do you find it necessary to stop and rest after activity? If so, how long must you rest before you can again become active? How long can you exert yourself before you must rest?
  8. Is there a specific time of day when your symptoms are more noticeable?
  9. Do you cough up a large amount of sputum? How often or how much? What does it look like?
  10. Have you experienced fever, sweating during the night, or excessive fatigue?
  11. Have you noticed a weight loss or gain recently?
  12. Is there a family history of respiratory illness?
E. Physical exam—appropriate sequence
  1. Patent airway
  2. Respiratory rate, depth
  3. Inspection
    a. Accessory muscle use
    b. Cyanosis—circumoral, nail beds
    c. Jugular venous distension
    d. Chest size and configuration
  4. Palpation
    a. Chest wall tenderness
    b. Subcutaneous emphysema
  5. Percussion—at the lung bases bilaterally
  6. Auscultation—the upper and lower lobes; especially the right middle lobe where aspiration is most common
    a. Normal lung sounds
    b. Adventitious lung sounds
      (1) Crackles
      (2) Rhonchi
      (3) Wheezes
      (4) Pleural friction rub

IV. Pathophysiologic disorders

A. Laryngeal cancer

1. Definition—cancer of the larynx or voice box
2. Pathophysiology—slow growing, starting as a squamous cell carcinoma; initially a small hard patch leading to ulceration and abscessing of the area
3. Etiology—majority of clients with laryngeal cancer have a history of smoking or of voice abuse
4. Incidence—men are more likely to develop than women; over 10,000 cases per year
5. Assessment
   a. Ask the following questions
      (1) Have you experienced any change in your voice?
      (2) Have you had a sore throat that would not go away? Any hoarseness?
      (3) Have you noticed any sores in your throat that would not heal?
      (4) Have you noticed any difficulty breathing or swallowing?
   b. Clinical manifestations
      (1) Hoarseness longer than two weeks
      (2) Difficulty swallowing or breathing
      (3) Persistent cough, sore throat
      (4) Lump in throat or neck area
   c. Abnormal laboratory findings—none specific
   d. Abnormal diagnostic tests
      (1) Laryngoscopy and biopsy—identifies tumor presence, vocal cord changes; positive biopsy for malignancy
      (2) Laryngeal tomography—evaluates for extension of disease
      (3) CXR—shows metastasis into lung
6. Expected medical interventions
   a. Surgery—excision of small lesions; partial laryngectomy; total laryngectomy; radical neck dissection
   b. Radiation therapy—may be primary intervention with small lesions or palliative with advanced lesions
7. Nursing diagnoses—postoperative
   a. Ineffective airway clearance related to difficulty coughing effectively through artificial airway

     b.   Impaired verbal communication related to effects of recent surgery, presence of artificial airway

     c.   Anxiety related to altered communication and ventilation

8.   Client goals

     a.   Client will maintain a patent airway at all times as evidenced by clear upper airway sounds

     b.   Client will make all needs known using alternative method of communication (writing notes)

     c.   Client will have relaxed facial features and indicate feeling less anxious

9.   Nursing interventions

     a.   Acute care—postoperative

          (1)   Evaluate upper airway patency and suction tracheostomy as needed using strict sterile technique

              (a)   Instill 5 ml of sterile saline into tracheostomy to liquefy secretions. NOTE: This is a controversial intervention since some studies have reported the instillation of saline facilitates the introduction of organisms into the lower respiratory tract; infection risk is increased. Also, the risk of hypoxemia 3 to 5 minutes afterwards may result from saline instillation.

              (b)   Hyperoxygenate by ambu bag with 100% oxygen with three to five breaths

              (c)   Instill catheter into tracheostomy (no suction) until patient coughs or resistance is met

              (d)   Remove catheter, suction intermittently, rotating catheter

              (e)   Cleanse catheter with sterile saline

              (f)   Hyperoxygenate again, and repeat ×1 if needed; let client rest for several minutes before suctioning again

              (g)   Place in high fowlers position to decrease edema and facilitate breathing

          (2)   Administer humidified oxygen by tracheostomy collar or T-piece

              (a)   Monitor vital signs for shock

              (b)   Monitor neck dressings for bleeding and behind the neck for bloody drainage

             (c) Monitor continuous portable suction devices, such as Jackson Pratt drains or hemovacs, for drainage; empty when half full or every eight hours; measure drainage; record as output

             (d) Explore alternative means of communication (if not evaluated preoperatively) and implement those mutually agreed upon

             (e) Medicate for pain as needed

    b. Home care: regarding client education

        (1) Discharge materials to include an extra tracheostomy tube and obturator that is used for insertion of the trach tube should it come out

        (2) Teach how to liquefy secretions with hydration and to use sterile saline if hydration not effective or a mucous plug is present

        (3) Need for a bedside humidifier or vaporizer

        (4) Stoma cleaning; tracheostomy tube not required after stoma healed

        (5) Use stoma bib or scarves to cover stoma, to protect from contaminants or to catch mucus

        (6) Reinforcement to continue with speech therapy and to join a support group

        (7) Need to wear a medic-alert bracelet

        (8) Need to continue with postoperative arm and shoulder exercises

10. Evaluation protocol

    a. How do I know that my interventions were effective?

        (1) Does client's breathing feel easy?

        (2) Does client's tracheostomy tube need to be suctioned?

        (3) Are client's secretions easy to cough up?

    b. What criteria will I use to change my interventions?

        (1) Client reports feeling short of breath or increased shortness of breath

        (2) Client reports that their secretions are too thick

        (3) Client indicates a need to be suctioned more often

    c. How will I know that my client teaching has been effective?

        (1) Client is wearing a medic-alert bracelet

        (2) Client is following speech therapy interventions and/or attends support group meetings

        (3) Client demonstrates appropriate stoma cleaning technique

11. Older adult alert
   a. Upper airway cilia are less efficient in older clients, making airways harder to clear
   b. Lungs are less elastic in older adult clients, so coughing may be more difficult. They may require a stimulus to cough.

B. **Pneumonia**
   1. Definition—an acute inflammatory process of the parenchyma of the lung with a significant increase in interstitial and alveolar fluid
      a. Can involve one segment or several segments
      b. Can involve one lobe or several lobes
      c. Can involve one whole lung or both lungs
      d. Pneumonitis refers to the noninfectious inflammatory process of lung parenchyma
   2. Pathophysiology—infecting organisms are typically inhaled; organisms are transmitted to the lower airways and alveoli causing inflammation; organisms can also be transmitted to the lungs via the circulatory system and become lodged in the lungs causing inflammation
   3. Etiology—may be caused by bacteria, virus, mycoplasm, fungus, protozoa, or from aspiration or inhalation of chemicals or other toxic substances
   4. Incidence—major cause of hospitalization and death in the United States; responsible for over 10% of hospital admissions
   5. Assessment
      a. Ask the following questions
         (1) Have you been having difficulty breathing?
         (2) Are you having pain? Where?
         (3) Do you have a cough? If yes, are you coughing up anything from your lungs when you cough? What does it look like?
         (4) Have you been running a fever? How high has your fever gone?
         (5) Have you been feeling tired?
      b. Clinical manifestations
         (1) High fever—usually sudden rise of 102° F or greater, chills, diaphoresis
         (2) Sinus tachycardia
         (3) Dyspnea
         (4) Bronchial breath sounds over area of pneumonia
         (5) Cough, increased sputum production
         (6) Chest pain over area of pneumonia

      (7) Headache

      (8) Fatigue

  c. Abnormal laboratory findings

      (1) Sputum culture—positive for organism infecting lungs

      (2) Blood cultures—may show organism in blood if client has progressed to stage of bacteremia

      (3) CBC—elevated WBC count >10,000

      (4) ABGs—decreased PO_2

  d. Abnormal diagnostic tests

      (1) CXR—areas of pneumonia appear as white opaque area; known as areas of consolidation

      (2) Bronchoscopy—areas infected are directly visualized; exudate can be cleared from area; sputum cultures can be taken

6. Expected medical interventions

  a. Antibiotic therapy based on sputum culture and sensitivity, administer antibiotics known to be bactericidal to infecting bacteria

  b. Hospitalization only if client's health warrants in-hospital care

7. Nursing diagnoses

  a. Ineffective airway clearance related to thick tenacious sputum

  b. Ineffective breathing pattern—tachypnea related to chest pain, airway inflammation

  c. Impaired gas exchange related to exudate in alveoli

  d. Activity intolerance related to hypoxemia and fatigue

8. Client goals

  a. Client will maintain open and clear airway as evidenced by clear upper airway sounds

  b. Client will maintain respiratory rate (RR) between 14 to 20 breaths per minute (BPM)

  c. Client will maintain PO_2 above 80 mm Hg without supplemental oxygen

  d. Client will complete physical care without frequent rest periods

9. Nursing interventions

  a. Acute care

      (1) Auscultate lungs every two hours for changes in lung sounds

      (2) Assess any sputum expectorated for change in color, consistency, odor

      (3) Monitor ABGs or pulse oximetry for hypoxemia

        (4) Elevate head of bed to improve respiratory excursion

        (5) Turn, cough, deep breathe every two hours; ambulate as tolerated

        (6) Position on back and unaffected side to increase ventilation of affected lung

    b. Home care regarding client education

        (1) Continue coughing and deep breathing exercises every two hours

        (2) Finish *all* antibiotics at prescribed intervals

        (3) Call physician for new onset of fever, chest pain, hemoptysis

10. Evaluation protocol

    a. How do I know that my interventions were effective?

        (1) Is client breathing easier?

        (2) Has client chest pain improved or been relieved?

        (3) Is client coughing up less sputum and has the color changed?

        (4) Other evaluations will be objective

            (a) Lung sounds will improve, adventitious breath sounds will disappear, lungs will be clear

            (b) Respiratory rate will decrease to rate of 14 to 20

            (c) Work of breathing will decrease, accessory muscle use will disappear

            (d) Temperature will return to normal

    b. What criteria will I use to change my interventions?

        (1) Dyspnea has not improved, or has increased

        (2) Chest pain has not improved

        (3) Sputum is increasing in amounts, color has not changed

        (4) Tachycardia and febrile state continues

    c. How will I know that my client teaching has been effective?

        (1) Client is coughing and deep breathing every two hours

        (2) Client is taking antibiotics every four hours as ordered

        (3) Client is able to state conditions that the physician should be made aware of

11. Older adult alert

    a. Older adults are at very high risk for pneumonia; all concerns should be further evaluated

    b. Be concerned about any changes in orientation. This may be a first indication of pneumonia in older adults.

     c. Be cautious in fluid administration. Hydrate older adults, but do not over-hydrate because overhydration may initiate CHF.

C. **Tuberculosis (TB)**

  1. Definition—a chronic, infectious granulomatous pulmonary disease

     a. Drug responsive strains

     b. Drug resistant strains

  2. Pathophysiology—the mycobacterium tubercle is transmitted in droplets of infected clients expelled during sneezing, coughing, or laughing; clients inhale infected droplets and bacillus invades lung tissue; clients usually require continued exposure to become infected

     a. Primary infection—bronchopneumonia begins at area of bacillus invasion; bacilli may spread via the lymphatic system; necrotic degeneration occurs at site of infection (caseation) causing cavities filled with necrotic tissue to eventually liquify; the liquified material drains out of the cavity, leaving an air-filled cavity which calcifies and can be seen on CXR; primary infection causes a sensitivity to the tuberculin bacillus which, in turn, causes an allergic reaction if the bacillus is introduced into the body again

     b. Secondary infection—active TB; primary infection sites may harbor latent bacilli for many years that become reactivated

  3. Etiology—inhalation of an acid-fast bacillus (AFB); mycobacterium tuberculosis

  4. Incidence—new cases annually greater than 3 million worldwide; a long decline occurred following the discovery of antitubercular drug therapy in the 1940s; a new resurgence has occurred with the immigration of people from third world nations and with the outbreak of the human immunodeficiency virus (HIV)

  5. Assessment

     a. Ask the following questions

        (1) Are you suffering from night sweats?

        (2) Have you lost weight?

        (3) Have you been having low grade fevers? (99° to 100° F)

        (4) Have you been having increasing difficulty breathing?

        (5) Have you had chest pain? Where?

   (6) Have you been coughing? Have you been coughing anything up when you cough? What does it look like?

  b. Clinical manifestations

   (1) Night sweats

   (2) Weight loss

   (3) Anorexia

   (4) Fatigue

   (5) Dyspnea

   (6) Productive cough

   (7) Pleuritic chest pain, caused by inflammation of the pleura, felt in the outer aspects of the lungs

  c. Abnormal laboratory findings

   (1) Sputum culture—positive for acid-fast bacilli; takes about 2 to 3 weeks for results

   (2) Skin testing—purified protein derivative (PPD) preferred method; induration or wheal greater than 10 mm is a positive result; checked 48 to 72 hours after placement of intradermal test on inner forearm

   (3) CBC—WBC may be elevated

  d. Abnormal diagnostic tests

   (1) CXR—may see calcification of original site of infection; infiltrates in the parenchyma

   (2) Pleural needle biopsy—caseation necrosis; positive for granulomas

6. Expected medical interventions

  a. Preventative therapy: isoniazid therapy for 9 to 12 months in clients with positive PPD but no radiologic changes or symptoms

  b. Three or more tuberculosis chemotherapeutic drugs; combination of first and second line drugs; 9 to 12 months for responsive strains

  c. Five or more tuberculosis chemotherapeutic drugs for resistant strains; first and second line drugs for as long as two years

  d. Respiratory isolation until sputum cultures are clear of bacilli (approximately two weeks after medication is started). NOTE: Documentation of this diagnosis must be reported to the public health department.

7. Nursing diagnoses

  a. Ineffective airway clearance related to thick tenacious secretions

      b. Ineffective breathing pattern related to airway inflammation

      c. Altered nutrition—less than body requirements related to anorexia and fatigue

      d. Anxiety related to social isolation secondary to isolation protocols

8. Client goals

      a. Client will maintain clear airway as evidenced by clear upper airway sounds

      b. Client will maintain respiratory rate (RR) between 16 to 24

      c. Client will demonstrate weight gain of ½ lb/week until ideal body weight is achieved

      d. Client will state that anxiety is decreased

9. Nursing interventions

      a. Acute care—infectious period

         (1) Maintain respiratory isolation

            (a) Private room with negative pressure ventilation—when door opens air rushes into room instead of air rushing out of room; restricts bacilli to client's room

            (b) Increased air circulation in room to dilute number of airborne bacilli

            (c) Door to room must remain closed at all times

            (d) Personnel and visitors wear masks if client is coughing and does not cover mouth effectively

            (e) Gowns—only if anticipation for contamination of clothes with sputum

            (f) Articles in the room—rarely implicated in transmission, but should be cleansed, disinfected, or discarded

            (g) Instruct client to cover mouth and nose with a tissue when laughing, coughing, and sneezing

            (h) Instruct client—must wear mask when removed from isolation and change it frequently, usually every two hours

            (i) Allow sunlight to enter isolation room because it kills bacilli

            (j) Burn tissues

            (k) Wash hands before and after entering room; after direct client care

         (2) Institute chemotherapeutic drug regime; include education about medications

        (a)   All daily medication must be taken as ordered, for the amount of time specified by the physician to arrest the disease

        (b)   Do not stop medication for any reason

        (c)   Report all adverse reactions to the physician

           (i)   GI disturbances

           (ii)   Stabbing pain or numbness in extremities

           (iii)   Loss of vision

        (d)   Clients should not allow themselves to run out of medication

    (3)   Diversional activities while in respiratory isolation

  b. Home care regarding client education

    (1)   The importance of continuing medications that are ordered, exactly as they are ordered

    (2)   The disease is infectious, but not transmitted on articles; do not discard any articles

    (3)   Hands must be washed after handling anything in contact with sputum

    (4)   Adequate nutrition must be maintained

    (5)   Client must never have another PPD; could cause anaphylactic reaction; chest x-rays should be used to evaluate disease; usually done every few years or when suspected symptoms appear

    (6)   Medication can be obtained from the public heath department

10. Evaluation protocol

  a. How do I know that my interventions were effective?

    (1)   Client stays in isolation room; wears mask when in contact with other people

    (2)   Client covers mouth with tissue when coughing, laughing, or sneezing

    (3)   Client indicates what medications should be taken and how often

  b. What criteria will I use to change my interventions?

    (1)   Client visits in room without use of a mask or washing hands after contact with sputum in the infectious stage

    (2)   Client leaves room without the use of a mask

    (3)   Client states the medication needs to be taken for a few weeks

    (4)   Client asks to take all pills in the morning

    c. How will I know that my client teaching has been effective?
- (1) Client demonstrates handwashing technique following the handling of anything in contact with sputum
- (2) Client thoroughly cleans eating utensils; uses dishwasher if available due to the long contact with very hot water
- (3) Client describes adverse reactions that should be brought to the attention of the physician or public health department
- (4) Client shows nurse a chart with indicated times for medication administration
- (5) Client indicates why it is important to not skip medication
- (6) Client specifies where medication can be obtained

11. Older adult alert
  - a. The older clients may become confused with multiple drug therapies and may not follow regimen correctly. These clients may need assistance to ensure proper administration.
  - b. Nutrition and fluid intake should be assessed frequently to ensure anorexia has passed and client's nutrition is optimal

D. **Adult respiratory distress syndrome (ARDS); noncardiogenic pulmonary edema**
  1. Definition—a disorder that follows insult to the body or the lungs directly
     - a. Increased pulmonary capillary permeability, resulting in noncardiogenic pulmonary edema
     - b. Massive interstitial fluid accumulation
     - c. Atelectasis; decreased lung tissue compliance
  2. Pathophysiology—lung injury leading to increased pulmonary capillary permeability; shift of fluid from vascular space to alveoli, interstitial space, and pleural space (noncardiogenic pulmonary edema); poor lung expansion, decreased lung compliance, and hypoxemia; type II pneumocytes are damaged with initial injury so that surfactant production is decreased (increased surface tension in alveoli)—atelectasis—hypoxemia
  3. Etiology—two categories
     - a. Pulmonary—aspiration, lung trauma, inhaled toxins, any type of pneumonia

    b. Nonpulmonary—multiple trauma, sepsis, any type of shock, fluid overload, eclampsia, head injury, pancreatitis, fat emboli, disseminated intravascular coagulation, transfusion reaction, high altitude, uremia

4. Incidence—over 100,000 cases occur each year, with most often a 40 to 50% mortality rate

5. Assessment
    a. Ask the following questions
        (1) Are you having difficulty breathing?
        (2) Do you know where you are, who you are and what the date is?
    b. Clinical manifestations
        (1) Changes in level of consciousness or orientation; initial restlessness, anxiety, irritability
        (2) Increased respiratory rate
        (3) Increased work of breathing, labored respirations
        (4) Use of accessory muscles, retractions
        (5) Crackles and rhonchi throughout lung fields (usually later in the process)
        (6) Cyanosis (late stage)
        (7) If on a ventilator, repeated high-pressure alarms without usual findings of increased resistance in airways from things such as increased secretions, fighting ventilator, or kinked tubes
    c. Abnormal laboratory findings—ABGs—PO_2 <80 mm Hg even with increased oxygen administration; PCO_2 initially shows respiratory alkalosis (low PCO_2 <35) due to increased respiratory rate, then respiratory acidosis as the client becomes fatigued (high PCO_2 >45); metabolic acidosis will appear as hypoxemia progresses due to anaerobic metabolism and lactic acid production
    d. Abnormal diagnostic tests
        (1) CXR—may be normal initially, slowly changing to indicate progressive pulmonary infiltrates; eventually will show a *snowstorm effect, whiteout effect,* or also called a *ground glass-like appearance*; massive pulmonary infiltrates
        (2) Pulmonary function studies—show decreased compliance or decreased elasticity of lungs

6. Expected medical interventions
    a. Mechanical ventilation with use of positive end expiratory pressure (PEEP) and positive pressure support (PPS) to

increase oxygen exchange across alveolar membrane; PEEP may range from 5 to 20 cm; PPS usually 5 cm

    b. Medications—sedation and pharmacologic paralysis to maintain optimal mechanical ventilation

    c. Steroid use is controversial

    d. Nutritional support via enteral or parenteral routes

7. Nursing diagnoses

    a. Impaired gas exchange related to changes in alveolar capillary membrane and fluid in alveoli

    b. Ineffective breathing pattern related to decreased lung compliance

    c. Activity intolerance related to hypoxemia caused by changes in alveolar capillary membrane

    d. Fear related to unknown outcome, decreased ability to maintain adequate ventilation, and effects of therapy

8. Client goals

    a. Client will maintain PO_2 >60 mm Hg and a PCO_2 35 to 45 mm Hg

    b. Client will maintain respiratory rate (RR)(RR) between 18 to 22 with no accessory muscle use

    c. Client will tolerate moving in bed without causing a decrease in SaO_2

    d. Client will show relaxed facial expressions or indicate fear is decreased

9. Nursing interventions

    a. Acute care—clients are usually transferred to critical care

        (1) Maintain airway patency through suctioning as necessary

            (a) Monitor lung sounds at least every 1 to 2 hours

            (b) Maintain ventilator settings as per physician orders

            (c) Evaluate and support vital signs as necessary—minimum of hourly vital signs; may require use of vasopressor therapy to maintain BP

            (d) Sedate and paralyze client as necessary—paralyzing agents such as norcuron are used to decrease the oxygen consumed by the client fighting to breathe; paralysis is total—client will be unable to even open eyelids; imperative to administer sedation at all times with paralyzing agent, as the paralyzing drug offers *no* sedation—only *paralysis*

    (e) Maintain nutritional status either through enteral feedings or total parenteral nutrition (TPN)

    (f) Provide alternate form of communication while client is on ventilator, such as a writing board or alphabet board

  b. Home care—the needs of the client at home will be based on the specific condition of the client. The major focuses will be education regarding

   (1) Respiratory care

   (2) Medications

   (3) Nutritional support

10. Evaluation protocol

  a. How will I know that my interventions were effective?

   (1) Client will have improved ABG results

   (2) Client will exhibit a reduced work of breathing; decreased accessory muscle use

   (3) Client will exhibit stable vital signs with near normals of baseline

  b. What criteria will I use to change my interventions?

   (1) ABG results not within prescribed parameters

   (2) Work of breathing is increased or unchanged

   (3) Vital signs are >20% of baseline

  c. How will I know that my client teaching has been effective?

   (1) Client effectively communicates needs

   (2) Client tries to work with the health care staff with things such as coughing

11. Older adult alert

  a. Older adults have decreased lung elasticity as a course of normal aging. ARDS will decrease elasticity even further and make the syndrome even more difficult to manage than in younger adults.

  b. Many older adult clients have decreased auditory acuity; if intubated and on a ventilator, the decreased auditory acuity will make communication with older clients even more difficult

E. **Chronic obstructive pulmonary disease (COPD)**

 1. Definition—a group of chronic, obstructive airflow diseases of the lungs involving the four diseases; also called chronic airway limitation (CAL)

  a. Chronic bronchitis

  b. Emphysema

     c. Asthma

     d. Bronchiectasis

2. Pathophysiology

    a. Chronic bronchitis

       (1) Hypertrophy and hypersecretion of mucous producing cells of the bronchi cause an increase in sputum production

       (2) Increased mucous causes a decrease in airway lumen size and eventually this mucous becomes colonized with bacteria

       (3) Bronchial wall becomes scarred and fibrotic in response to chronic infection which leads to stenosis and airway obstruction (Figure 6-1)

    b. Emphysema

       (1) Enlargement of air spaces distal to airways that conduct air to the alveoli

       (2) Enlarged spaces cause a breakdown in the alveoli walls which will cause an increase in airway size on inspiration, but a decrease in alveolar membrane for gas exchange

       (3) Small airways collapse on exhalation causing air trapping in the alveolar spaces

       (4) All of this is a product of the destruction of elastin in the distal airways and alveoli

    c. Asthma—two types, both resulting in bronchoconstriction

       (1) Intrinsic—no specific cause; usually adult onset

       (2) Extrinsic—response to specific allergen (Table 6-1)

    d. Bronchiectasis

       (1) Chronic dilation of the bronchi

       (2) Eventual breakdown of elastic and muscular layers of the bronchi

       (3) Seen as a result of chronic infections and/or inflammation

3. Etiology

    a. Introduction of irritants (smoking), infections, and allergens into the respiratory system

    b. May be a genetic deficiency of Alpha-1-antitrypsin (responsible for preventing breakdown of lung elastin) which can lead to emphysema

4. Incidence—greater than 10% of the older adult population have some form of COPD

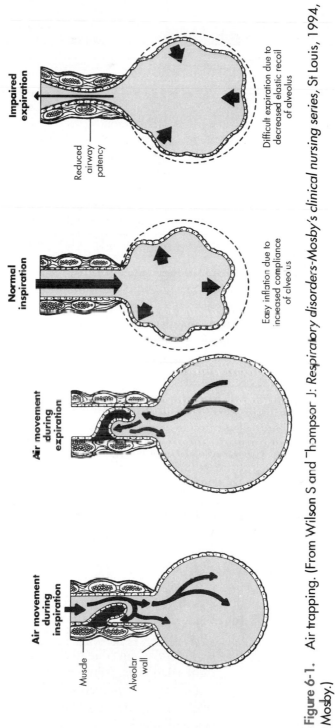

Figure 6-1. Air trapping. (From Wilson S and Thompson J: *Respiratory disorders-Mosby's clinical nursing series,* St Louis, 1994, Mosby.)

Air movement during inspiration

Muscle

Alveolar wall

Air movement during expiration

Normal inspiration

Easy inflation due to increased compliance of alveolus

Impaired expiration

Reduced airway patency

Difficult expiration due to decreased elastic recoil of alveolus

Table 6-1. Intrinsic Versus Extrinsic Asthma

Characteristic	Extrinsic	Intrinsic
Allergens as precipitants	Yes	No
Immediate skin test	Positive	Negative
Elevated IgE	Common	Uncommon
Eosinophilia	Yes	Yes
Childhood onset	Common	Uncommon
Other Allergies	Common	Uncommon
Family history of multiple allergies	Common	Uncommon
Hyposensitization therapy	Helpful	Equivocal
Typical attack	Acute and self-limiting	Often fulminant and severe
Relationship of attack to infection	May be present	Common

5. Assessment
   a. Ask the following questions
      (1) Do you have difficulty breathing? Do you have difficulty all the time or is it caused by exertion?
      (2) Do you cough frequently? Do you bring up a large amount of sputum when you cough? How much? What does it look like?
      (3) Do you cough up more sputum when you are more active?
      (4) Have you noticed a weight loss over the last year?
      (5) Do you feel tired quite often?
      (6) Are your activities impaired by your shortness of breath or your fatigue?
      (7) Do you have many respiratory infections? Over what period of time?
   b. Clinical manifestations—all conditions are manifested by prolonged expiration; a change in the normal inspiratory: expiratory ratio of 1:2 to 1:>2
      (1) Chronic bronchitis
         (a) Productive cough
         (b) Dyspnea, especially on exertion
         (c) Wheezing, rhonchi
         (d) Cyanosis—*blue bloater*
         (e) Peripheral edema due to cor pulmonale— right-sided heart failure caused by pulmonary insufficiency from increased pulmonary vascular resistance, pulmonary hypertension; noncardiogenic
         (f) Clubbed fingers

    (2) Emphysema

        (a) Dyspnea with exertion progressing to dyspnea at rest

        (b) Accessory muscle use

        (c) Increase anterior-posterior diameter of the chest

        (d) Wheezes

        (e) Overall emaciation

        (f) Pink color associated with dyspnea—*pink puffer*

        (g) Peripheral edema due to cor pulmonale

        (h) Clubbed fingers

    (3) Asthma

        (a) Dyspnea

        (b) Tight feeling in chest

        (c) Nonproductive cough

        (d) Inspiratory and/or expiratory wheezes

        (e) Clubbed fingers

    (4) Bronchiectasis

        (a) Dyspnea

        (b) Cough with large amount of sputum production

        (c) Accessory muscle use

        (d) Weight loss

        (e) Emaciation

        (f) Fever

        (g) Clubbed fingers

  c. Abnormal laboratory findings

    (1) ABGs—decreased PO_2, increased PCO_2 as disease processes progress; commonly PO_2 is 60 to 80 and PCO_2 50 to 60

    (2) CBC—polycythemia when client becomes chronically hypoxemic

    (3) Sputum culture—may indicate chronic bacterial infection

  d. Abnormal diagnostic tests

    (1) CXR—flattened diaphragm, increased lung markings, cardiac enlargement, lung hyperinflation

    (2) Pulmonary function tests—decreased forced expiratory volume in one second (FEV1); total lung capacity, residual volumes; may be increased due to air trapping

6. Expected medical interventions

  a. Oxygen when needed to maintain a PO_2 >60 mm Hg or during exercise; PO_2 ≤80 since >80 may result in respiratory depression

   b. Drug therapy—bronchodilators, mucolytics, expectorants;
       oral and nebulizer routes
   c. Physical therapy—postural drainage and chest percussion
       to assist with sputum expectoration
   d. Mechanical ventilation when conservative medical
       interventions fail
7. Nursing diagnoses
   a. Ineffective airway clearance related to thick tenacious
       secretions and fatigue
   b. Ineffective breathing pattern related to fatigue and
       obstruction of the bronchial tree
   c. Impaired gas exchange related to changes in
       the alveolar-capillary membrane and increased
       sputum production
   d. Activity intolerance related to hypoxemia and fatigue
   e. Altered nutrition—less than body requirements related to
       increased metabolic demands, fatigue, and anorexia
   f. Anxiety or fear related to inability to breathe effectively
8. Client goals
   a. Client will be able to effectively clear airway as evidenced by
       stating that airway feels clear and respirations are not labored
   b. Client will have an effective breathing pattern as evidenced
       by a rate within 10% of baseline for the client and use of
       only abdominal muscles
   c. Client will maintain a PO_2 of >60 mm Hg or within 10% of
       baseline; and a PCO_2 <60 mm Hg or within 10% of baseline
   d. Client will demonstrate increase in activity with decrease
       in dyspnea or fatigue as stated by client
   e. Client will maintain present weight or if under weight, gain
       ½ lb/week
   f. Client will state feeling less anxious or fearful with each
       episode of dyspnea
9. Nursing interventions
   a. Acute care
       (1) Assess
            (a) Patency of airway, suction if cough ineffective or
                 not present
            (b) Respiratory rate, pattern, and depth
            (c) Accessory muscle use
            (d) Lung sounds for changes, increased or
                 decreased rhonchi, crackles, wheezes; in severe
                 asthma attacks the sudden absence of wheezing

is ominous and indicates that the small airways
are totally collapsed
    (e) Skin color changes
        (i) Rubor = hypercapnia = PCO_2 >45
        (ii) Cyanosis or gray = hypoxemia = PO_2 <80
    (f) ABGs as drawn
    (g) Effectiveness of bronchodilator therapy
    (h) Anxiety if increased or diminished; increased
anxiety commonly indicates increased
respiratory distress
  (2) Monitor oxygen administration
    (a) REMEMBER!!! Normal drive to breathe is an
elevated CO_2
    (b) REMEMBER!!! Some clients with COPD have
an altered drive to breathe leading to
hypoxemia—increasing PO_2 with supplemental
oxygen administration may suppress their drive
to breathe and cause apnea; Note: With any
decrease in RR <20% of client baseline the
oxygen might need to be discontinued. COPD
drive is usually PO_2 <80.
    (c) Oxygen administration usually maintained with a
nasal cannula at one to two liters of oxygen per
minute (approximately 24% oxygen as opposed
to 21% oxygen in room air)
  (3) Monitor fluid intake to ensure appropriate hydration
to keep secretions thin
 b. Home care regarding client education
  (1) Respiratory maintenance techniques
    (a) Avoid irritants, especially smoking; suggest use
of nicotine patch to assist in quitting
    (b) Use appropriate technique for pursed lip
breathing
        (i) Inhale through nose counting to two and
pausing for one count
        (ii) Exhale slowly through pursed lips, as if
blowing a kiss or blowing into a straw,
while counting to four
    (c) How to cough effectively
        (i) *Do not force a cough*—may be damaging
to airways
        (ii) Take three deep breaths

(iii) Bear down against throat—feel pressure against throat

(iv) Cough will occur as pressure rises in throat and chest area

(d) Appropriate technique for use of abdominal muscles for breathing

(i) Abdomen should rise with inspiration

(ii) Abdomen should fall with exhalation

(e) How to balance rest and activity at home

(i) Activities no longer than 20 minutes

(ii) Rest at least 30 minutes between activities

(f) Meals should be small, frequent, high calorie, high carbohydrate and with no gas-forming foods; this prevents gastric bloating which could put pressure on the diaphragm and impede ventilation; avoid *large*, high carbohydrate meals since carbohydrates when digested give off more CO_2 than other substances and would result in an increased workload of breathing. NOTE: Carbohydrates are needed for adequate energy to breathe; give in frequent, small amounts.

(g) How to use inhalers correctly

(i) Deep breathe and exhale slowly

(ii) On second deep breath with inhaler within about 1 inch of mouth, push down to release medication; keep mouth wide open to facilitate aerosol medication movement into lungs instead of the back of the throat; if a spacer is used, lips may be put loosely around opening

(iii) Hold breath as long as possible; exhale slowly

(h) How to tell amount of medication left in inhaler—put canister in water

(i) If it floats it is empty

(ii) If it sinks it is full

(i) Avoid known allergens

(j) Avoid other people with upper respiratory illnesses

(k) Seek treatment for upper respiratory illness immediately, within 24 hours of initial onset

(l) Keep humidity in the home at least at 40% with use of a humidifier

        (2) Home care equipment—make sure arrangements have been made for oxygen and for nebulizer equipment in the home if necessary

        (3) Discuss necessary changes in sexual fulfillment, such as change in positions or the use of bronchodilators before sexual intercourse; suggest and refer to a sexual counselor to further assist if necessary

10. Evaluation protocol

   a. How do I know that my interventions were effective?

      (1) Does client feel short of breath? Has it improved?

      (2) Was client able to complete bathe independently this morning? Did client become short of breath while bathing?

      (3) Is client using oxygen? Is client using it just with activity or all the time?

      (4) Has client been feeling anxious? Has client been feeling less anxious?

   b. What criteria will I use to change my interventions?

      (1) Increased shortness of breath at rest

      (2) Decreased activity level due to increased shortness of breath

      (3) Sputum that is difficult to expectorate

      (4) Lung sounds that are deteriorating

      (5) ABGs that are deteriorating

   c. How will I know that my client teaching has been effective?

      (1) Client demonstrates appropriate pursed lip breathing technique

      (2) Client demonstrates appropriate abdominal breathing technique

      (3) Client demonstrates appropriate use of inhalers or nebulizer equipment

      (4) Client is drinking high calorie supplements, eating small meals, and is not eating gas-forming foods

11. Older adult alert

   a. The majority of clients affected with COPD are in the population classified as older adults

   b. In older clients the thoracic muscles have become weaker, meaning they will be unable to tolerate the increased work of breathing required of COPD

   c. There are less alveoli in older adult clients so that oxygen exchange will be even more impaired in older adult clients with COPD

       d. The weaker thoracic muscles will also make coughing more difficult for older adult clients; thus, retained secretions will be a problem in many instances

F. **Lung cancer**
  1. Definition—a malignancy of the lower respiratory tract
  2. Pathophysiology—uncontrolled growth of undifferentiated cells which begin to invade surrounding tissues
    a. Adenocarcinoma—most common; originates in peripheral lung tissue
    b. Squamous cell carcinoma—originates in bronchial epithelium
    c. Small cell carcinoma (oat cell)—originates in cells of the airways
    d. Large cell carcinoma—originates peripherally in the lung; multiple masses occur
  3. Etiology—tobacco smoke is the major cause (approximately 80%) of lung cancer; exposure to asbestos and radon are also factors
  4. Incidence—has been growing significantly over the last 10 years
  5. Assessment
    a. Ask the following questions
      (1) Do you experience a cough? Do you produce sputum with your cough? How much? What does it look like?
      (2) Do you ever feel short of breath?
      (3) Do you ever cough up blood?
      (4) Do you ever experience hoarseness?
      (5) How many pillows do you sleep on at night?
      (6) Have you lost a noticeable amount of weight in the past couple of months?
    b. Clinical manifestations
      (1) Chronic cough; productive or nonproductive
      (2) Dyspnea
      (3) Hoarseness
      (4) Chest tightness or pain
      (5) Hemoptysis—blood in sputum
      (6) Shoulder or arm pain
      (7) Frequent occurrences of bronchitis or pneumonia
      (8) Superior cava syndrome—edema of the face, neck, arms, and upper torso when the lung tumor presses on the superior vena cava

      c. Abnormal laboratory findings—sputum for cytology: malignant cells identified

      d. Abnormal diagnostic tests

         (1) CXR—nodule or lesion identified

         (2) CT scan—nodule or lesion identified and position pinpointed in chest

         (3) Lung scan—identifies size, shape, and actual position of lesion

         (4) Brain and Bone Scans—identify metastasis

6. Expected medical interventions

      a. Surgery—lobectomy, pneumonectomy, wedge resection, segmental resection if lesion is operable

      b. Radiation therapy—may be sole therapy if client has an inoperable tumor; can be used also preoperatively and postoperatively to decrease lesion size

      c. Antineoplastic Therapy—used for small cell carcinoma

7. Nursing diagnoses

      a. Ineffective airway clearance related to thick tenacious sputum and chest muscle weakness

      b. Ineffective breathing pattern related to chest pain and muscle weakness

      c. Impaired gas exchange related to impaired ventilation secondary to invasive tumor

      d. Altered nutrition—less than body requirements related to anorexia

      e. Anxiety related to difficulty breathing and fear of death

8. Client goals

      a. Client will maintain a patent airway as evidenced by clear upper airway sounds

      b. Client will maintain respiratory rate (RR) between 18 to 22 with appropriate breath sounds in bases

      c. Client will maintain PO_2 and PCO_2 within 10% of client baseline

      d. Client will remain at present weight without any further loss

      e. Client will state that anxiety has reached a manageable level and does not prevent maintenance of an active life

9. Nursing interventions

      a. Acute care

         (1) Assess

            (a) Airway patency at least every one to two hours; suction if cough not effective or not coughing with secretions present

(b) Respiratory rate and depth at least every two to four hours

(c) Lung sounds for changes, especially wheezing which may reflect impaired, narrowed lower airways

(d) ABGs for deterioration

(e) Accessory muscle use

(f) Sputum—evaluate color, odor, and consistency; hemoptysis

(g) Hydration status

(2) For postoperative thoracotomy clients assess all of the above

(a) In addition, assess

(i) Chest tube patency and drainage; immediate postoperatively expect 150 cc per hour of sanguinous drainage, decreasing in amount and changing from sanguinous to serosanguinous or serous drainage within 48 hours; unlikely to have bubbling in water seal chamber; note continuous bubbling in suction control chamber if connected to suction of usually 20 cm H_2O; chest tubes usually removed three to six days postop

(ii) Chest wall for subcutaneous emphysema— air trapped in subcutaneous tissue—feels like crumpled plastic wrap under the skin; check around chest tube insertion site first, then shoulder and neck areas

(iii) Dressing for bleeding; check behind client's back for blood

(iv) Pain—adequate pain medication will allow client to turn, cough, and deep breathe more effectively

(b) Turn, cough, and deep breathe client every two hours after pain medication; deep breathing frequently accomplished through use of incentive spirometer mechanisms. REMEMBER: When positioning a client on a side, the lung up in the air (upward) is the one ventilated most effectively. The lung the client is lying on is compressed and not as effectively ventilated.

      (c) Specific positioning guidelines
          (i) Pneumonectomy—on back and operative side ONLY; placing client on unoperative side prevents adequate expansion of remaining lung; remember the good lung is on the unoperative side; it now receives all the blood from the heart so adequate perfusion is less of a concern; engorgement of the lung may occur; right heart failure may also be a problem; increased risk of mediastinal shift—mediastinum can shift toward remaining lung due to lack of anchoring tissue on empty cavity side especially in the first few days after surgery
         (ii) All other thoracotomies—turn to back and unoperative side ONLY; may tilt to operative side—lying on operative side prevents reexpansion of lung tissue remaining on operative side, may cause compression of chest tubes, and is more uncomfortable to client
    (d) Assist with active and passive range of motion for arm on the operative side to prevent tightening of shoulder muscles
    (e) Encourage semifowlers position for optimal ventilation of remaining lung tissue

b. Home care regarding client education
  (1) Postoperative needs
    (a) Incisional care—frequency, technique, observations that are normal and those necessary to report to physician
    (b) Activity limitations—varies with individuals
    (c) Specific assessment factors the client needs to report or discuss with physician
    (d) Need to continue postoperative coughing and deep breathing exercises with use of incentive spirometer at home
    (e) Need to continue arm exercises
  (2) Nonsurgical clients
    (a) Need to weigh themselves weekly
    (b) Eating pattern of small frequent meals

   (c) Suggestion to use antiemetics before meals
   (d) Discuss how to balance rest and activity
   (e) Instruct how to have physician ordered oxygen delivered to the home and used in the home
   (f) Instruct clients and significant others about use of nebulizer therapy
   (g) Potential need to have adequate fluid intake to liquefy secretions

 10. Evaluation protocol
  a. How do I know that my interventions were effective?
   (1) Does client feel short of breath? Is it more or less than it was two hours ago?
   (2) Is client's sputum difficult to cough up?
   (3) Is client having chest or incisional pain?
   (4) Is client feeling anxious? More anxious than yesterday?
  b. What criteria will I use to change my interventions?
   (1) Increased or unresolved shortness of breath
   (2) Thick tenacious sputum that is difficult to expectorate
   (3) Increased or unresolved chest or incisional pain
   (4) Client describing anxiety that prevents activity
  c. How will I know that my client teaching has been effective?
   (1) Client demonstrates correct wound care technique
   (2) Client states conditions that should be reported to physician
   (3) Client demonstrates correct use of oxygen and nebulizer equipment
   (4) Client describes small meals that are prepared and the use of an antiemetic before meals
   (5) Client shows a chart of weekly weights taken in the home with evaluation of gain or loss

 11. Older adult alert
  a. The cough is weak in older clients due to a decrease in chest wall muscle strength. These clients are at a greater risk for atelectasis and pneumonia than younger people.
  b. Older clients who are postoperative for thoracic surgery are at greater risk for hypoxemia due to loss of lung tissue and normal decrease of functioning alveoli due to the aging process

G. **Chest/lung trauma**
 1. Definition—injury that occurs to chest wall and/or the lung as a result of a blunt or nonpenetrating impact or penetrating impact to the chest
  a. Rib fracture—break in the integrity of the rib

  b. Flail chest—multiple rib fractures that leave an area of the chest wall unstable, with a need for impeding ventilation

  c. Pneumothorax—air entering the space between the visceral and parietal pleura; absent breath sounds

  d. Hemothorax—blood entering space between visceral and parietal pleura; absent breath sounds; potential signs of shock; *pneumothorax and hemothorax can be a consequence of rib fracture and flail chest*

  e. Tension pneumothorax—air entering the pleural space and becoming trapped to the point of causing increased thoracic pressure and mediastinal content shift; commonly acute tracheal deviation to the side opposite of pneumothorax; medical emergency due to disruption of cardiac output and respiratory embarrassment

2. Pathophysiology—there is normally negative pressure (suction) between the visceral and parietal pleura; any injury that allows air or positive pressure to enter the pleural space will prevent the lung from remaining inflated

  a. Injury that allows blood to enter the pleural space may also prevent the lung from remaining inflated

  b. Tension pneumothorax—air enters the pleural space through a hole in the lung, such as when a bleb (a fragile thin walled alveoli) ruptures, and then becomes trapped in the thorax causing an increase in pressure; this pressure pushes the heart, vena cavas, and aorta out of position; resulting in poor venous return to the heart which leads to poor cardiac output (Figure 6-2)

3. Etiology—most common cause for blunt chest trauma is a motor vehicle accident and falls; penetrating trauma is commonly due to gunshot or knife injuries

4. Assessment

  a. Ask the following questions

    (1) Are you having difficulty breathing?

    (2) Do you have pain in your chest? Point to your pain with one finger.

  b. Clinical manifestations

    (1) Some degree of shortness of breath

    (2) Chest pain at point of injury

    (3) Tachycardia

    (4) Anxiety—may be extreme

  c. Abnormal laboratory findings—ABGs—decreased PO_2, initially decreased PCO_2 related to tachypnea followed by increased PCO_2 as the ability to hyperventilate is lost

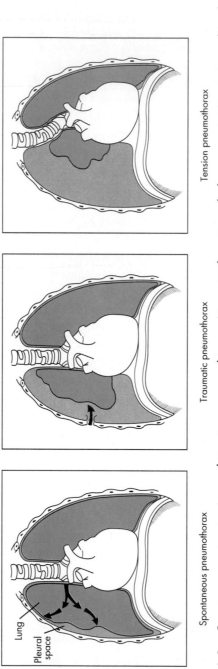

Spontaneous pneumothorax   Traumatic pneumothorax   Tension pneumothorax

Figure 6-2. Spontaneous, traumatic, and tension pneumothorax. (From Wilson S and Thompson J: *Respiratory disorders- Mosby's clinical nursing series*, St Louis, 1994, Mosby.)

190

d. Abnormal diagnostic tests—CXR—will indicate percentage of pneumothorax and amount of space occupied by blood in the pleural space with a hemothorax; also will identify rib fractures and flail chest

5. Expected medical interventions
   a. Rib fractures—rest, heat to area, and pain relief
   b. Flail chest—chest tube with water seal drainage if a hemothorax or pneumothorax exists with flail chest; may require mechanical ventilation to support ventilation
   c. Pneumothorax—chest tube insertion and water seal drainage; locate in anterior upper thorax to remove air
   d. Hemothorax—chest tube insertion and water seal drainage; locate lower thoracic area to drain blood from chest; may require blood administration to replace lost blood

6. Nursing diagnoses
   a. Ineffective breathing pattern related to decreased lung expansion
   b. Impaired gas exchange related to decreased alveolar membrane surface available for gas exchange
   c. Anxiety related to inability to ventilate effectively

7. Client goals
   a. Client will maintain RR between 20 to 24
   b. Client will maintain a PO_2 between 80 to 100 mm Hg; PCO_2 between 35 to 45 mm Hg
   c. Client will state feeling less anxious

8. Nursing interventions
   a. Acute care
      (1) Assess
          (a) Airway patency
          (b) Respiratory rate, depth, and character
          (c) Lung sounds for abscence
          (d) Chest for rise and fall of chest symmetrically with respirations
          (e) ABGs
          (f) Chest wall for subcutaneous emphysema especially with rib fractures and flail chest
      (2) Maintain semifowlers position to assist with ventilatory effort
      (3) Medicate for pain
      (4) Appropriate care for pleural chest tubes with water seal drainage (Figures 6-3 and 6-4)—sequence of chambers from client to system

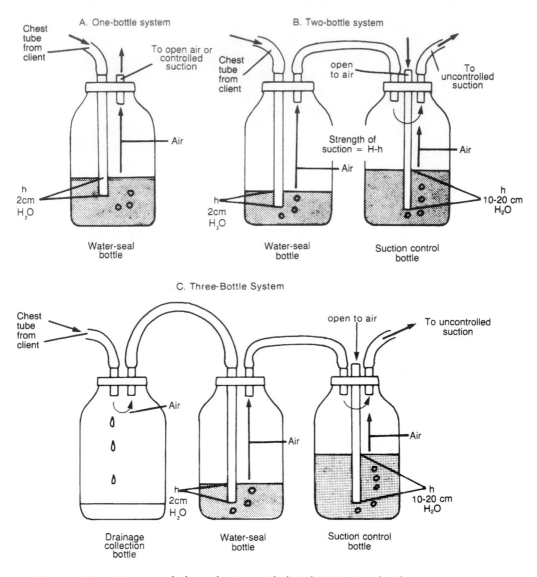

A. One-bottle system

Chest tube from client

To open air or controlled suction

Air

h
2cm
H_2O

Water-seal bottle

B. Two-bottle system

Chest tube from client

open to air

To uncontrolled suction

Strength of suction = H-h

Air

Air

h
2cm
H_2O

h
10-20 cm
H_2O

Water-seal bottle

Suction control bottle

C. Three-Bottle System

Chest tube from client

open to air

To uncontrolled suction

Air

Air

Air

h
2cm
H_2O

h
10-20 cm
H_2O

Drainage collection bottle

Water-seal bottle

Suction control bottle

Figure 6-3. Water seal chest drainage (*h*=height). **A,** One-bottle system. **B,** Two-bottle system. **C,** Three-bottle system. (From *AJN/Mosby Nursing board review,* ed 9, St Louis, 1994, Mosby.)

    (a)   Collection bottle-chamber—collects drainage from chest and allows measurement of drainage

    (b)   Water seal bottle-chamber—seals end of chest tube with 2 cm of water so that air cannot enter chest tube and eventually thoracic cavity

        (i)   Normal function—water will fluctuate with respirations and may bubble on exhalation

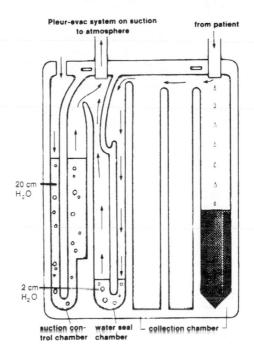

Pleur-evac system on suction
to atmosphere

from patient

20 cm
H₂O

2 cm
H₂O

suction con-
trol chamber

water seal
chamber

collection chamber

Figure 6-4. Pleur-Evac system. A Pleur-Evac unit consists of three chambers comparable to a three-bottle water seal drainage system. The suction control chamber is equivalent to bottle no. 3—the suction control bottle. The water seal chamber is equivalent to bottle no. 2—the water seal bottle. The collection chamber corresponds to bottle no. 1—the drainage collection bottle. (From *AJN/Mosby Nursing board review*, ed 9, St Louis, 1994, Mosby.)

when air escapes from a significant pneumothorax; not found with hemothorax
  (ii) Abnormal function—continuous bubbling indicates air is leaking into the system
(c) Suction control bottle-chamber—filled to level of ordered suction with sterile water; normal suction is –20 cm H₂O
  (i) Normal function—should gently bubble continuously when suction is on; suction source attached to chamber or bottle
  (ii) Abnormal functioning—intermittent or no bubbling; check that suction is turned on, not disconnected or tubing kinked
(d) Make certain all connections are taped to prevent air leaks
(e) Tubing should be free draining without kinks

       (f) Drainage system must be below level of insertion site on chest wall at all times

       (g) Have clamps with rubber tips at bedside for emergency situation only—clamping for extended periods especially with a large leak from a pneumothorax may cause a tension pneumothorax; chest tube must be clamped during change of water seal drainage collection system

       (h) Encourage turning, coughing, and deep breathing to prevent atelectasis

  b. Home care regarding client education

    (1) Chest tube insertion site care and signs of infection at site

       (a) If dressing in place, do not remove until physician evaluates site

       (b) If no dressing, clean with soap and water; watch for and report redness, swelling, or any kind of drainage from area

    (2) Need for follow-up care to evaluate for further pulmonary impairment

    (3) Guidelines to increase activity as able

    (4) Need to balance rest and activity

9. Evaluation protocol

  a. How do I know that my interventions were effective?

    (1) Is client having difficulty breathing?

    (2) Has client's chest pain diminished?

    (3) Objective evaluation

       (a) Equal lungs sounds

       (b) Bilateral chest movement

       (c) Decreased chest tube drainage with change of color from sanguinous to serosanguinous to serous

  b. What criteria will I use to change my interventions?

    (1) Increased dyspnea with activity or at rest, or dyspnea not improved

    (2) Increased chest pain or unrelieved chest pain with prescribed medications

    (3) Lung sounds remain absent in one area of chest

    (4) Unilateral chest movement

    (5) Significant serosanguinous chest tube drainage, >50 cc/h after the first eight hours

  c. How will I know that my client teaching has been effective?
    (1) Client demonstrates correct chest tube site care
    (2) Client keeps scheduled follow-up visits with physician
    (3) Client walks ½ a block more each day
 10. Older adult alert
  a. Older adults are at high risk for infection due to decreased immune response; chest injuries should be evaluated carefully for signs of infection; a 99° F temperature may indicate an initial infection
  b. Cough will be impaired due to decreased muscle strength, so older adults are at great risk for atelectasis and pneumonia following chest injuries

H. **Pneumoconioses**
 1. Definition—occupational lung disorder related to inhalation of particulate matter during working schedule; three most common disorders are silicosis, asbestosis, and coal workers pneumoconioses
 2. Pathophysiology—silicone and asbestos when inhaled produce an inflammatory and fibrotic type of reaction resulting in emphysematous type of lung disorder; coal dust inhaled over many years is deposited in the alveoli and becomes very difficult to clear; eventually interferes with alveolar membrane function
 3. Etiology—inhalation of silicone from ceramic or building material; asbestos when manufactured into fireproofing products; coal dust from prolonged exposure during coal mining
 4. Assessment, diagnoses, interventions and evaluations of these clients will be identical to the client with chronic obstructive pulmonary disease. Please refer to COPD pp. 178-183 number 5 through 11 for discussion of nursing care.

I. **Pulmonary embolism**
 1. Definition—blockage of a branch of the pulmonary artery by a thrombus, piece of fatty tissue, a piece of tumor, air, or a particle of amniotic fluid; blood is prevented from entering the lungs for gas exchange
 2. Pathophysiology—the embolism is freed from the point of origin, travels to the pulmonary artery and becomes lodged in one of the branches; the larger the embolism the larger the obstruction in the pulmonary artery; ventilation > perfusion:

the lungs are appropriately ventilated but blood is unable to come in contact with oxygen rich alveoli due to the embolism; blood is shunted to left side of heart unoxygenated and client becomes hypoxemic

3. Incidence—over 6000 cases per year in the United States, with a mortality rate of over 35%

4. Etiology—thrombus formation usually originates in veins of legs or pelvis

   a. Follows prolonged bedrest, venous stasis, dehydration, or some other cause of increased coagulability

   b. Fat embolism follows fracture of the long bones—typically the femur

   c. Air embolism may occur via a central venous catheter or during cardiopulmonary bypass

   d. Amniotic embolism follows childbirth

   e. Tumor embolism is associated with a malignancy

5. Assessment

   a. Ask the following questions

      (1) Are you having difficulty breathing?

      (2) Do you have chest pain? Point to where it hurts the most with one finger.

      (3) Have you experienced any fever?

   b. Clinical manifestations

      (1) Sudden onset dyspnea

      (2) Anxiety, fear, feeling of impending doom

      (3) Sinus tachycardia, dysrhythmias

      (4) Fever >100° F

      (5) Crackles, pleural friction rub; localized or generalized dependent on magnitude of embolism

      (6) Pleuritic chest pain

   c. Abnormal laboratory findings—ABGs—PO_2 <80 mm Hg; PCO_2 initially decreased due to tachypnea, but may rise >45 mm Hg as client tires

   d. Abnormal diagnostic tests

      (1) Ventilation-perfusion lung scan (definitive for diagnosis)—ventilation with radioactive gas shows normal ventilation; injection with radioactive dye shows areas of lung not appropriately perfused

      (2) CXR—may show some decrease in vascular markings on effected area of lung

6. Expected medical interventions

   a. Bedrest for two to three days followed by slow increase in mobility

    b.   Anticoagulation with continuous heparin drip, usually for 7 to 10 days; maintaining therapeutic activated partial thromboplastin time (APTT) of 1.5 to 2 times the normal

    c.   Oral anticoagulant therapy begun three days before heparin is stopped to allow time for oral anticoagulant to reach therapeutic level; prothrombin time (PT) of 1.5 to 2 times normal; maintained for at least six months

    d.   Surgical intervention—vena cava umbrella for repeated incidence of pulmonary embolism

    e.   Thrombolytic therapy—streptokinase or urokinase in the face of massive pulmonary embolism; medication is directly injected into the pulmonary artery which contains the clot

7. Nursing diagnoses

    a.   Impaired gas exchange related to ventilation-perfusion abnormality

    b.   Ineffective breathing pattern related to chest pain, hypoxemia, and anxiety

    c.   Chest pain related to inflammatory process initiated by embolism

    d.   Anxiety related to difficulty breathing and fear of death

8. Client goals

    a.   Client will maintain PO_2 and PCO_2 within 10% of client baseline

    b.   Client will maintain respiratory rate (RR) within 20 to 24

    c.   Client will state chest pain has diminished

    d.   Client will state anxiety has decreased to a manageable level and the feeling of doom is gone

9. Nursing interventions

    a.   Acute care

        (1) Immediate care

            (a) Vital signs every 15 minutes until within 10% of baseline for client; may require vasopressor therapy for support

            (b) Evaluate neurologic status every one to two hours for changes related to hypoxemia

            (c) Evaluate lung sounds every one to two hours for changes—increased respiratory effort at rest, increased crackles, onset of wheezing, rhonchi

            (d) Evaluate SaO_2 and ABGs, parameters as ordered for increased hypoxemia

            (e) Administer oxygen as per order—usually ordered to keep SaO_2 >90%

      (f)   Medicate for pain as vital signs permit; morphine sulfate relieves feelings of anxiety and promotes bronchial dilation

      (g) Monitor for indications of right-sided heart failure, acute cor pulmonale

         (i)   Distended neck veins at >35 degree elevation of HOB

         (ii) CVP >10 cm H_2O or >8 mm Hg

         (iii) Right ventricular gallop

         (iv) Peripheral edema, sacral, ankles or feet

  b. Ongoing care

     (1) Monitor for sign of excessive anticoagulation—blood in stool, urine, gums, bruising, petechiae especially over chest wall

     (2) Avoid intramuscular injections due to anticoagulant therapy

     (3) Wean off of oxygen as soon as possible with physician orders and the use of SaO_2 monitoring

  c. Home care regarding client education

     (1) Instructions regarding anticoagulant therapy

       (a) Clients understand any abnormal or excessive bruising or bleeding may be an indication of overanticoagulation; notify physician immediately

       (b) Use a soft toothbrush

       (c) Know how often to have prothrombin time drawn to evaluate maintenance dose of anticoagulant

       (d) Clients need to notify all caregivers that they are taking an anticoagulant; may want to obtain a medic-alert bracelet

       (e) Clients know what foods should not be eaten and will interfere with anticoagulants, such as green leafy vegetables

10. Evaluation protocol

  a. How do I know that my interventions were effective?

     (1) Is client still having difficulty breathing?

     (2) Has client's chest pain gone away or improved?

     (3) Objective assessment

       (a) Vital signs are stable

       (b) Neurologic status is stable

       (c) SaO_2 or ABGs indicates hypoxemia has resolved

       (d) APTT is at therapeutic level

      b. What criteria will I use to change my interventions?
- (1) Unstable vital signs
- (2) Deterioration in neurologic status
- (3) SaO_2 or ABGs indicates continued hypoxemia
- (4) APTT not in therapeutic range

      c. How will I know that my client teaching has been effective?
- (1) Client indicates that PT must be drawn weekly
- (2) Client takes oral anticoagulant daily, at the same time each day
- (3) Client purchases soft bristled toothbrush, or, if wearing dentures, client checks gums daily for bleeding
- (4) Client indicates no excessive bruising or evidence of bleeding

11. Older adult alert

      a. Older adults are at great risk for pulmonary embolism as a result of decreased cardiac output they experience in the process of aging. They are also at risk as a result of proneness to venous stasis from decreased exercise or walking and from decreased tone in venous walls.

      b. Older adults can become dehydrated very quickly as a result of diuretic therapy and poor nutritional habits. This also increases their risk of pulmonary embolism.

REVIEW QUESTIONS

1. When assessing a client who has experienced a pulmonary embolism, the nurse would expect to see what type of respiratory pattern?
   a. Rate >30 per minute
   b. Apnea
   c. Accessory muscle use
   d. Rapid and shallow

2. A client with newly symptomatic COPD is being started on a bronchodilator. The nurse's understanding of the action of this drug will help the nurse to understand that the expected effect in this client will be
   a. Decreased respiratory rate
   b. Decreased work of breathing
   c. Help in clearing secretions
   d. Help in liquefying secretions

3. A client with asthma informs the nurse that the Cromolyn is carried with him wherever he goes in case he has an asthma attack. The best intervention in relation to this statement is to
   a. Praise him for thinking ahead in preventing a problem
   b. Instruct him that this drug works over a long period of time to decrease airway secretions
   c. Instruct him that there is no reason to carry it with him because it is used only for emphysema
   d. Instruct him that this drug is used prophylactically to prevent asthma, not to stop an acute attack

4. A common assessment finding associated with pneumonia is
   a. Accessory muscle use
   b. Bronchial breath sounds over area of pneumonia
   c. Dry, hacking cough
   d. Night sweats

5. A nurse has placed a purified protein derivative skin test on a client suspected of having tuberculosis. The nurse understands a check of this site must be done in
   a. 4 hours
   b. 24 hours
   c. 24 to 48 hours
   d. 48 to 72 hours

6. A client has been diagnosed with Adult Respiratory Distress Syndrome (ARDS). In the early stages of the illness expected findings on the ABGs are
   a. Low PO_2, low PCO_2
   b. Low PO_2, high PCO_2
   c. High PO_2, low PCO_2
   d. Normal PO_2, normal PCO_2

7. Clients with ARDS would have which one of these nursing diagnoses placed on their nursing care plan?
   a. Ineffective airway clearance related to thin secretions and fatigue
   b. Ineffective breathing pattern related to hypoxia
   c. Impaired gas exchange related to changes in the alveolar capillary membrane
   d. Activity intolerance related to anxiety

8. A client with emphysema is complaining to the food service supervisor because he is not given a choice of cabbage which he enjoys eating. The nurse's best intervention is to
   a. Explain that this is a gas-forming food and he cannot have that type of food
   b. Explain to food service that he can have whatever he wants
   c. Ask his wife to bring him food from home if the food service group will not give it to him
   d. Instruct client that gas-forming foods produce more gas which then pushes up on his diaphragm and makes it even more difficult to breathe

9. The nurse would expect a client with a tension pneumothorax to display what types of assessment findings?
   a. Chronic cyanosis and hypotension
   b. Sustained bradypnea and hypotension
   c. Boring chest pain and diaphoresis
   d. Acute dyspnea and tachycardia

10. When discharging clients who have been hospitalized for 10 days due to pulmonary embolism, appropriate education *must* include
    a. To eliminate green leafy vegetables from their diet
    b. To eliminate all green vegetables from their diet
    c. That they must have a PT drawn every week
    d. They should take only aspirin for fever or pain

ANSWERS, RATIONALES, AND TEST-TAKING TIPS

Rationales	Test-Taking Tips

1. Correct answer: d

The best answer in this group is rapid, shallow respirations. The pain of pulmonary embolism will cause the client to not want to breathe deeply, but will have to breathe more rapidly to maintain oxygenation.

Key word in the question is "respiratory pattern" and the only response that describes a "pattern" is response *d*.

2. Correct answer: b

Bronchodilators enlarge the diameter of the airways which allows for easier passage of air, and thus indirectly will decrease respiratory rate and decrease work of breathing.

The key words in the stem are "action of the drug." Mucomyst liquifies secretions. Narcotics decrease respiratory rate. Clearing secretions is done best by a strong cough effort.

3. Correct answer: d

Cromolyn has no use in the face of an acute asthma attack. It is used only to prevent an attack.

The approach to select the correct response is to eliminate choices, then the only response left is the correct one. An important clue in the stem is the stated client situation "asthma attack." In response *a*, the word "preventing" contradicts the stated need by the patient and also the word "problem" is too general to relate to the situation of an asthma attack. In response *b*, the verbiage "over a long period of time" contradicts the given situation of asthma attack. In response *c,* to eliminate it as a choice, remember that there is no drug to treat emphysema, only drugs to treat the effects of emphysema. The only response left is *d*, the correct response.

4. Correct answer: b

Bronchial breath sounds, normally heard over the trachea, can be heard over the area of consolidation in a client with pneumonia. They are sounds transmitted from the trachea mainstem bronchus over the area filled with exudate. This client typically will not be using accessory muscles, but breathing rapidly and shallowly from pain. A productive cough is a usual finding. Night sweats are seen in clients with tuberculosis, AIDS, Hodgkin's, or menopause.

The technique of matching words in the question and response works here—match pneumonia in question and the response with pneumonia. Remember to use this technique only if you have no educated guess to narrow the responses.

5. Correct answer: d

PPDs must be checked in 48 to 72 hours for accurate evaluation. A positive finding is an induration of >10 mm. Erythema >10 mm may be a finding but is not considered a positive result.

Remember the T in TB test requires at least Two days to Three days for the check of a response.

6. Correct answer: a

PO_2 will be low as a result of the hypoxemia of the syndrome; the PCO_2 will be low due to the rapid respiratory rate associated with the hypoxemia.

The time "in the early stages" is important to note. The patient will be blowing off a lot of CO_2 yet because of the congestion there will be little O_2 exchanged.

7. Correct answer: c

This is the best stated nursing diagnosis—ineffective airway clearance would be related to thick secretions; ineffective breathing pattern

Recall ARDS as a problem is located at the alveolar capillary membrane.

would be related to hypoxemia; activity intolerance would be related to fatigue.

8. Correct answer: d

Response *a* reflects rigidity with emphasis on rules, not client needs and is not the best approach. Response *d* gives the most thorough explanation.

Responses *b* and *c* can be clustered under the approach that the client can eat whatever he wants. How the question is asked gives the clue that this is not a correct approach to the problem of diet. With responses *a* and *d* left, *a* reflects rigidity and *d* relates the reason for restriction to breathing difficulty. The client will more easily understand this explanation.

9. Correct answer: d

The best answer is acute dyspnea and shortness of breath; chest pain is not that common, nor is diaphoresis; cyanosis is a very late sign, and bradypnea would not be seen; rather tachypnea and tachycardia are more commonly seen.

The key words in response a "chronic," response *b* "sustained," and response *c* "boring" can be clustered to eliminate these as correct answers. The word "acute" in response *d* is a clue that this is the correct response since tension pneumothorax is more commonly an acute situation.

10. Correct answer: a

Green leafy vegetables may render the coumadin ineffective; not all green vegetables have this effect. They must have a PT drawn every week initially and not throughout the course of therapy. Clients must not take aspirin with the coumadin since ASA increases the risk of bleeding.

The absolute words "all" in response *b*, "every" in response *c*, and "only" in response *d* are clues that these are incorrect responses.

The Gastrointestinal System

STUDY OUTCOMES

After completing this chapter, the reader will be able to do the following:

▼ Identify major anatomic components and functions of the gastrointestinal (GI) system.

▼ Identify assessment findings of clients with alterations of the gastrointestinal system.

▼ Choose appropriate nursing diagnoses for the gastrointestinal disorders discussed.

▼ Implement appropriate nursing interventions for the client with a gastrointestinal disorder.

▼ Evaluate the progress of the client with a gastrointestinal disorder for establishment of new nursing interventions based on evaluation findings.

KEY TERMS

Absorption	Small particles of digested food that cross the membranes of the intestines and enter the blood stream.
Digestion	Breaking down of proteins, polysaccharides, and fat, through the action of acids and enzymes secreted into the GI tract.
Dysphagia	Difficulty swallowing.
Motility	The action of peristalsis.
Peristalsis	Rhythmic contraction of the smooth muscles of the GI tract responsible for movement of solid matter through the tract.
Secretion	Release of a chemical substance from gland cells of the GI system.

CONTENT REVIEW

I. **The gastrointestinal system is responsible for the ingestion and digestion of food, the absorption of nutrients, and the storage and elimination of waste products**

II. **Structure and function**
   A. Mouth (buccal cavity)—mastication or chewing of food breaks down food into smaller particles to make digestion easier; lubrication of food also occurs in mouth with introduction of the enzyme ptyalin
   B. Esophagus—muscular tube responsible for propelling food from mouth to stomach through peristalsis
   C. Stomach—J-shaped organ found in upper abdomen responsible for continuation of digestive process
      1. Four stomach areas
         a. Fundus—left upper stomach
         b. Body—main section
         c. Cardia—base of the esophagus
         d. Antrum—right lower section, just above the pylorus
      2. Secretions
         a. Hydrochloric acid
         b. Intrinsic factor
         c. Pepsin

        d. Pepsinogen

        e. Lipase

        f. Bile

        g. Mucous, to protect the walls of the stomach from autodigestion

    3. Endocrine cells of the stomach secrete gastrin which controls gastric secretions and motility

D. **Pancreas—called an accessory organ, found behind the stomach; secretes a liquid rich in sodium bicarbonate to decrease acidity of gastric contents as well as trypsin, chymotrypsin, lipase, and amylase; these secretions enter from the pancreatic duct into the duodenum**

E. **Liver—right side of upper abdominal cavity, just under the diaphragm; made up of microscopic lobules, each with a central venule and surrounded by the hepatic artery**

    1. Maintains blood glucose and amino acid levels by removing excesses from the portal circulation and secreting glucose if level drops

    2. Synthesizes blood glucose, proteins, amino acids, and fats

    3. Produces and secretes bile and bile salts necessary for digestion of fat

    4. Bile is delivered and then stored in the gallbladder, which is situated beneath the liver

F. **Small intestine**

    1. Three distinct areas—the duodenum, the jejunum, and the ileum, which are positioned anatomically as listed

    2. Mucosa of the small intestines is covered with millions of finger like projections called villi—responsible for absorption of food particles after further digestion in the small intestines

    3. Brush border, made up of microvilli, line the outer surface of the villi and are responsible for majority of enzyme or digestive activity in the small intestines

    4. Enzymes available at the brush border are peptidase, sucrase, lactase, and maltase

    5. Contents of the small intestines are constantly churned by peristalsis of the wall of the small intestines, allowing more food particles to have contact with the villi and thus be further digested and absorbed

G. **Large intestine**
1. Five distinct areas—ascending colon, transverse colon, descending colon, sigmoid colon, and rectum, which are positioned anatomically as listed
   a. Ascending colon—right side of abdomen; accepts contents of the ileum and pushes them forward in the colon
   b. Ileocecal valve between the ileum and cecum, or beginning pouch of the colon, prevents backflow of material into the ileum
   c. Contents are continuously pushed through the transverse colon, which lies horizontally just below the stomach
   d. Contents continuously pushed through the descending colon on left side of abdomen
   e. Absorbed throughout this trip are water, urea, and electrolytes
   f. Intestinal contents are then pushed into the sigmoid colon, so called because of its S-shape
   g. Contents first enter the rectum and then are expelled through the anus
2. Feces is stored in distal half of colon until defecation occurs; feces is composed of ¾ water, ¼ solid matter comprising food residue, digestive enzymes, bile pigments, and mucus

III. Targeted concerns
A. **Pharmacology—priority drug classifications**
1. Antacids—neutralize gastric acid
   a. Expected effects—relief of gastric pain, indigestion, and gastroesophageal reflux
   b. Commonly given drugs
      (1) Aluminum hydroxide (Amphojel)
      (2) Calcium carbonate (Tums)
      (3) Magnesium hydroxide (Milk of Magnesia)
   c. Nursing considerations
      (1) Antacids can alter the absorption of other medications if taken concurrently or within one hour of other medications
      (2) Shake preparations well before taking
      (3) Follow with a glass of water to ensure medication has entered the stomach
      (4) Commonly taken one hour after eating and at bedtime

2. Combination antacids—composed of a combination of aluminum and magnesium
   a. Expected effects—same as above
   b. Commonly given drugs
      (1) Magaldrate (Riopan)
      (2) Aluminum and magnesium hydroxide (Maalox)
      (3) Aluminum, magnesium, and simethicone (Mylanta)
   c. Nursing considerations—same as above; used by clients who have experienced diarrhea or constipation with single agent antacids
3. Antidiarrheal agents—slows intestinal motility and peristalsis
   a. Expected effect—decreased episodes of diarrhea
   b. Commonly given systemically acting drugs
      (1) Diphenoxlate hydrochloride with atropine sulfate (Lomotil)
      (2) Loperamide (Immodium)
      (3) Camphorated tincture of opium (Paregoric)
   c. Nursing considerations
      (1) Hold drug and call physician if abdomen becomes distended and bowel sounds decrease
      (2) Encourage client to ensure that fluid intake is increased to at least 2000 ml/day during this period to prevent dehydration
      (3) Caution client that these medications may cause drowsiness
4. Antiemetics—most agents act on chemoreceptor trigger zone in brain to prevent or decrease nausea and vomiting
   a. Expected effects—decreased or inhibited nausea and vomiting
   b. Commonly given drugs
      (1) Prochlorperazine (Compazine)
      (2) Trimethobenzamide (Tigan)
      (3) Metoclopramide (Reglan)—also acts by increasing motility of the GI tract and to empty the stomach and increasing tone of the esophageal-gastric sphincter
   c. Nursing considerations
      (1) Warn clients that they may feel sleepy and to not drive or use machinery for six to eight hours after taking medication

        (2) Instruct clients to not use alcohol while taking these drugs since alcohol enhances the drowsiness effect

5. Inhibitor of gastric acid secretion (Histamine$_2$ Receptor Antagonists-Proton Pump Inhibitors)—inhibits release of hydrochloric acid by occupying the histamine receptor in the gastric mucosa
   a. Expected effect—decreased gastric acid secretion
   b. Commonly given drugs
      (1) Cimetadine (Tagamet)
      (2) Ranitidine (Zantac)
      (3) Famotidine (Pepcid)
      (4) Omeprazole (Prilosec)—proton pump inhibitor
   c. Nursing considerations
      (1) May cause dizziness, headache
      (2) Warn client medications may cause constipation
      (3) Commonly clients take these medications 30 minutes before or just prior to meals and at bedtime
6. Laxatives—used to treat or prevent constipation or to prepare the bowel for examinations
   a. Expected effects—bowel evacuation and bowel normalization
   b. Commonly given drugs
      (1) Bulk forming agents
         (a) Psyllium (Metamucil)
         (b) Methylcellulose (Citrucel)
         (c) Bran
      (2) Emollients—adds additional fluid and fat to stool thus softening the stool
         (a) Docusate sodium (Colace)
         (b) Docusate calcium (Surfak)
      (3) Irritants—increases peristalsis
         (a) Cascara (Cas-Evac)
         (b) Senna (Senokot)
         (c) Bisacodyl (Dulcolax)
      (4) Lubricants—lubricates the intestines—mineral oil
      (5) Saline osmotics—increases water in the stool, distends bowel, and increases peristalsis
         (a) Milk of Magnesia
         (b) Magnesium sulfate
         (c) Magnesium citrate—commonly used as a prep before lower GI x-rays

      (d) Lactulose (Cephulac)—commonly used in liver disease when serum ammonia levels are elevated

  c. Nursing considerations

      (1) Assess abdomen for bowel sounds, distension, and tenderness before administration; evaluate for intestinal obstruction

      (2) Encourage client to increase fluid intake, roughage, and bulk in diet to normalize bowel elimination

      (3) Educate client about the impact of adequate exercise, fluid, and dietary fiber

7. Anticholinergics—inhibits the action of acetylcholine

  a. Expected effects—decreases GI secretions, decreases colon spasms

  b. Commonly given drugs

      (1) Propantheline (Pro-Banthine)

      (2) Dicylcomine (Bentyl)

  c. Nursing interventions

      (1) Warn client that drugs may cause drowsiness and blurred vision; caution against driving or using machinery until effects have subsided

      (2) Encourage client to increase fluid, bulk, and roughage in diet to counteract constipating effect of drug

8. Mucosal healing agents—adhere to ulcer to protect from acid; stimulates release of prostaglandins which increase protection of mucosal layer; absorbs pepsin

  a. Expected effect—protects inflammed mucosa from acid

  b. Commonly given drug—sulcralfate (Carafate)

  c. Nursing interventions

      (1) Educate client to take on an empty stomach, usually 45 to 60 minutes before eating

      (2) Inform client to avoid antacids within 30 minutes of taking drug

      (3) Inform client that medication works best if dissolved in a small amount of liquid and is then taken rather than swallowing the pill whole

B. **Procedures**

  1. Abdominal x-ray—shows intestinal gas, fluid, masses, and size and position of organs

  2. Ultrasonography—sound waves used to produce images of abdominal contents, usually used for gallbladder visualization

    3. CT scan—x-ray images taken at several angles, then synthesized by a computer to produce an accurate picture of the structure that is assessed; contrast material may be used orally, rectally, or intravenously

    4. MRI scan—uses magnetic field to produce images of areas assessed

    5. Endoscopy—direct visualization of an area of gastrointestinal tract with a fiberoptic scope; prefix denotes area being visualized

       a. Esophagogastroduodenoscopy (EGD)—esophagus, stomach, and duodenum

       b. Proctosigmoidoscopy—rectum and sigmoid colon

       c. Colonoscopy—entire length of colon

       d. Endoscopic retrograde cholangiopancreatography (ERCP)—esophagus, stomach, and duodenum visualized; dye injected into pancreatic and bile ducts and x-rays taken

    6. Barium swallow—client swallows thickened barium, assumes several positions on x-ray table; serial x-rays taken

    7. Barium enema—barium introduced into large intestines through an enema; client placed in several positions and x-rays taken

       a. Water soluble contrast studies (Gastrografin) used the same way as barium, but is safer in the client who may be suffering from a perforation

    8. Oral cholecystography—oral ingestion of a radiopaque dye is administered to client and then x-rays are taken of the gallbladder

    9. Stool analysis—used to identify abnormal constituents such as blood, pathogens, or fats

    10. Schilling test—evaluates small bowel absorption of vitamin B_{12} and possible lack of intrinsic factor

C. Psychosocial

    1. Anxiety—an uncomfortable feeling associated with an unknown direct cause; common in this client as a result of sometimes vague symptoms with unknown causes

    2. Social isolation—common in the client with a chronic illness of the GI tract as a result of the sometimes unpredictable nature of the symptoms and the inability to tolerate many foods

3. Fear—an uncomfortable feeling associated with a known cause; in these clients the causes range from abdominal pain to nausea and rectal bleeding
4. Lifestyle changes—apparent especially in the client who must learn to cope with an ostomy
5. Body-image disturbances—may be seen in the client who must learn to cope with an ostomy
6. Substance use—ingestion of alcohol may be more common in clients with GI dysfunction and may result in lifestyle or work problems

D. **Health history—question sequence**
1. What is your height and weight?
2. What specifically about your eating, stomach, or bowels has been bothering you lately?
3. Do you have any pain or sores in your mouth? Do you have any difficulty chewing?
4. When did the problem **first** occur?
5. How often do you have this problem? Does it occur in relation to eating, activity, or having a bowel movement?
6. If the problem is pain, can you point to the pain?
7. Can you describe the pain? Is it sharp, burning, or dull? When does it occur in relation to your daily activities such as work, rest, or meals?
8. On a scale of 0 to 10 where would you rate your pain?
9. Is there anything you do or eat that makes the pain worse or better?
10. What relieves the pain?
11. Do you notice any other symptoms when you are having your discomfort?
12. Are you following a special diet?
13. Are you being treated by a physician for any other medical problems?
14. Are you presently taking any medications that the physician has prescribed?
15. Are you presently taking any medications that you buy without a prescription?
16. Have you ever had surgery of the GI tract?
17. Do you have any allergies to foods or medications?

E. **Physical exam—appropriate sequence**
1. Airway, breathing, circulation—vital signs
2. Height and weight
3. Inspection of oral cavity

4. Inspection of abdomen
5. Auscultation of abdomen—bowel sounds in all four abdominal quadrants; normal frequency of 5 to 35 sounds per minute in an irregular manner
6. To determine absence of bowel sounds—listen at least five minutes in each quadrant
7. Auscultate for bruits—none should be heard
8. Abdominal percussion—each quadrant
9. Abdominal palpation—each quadrant

IV. Pathophysiologic disorders

A. Oral candidiasis (thrush)
   1. Definition—overgrowth of the normal oral flora with *candida albicans*, a fungus
   2. Pathophysiology—disruption of the normal balance of oral flora allows the *candida albicans* to become overgrown
   3. Etiology—immunosuppression or extended use of antibiotics
   4. Incidence—common in the client who is immunosuppressed, has diabetes, or is on extended use of antibiotics
   5. Assessment
      a. Ask the following questions
         (1) Do you have any pain in your mouth?
         (2) Have you noticed any bleeding in your mouth?
         (3) Are you presently taking an antibiotic?
         (4) Do you have any strange sensations in your mouth?
      b. Clinical manifestations
         (1) Patchy white areas on tongue and oral mucous membranes, resembling milk curds
         (2) Patches adhere to mucous membranes; not easily removed
   6. Expected medical intervention—oral Nystatin; swish medication in mouth then swallow
   7. Nursing diagnosis—pain related to impaired oral mucous membranes
   8. Client goal
      a. Client will state mouth pain has decreased or been relieved
   9. Nursing interventions
      a. Acute care
         (1) Analgesics as needed for pain relief
         (2) Warm saline mouth washes with small amounts of hydrogen peroxide
         (3) Decrease diet to liquids or pureed foods

      b. Home care regarding client education
- (1) Dental hygiene to be followed at home
- (2) How to continue medication at home; correct administration
- (3) How to identify a new onset of infection

10. Evaluation protocol
    a. How do I know that the interventions were effective?
- (1) Is client's mouth pain relieved or improved?
- (2) Is client tolerating meals without excess pain?

    b. What criteria will I use to change my interventions?
- (1) Increased or nonrelieved mouth pain
- (2) Inability of client to tolerate food that is served

    c. How will I know that client teaching has been effective?
- (1) Client demonstrates correct oral hygiene technique
- (2) Client demonstrates correct technique for medication administration
- (3) Client identifies changes in oral mucosa to be brought to physician's attention

11. Older adult alert
    a. This is a common problem in older adults due to normal changes in the oral flora
    b. The use of dentures may aggravate any alteration in gum integrity

B. Gastroesophageal reflux disease (GERD)
1. Definition—regurgitation of stomach contents into lower esophagus
2. Pathophysiology—lower esophageal sphincter does not close appropriately in between swallowing; reflux of gastric contents very often leads to esophagitis; eventually the basal epithelial layer of the esophagus will thicken and lead to esophageal strictures
3. Etiology—alcohol, anticholinergic drugs, caffeine, increased estrogen levels
4. Assessment
    a. Ask the following questions
- (1) Do you ever feel a burning behind your breastbone?
- (2) When do you experience this burning?
- (3) Do certain foods aggravate this burning?
- (4) Do you ever notice a pain behind your breastbone?
- (5) How long does it last?
- (6) Does anything relieve this pain?

    b. Clinical manifestations
- (1) Heartburn—mid-sternal area
- (2) Heartburn or pain radiation into the back, neck, jaw, or both arms
- (3) Discomfort changes to an aching feeling
- (4) Usually relieved within three to five minutes
- (5) Relieved with liquid antacids

    c. Abnormal diagnostic tests
- (1) Barium swallow—shows evidence of reflux; changes in esophageal wall
- (2) Continuous ambulatory 24-hour esophageal pH monitoring—identifies acid reflux into esophagus and the amount refluxing
- (3) Esophagoscopy—presence of hiatal hernia, esophagitis

5. Expected medical interventions
- a. Antacids to neutralize stomach acid
- b. H_2 histamine receptor antagonists to decrease acid production
- c. Metoclopramide (Reglan) to increase lower esophogeal sphincter tone and decrease reflux

6. Nursing diagnoses
- a. Pain related to reflux of stomach contents into esophagus
- b. Diarrhea or constipation related to administration of antacids

7. Client goals
- a. Client will state pain had decreased or subsided
- b. Client will state diarrhea or constipation is controlled with a return to normal bowel habits

8. Nursing interventions—client education
- a. Diet modifications—restrict foods that are spicy, acidic, fatty, contain caffeine, or cause an increase in symptoms
- b. Eat slowly—chew each mouthful 20 to 30 times before swallowing
- c. Medication administration regime
- d. Small meals are encouraged every two hours
- e. Prevent stomach distention when eating—do not overeat, avoid swallowing air
- f. Sit in an erect position after meals for at least two hours
- g. Avoid wearing tight clothing around the abdomen

9. Evaluation protocol
- a. How will I know that client teaching has been effective?
  - (1) Client produces a food diary which indicates that appropriate foods were eaten

      (2) Client identifies specific foods or drinks that aggravate the symptoms

      (3) Client reports fewer episodes of heartburn or pain

      (4) Client reports a change in wardrobe to decrease tight-fitting abdominal clothing

      (5) Client reports appropriate medication administration

10. Older adult alert—older clients will have aggressive medical treatment for the prevention of surgery and the complications of impaction or perforation which occur more commonly in this population

C. **Hiatal hernia**

  1. Definition—protrusion of a portion of the stomach up into the thoracic cavity through an enlarged opening of the diaphragm near the lower esophagus

  2. Pathophysiology—muscle support is decreased around opening in diaphragm for the esophageal protrusion, and the stomach is permitted to move up through this weakness and into the thoracic cavity. Two types

    a. Type I—sliding hiatal hernia: a portion of the upper stomach and the gastroesophageal junction are displaced upward into the thorax

    b. Type II—rolling hiatal hernia: a portion, or all of the stomach is displaced upward into the thorax

  3. Etiology—aging, congenital muscle weakness, trauma or surgery at the level of the esophageal opening in the diaphragm

  4. Incidence—more common in the female population and the incidence increases with age

  5. The remainder of the information about hiatal hernia would be identical to the client with gastroesophageal reflux (refer to pp. 215-217)

D. **Peptic ulcer disease**

  1. Definition—a term used to depict the disorders known as gastric ulcer and duodenal ulcer

    a. Gastric ulcer—a break in the mucosa of the stomach

    b. Duodenal ulcer—a break in the mucosa of the duodenum

  2. Pathophysiology

    a. Gastric

      (1) Most found in distal half of stomach or in area of lower curvature

      (2) Failure of defense mechanisms of mucosa from gastric acid

(a) Inhibition of prostaglandin production such as caused by nonsteroidal antiinflammatory drugs (NSAIDs)

(b) Prostaglandins thought to be responsible for mediating a protection mechanism

  b. Duodenal

    (1) Increased parietal cell mass causes increased acid release

    (2) Increased gastrin that stimulates histamine, a powerful secretory mechanism for acid

    (3) Increased emptying time of the stomach increases acid load in the duodenum and lowers duodenal pH leading to not enough buffer in the duodenum to protect it

3. Etiology

  a. Gastric—nonsteroidal antiinflammatory drugs, alcohol, cigarette smoking all inhibit prostaglandin production and thus alter mucosal defense

  b. Duodenal—hypersecretion of hydrochloric acid, secondary to increased gastrin release and a decrease in duodenal pH, which allows pepsin to become more active and damage the mucosa

4. Assessment

  a. Ask the following questions (Table 7-1)

    (1) Where is your pain? Point to it.

    (2) Do you have your pain before or after you ingest food?

Table 7-1. Assessment of Peptic Ulcer Disease

Assessment Concerns	Gastric	Duodenal
Type of pain	Aching, burning, gnawing	Same
Placement of pain	Epigastric, slightly left	Epigastric, slightly right
Cause of pain	Food may cause pain	Empty stomach may cause pain
What relieves pain	Vomiting may help	Food or antacids
Eating effects	Anorexia, and weight loss	Normal appetite
Belching	Occurs	More common
Vomiting	Occurs	Uncommon

    (3) Is there anything you can take to relieve the pain?

    (4) Have you lost your appetite?

b. Clinical manifestations—(Table 7-2)

c. Complications

    (1) Bleeding

        (a) Gastric—manifested as hematemasis: vomiting blood

        (b) Duodenal—seen as melena or tarry stools

    (2) Perforation—penetration of ulcer through wall; severe abdominal pain, a board-like abdomen, emesis, fever most common findings

    (3) Gastric outlet obstruction—more common in ulcer in pyloric region; ulceration and healing repeatedly cause scar tissue which obstructs outlet

Table 7-2. Symptoms of Gastric Ulcers and Duodenal Ulcers

Symptom	Gastric Ulcers (%)	Duodenal Ulcers (%)
Anorexia	46-57	25-36
Belching*	48	59
Bloating*	55	49
Fatty food intolerance	–	14-72
Heartburn	19	27-59
Nausea	54-70	49-59
Pain		
Epigastric*	67	61-86
Radiation to back*	34	20-31
Frequently severe	68	53
Gnawing*	13	16
Episodic	16	56
At night	32-43	50-88
Increased by food	24	10-40
Food relief	2-48	20-63
Not related to food*	22-53	21-49
Relief with antacids*	36-87	39-86
Vomiting	38-73	25-57
Weight loss	24-61	19-45

Modified from Soll AH, Isenberg JI: Duodenal ulcer disease. In Sleisenger MH, Fordtran JS, editors: *Gastrointestinal diseases,* ed 3, Philadelphia, 1983, WB Saunders.

*Symptoms are similar for both types of ulcers.

    d. Abnormal diagnostic tests
       (1) Esophagogastroduodensocopy—visualization of ulcer
       (2) Barium swallow—identification of ulcer on x-ray
5. Expected medical interventions
    a. Antacids—neutralize acids; one hour after meals and at bedtime; up to seven doses daily if frequent meals eaten
    b. H_2 histamine receptor antagonist
    c. Mucosal healing agents—adhere to ulcer to protect from acid; stimulates release of prostaglandins which increase protection of mucosal layer
    d. Diet—remove from diet those foods that cause discomfort; frequent small feedings; milk stimulates gastric acid production
    e. Surgery
       (1) Billroth I and Billroth II (Figure 7-1)
       (2) Vagotomy and pyloroplasty—severing parasympathetic stimulation and opening of pylorus to compensate for resultant decrease in gastric emptying (Figures 7-2 and 7-3)
6. Nursing diagnoses
    a. Pain related to action of gastric acid against a gastric or duodenal ulcer
    b. Anxiety related to unknown cause of pain or unknown outcome or chronicity of illness
    c. Alteration in nutrition related to anorexia and nausea as evidenced by weight loss
7. Client goals
    a. Client will state pain has decreased or been relieved
    b. Client will state anxiety has decreased
    c. Client will demonstrate a weight within two pounds of baseline
8. Nursing interventions
    a. Acute care
       (1) Client with gastrointestinal bleeding
          (a) Monitor vital signs every 15 minutes to one hour until within 10% of baseline and stable
          (b) Evaluate for postural hypotension and sustained sinus tachycardia
          (c) Prepare for blood or blood product administration
          (d) Maintain a large bore IV—16 or 18 gauge needle
          (e) Monitor I&O

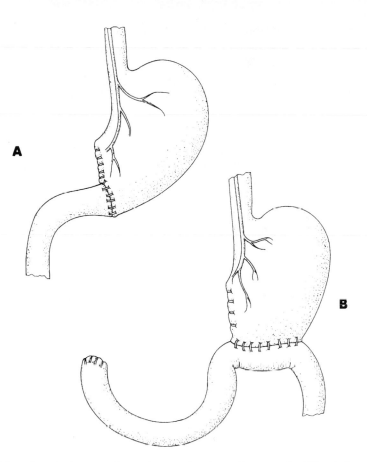

Figure 7-1. Surgical procedures in peptic ulcer disease. **A,** Billroth I procedure (gastroduodenostomy). **B,** Billroth II procedure (gastrojejunostomy). A vagotomy (severing of the vagus nerve) may be done to decrease acid production. (From Beare PG and Myers JL: *Principles and practice of adult health nursing,* ed 2, St Louis, 1994, Mosby.)

    (f)   Monitor urine output—every one to two hours

    (g)   Insertion of NG tube—gastric lavage usually if active bleeding

        (i)   Use tap water—best at room temperature

        (ii)   Lavage no longer than 30 minutes

       (iii)   Measure amount inserted and amount returned for accurate I&O, especially if not equal; i.e., 1200 ml returned in eight hours – 1000 ml inserted by lavage = 200 ml of actual gastric output

       (iv)   Allow instilled water to be removed by gravity

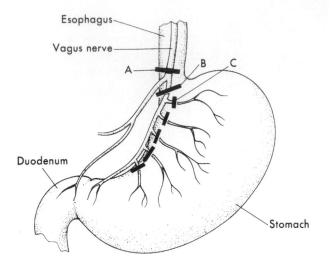

Figure 7-2. Vagotomy procedures. **A,** Truncal. **B,** Sective. **C,** Parietal cell vagotomy. (From Beare PG and Myers JL: *Principles and practice of adult health nursing*, ed 2, St Louis, 1994, Mosby.)

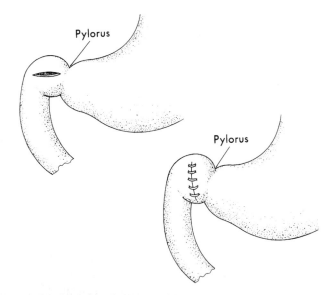

Figure 7-3. Pyloroplasty (Heinke-Mikulicz procedure). The pyloric outlet is widened and a vagotomy done to allow emptying of gastric contents. (From Beare PG and Myers JL: *Principles and practice of adult health nursing*, ed 2, St Louis, 1994, Mosby.)

    (2) Client who has undergone gastric surgery

        (a) Normal postoperative regime as described in Chapter 10, p. 315

        (b) Flush NG tube ONLY as per physician order—commonly every four hours with 30 ml of sterile normal saline

        (c) DO NOT REPOSITION NG TUBE—sits near anastomosis and repositioning may push through suture line

        (d) Evaluate NG drainage—should change from bright red to coffee brown to bile to a greenish characteristic over 24 to 48 hours

  b. Home care regarding client education

    (1) Dumping syndrome

        (a) Follows gastric surgeries

        (b) Caused by rapid gastric emptying

        (c) Food in duodenum and jejunum is hypertonic—pulls extravascular fluid toward it, further distending duodenum or jejunum; a diet high in carbohydrates aggravates the condition

        (d) Client feels nauseated, epigastric pain, vomiting, diarrhea, dizziness, tachycardia, orthostatic hypotension within 30 to 45 minutes after eating

        (e) Several hours after meal client experiences hypoglycemia due to increased insulin released in response to rapid gastric emptying

        (f) Prevention

            (i) Six small meals per day

           (ii) Low carbohydrates, high protein and fat diet

          (iii) Eat slow, chew each bite at least 20 to 30 times

          (iv) Do not drink fluid with meals—increases gastric emptying

           (v) Lay on left side for 30 minutes to one hour after meals to decrease emptying time

    (2) Specific medication regime

        (a) Sulcralfate (Carafate)—take on an empty stomach one hour before meals and bedtime

        (b) Do not take Carafate with antacids which inactivate Carafate, or 30 minutes before or after Carafate

9. Evaluation protocol
   a. How do I know that my interventions were effective?
      (1) Vital signs are stable ± 10% of baseline
      (2) Urine output is acceptable, at least 30 ml/hr
      (3) Gastric lavage has been effective, bloody drainage has decreased
      (4) Postoperative client's NG drainage returns to greenish drainage within 48 hours
      (5) No bleeding episodes
   b. What criteria will I use to change my interventions?
      (1) Vital signs not ± 10% of baseline
      (2) Urine output <30 ml/hr
      (3) Postoperative client experiences postoperative bloody drainage longer than 24 hours
   c. How will I know that my client teaching has been effective?
      (1) Client reports no episodes of dumping syndrome
      (2) Client reports medication administration is appropriate and effective
10. Older adult alert
   a. Many drugs prescribed for older adults can predispose them to peptic ulcers, such as the NSAID
   b. Older clients may not have early manifestations of peptic ulcer disease, and may present only when life-threatening manifestations occur such as GI hemorrhage

E. Cholecystitis/cholelithiasis
1. Definition—inflammation of the gallbladder; presence of calculi in the gallbladder
2. Pathophysiology—stone blocks bile drainage from gallbladder; gallbladder becomes inflamed and bile, being an irritant, causes inflammatory changes in wall of gallbladder
3. Etiology—majority of cholecystitis is caused by gallstones; two types
   a. Cholesterol stones—occur when bile becomes supersaturated with cholesterol
   b. Pigment stones—unknown origin
4. Incidence—more common in females; increased incidence after menopause; more common in pregnant women or within a few months after delivery; female sex hormones may play a role in the formation of gallstones
5. Assessment
   a. Ask the following questions
      (1) Are you experiencing pain? Point to your pain.

        (2) Does your pain coincide with food intake? If yes, any specific types of food?

        (3) Have you been running a fever?

        (4) Have you experienced any nausea, vomiting, or diarrhea?

    b. Clinical manifestations

        (1) Right upper quadrant pain—may radiate to right scapular area or shoulder

        (2) Pain follows ingestion of a high fat meal

        (3) Pain may be accompanied by anorexia, nausea, vomiting, and flatulence

        (4) If there is a stone lodged in the common bile duct, there may be mild jaundice, clay-colored stools, and tea-colored urine

    c. Abnormal laboratory findings

        (1) CBC—elevated WBC count

        (2) Serum bilirubin—may be elevated if obstruction of common bile duct

    d. Abnormal diagnostic tests

        (1) Ultrasound of gallbladder—identifies gallstones, thickened wall of gallbladder

        (2) Oral cholecystogram—identifies gallstones

        (3) Intravenous cholangiogram—identifies stones in the bile ducts

6. Expected medical interventions

    a. Fat reduction in the diet

    b. Dissolution of gallstones with medication—chenodeoxycholic acid (CDCA)

    c. Lithotripsy—done as outpatient

    d. Cholecystectomy—if stones removed from common bile duct or if common bile duct explored, T-tube must be placed (Figure 7-4); hospitalization usually required for three to five days

    e. Laparoscopic cholecystectomy—either done as outpatient or if in-hospital, stay is 24 to 48 hours

7. Nursing diagnoses

    a. Pain related to inflammation of the gallbladder or related to effects of surgery

    b. Ineffective breathing pattern related to pain associated with cholecystectomy incision

    c. Risk for fluid volume deficit related to nausea and vomiting

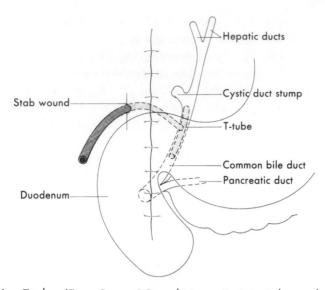

Figure 7-4. T-tube. (From Beare PG and Myers JL: *Principles and practice of adult health nursing,* ed 2, St Louis, 1994, Mosby.)

8. Client goals
   a. Client will state pain has decreased or been relieved
   b. Client will take 10 deep breaths every one to two hours and have clear breath sounds
   c. Client will have appropriate fluid volume as evidenced by I&O within ± 300 ml
9. Nursing interventions
   a. Acute care
      (1) Acute cholecystitis
         (a) Frequent vital signs as indicated by status
         (b) Give analgesics for pain
         (c) Maintain NPO status
         (d) Maintain NG patency if present
         (e) Maintain IV line and administer fluids as ordered to replace lost fluids
         (f) Do preoperative teaching if surgery is planned
         (g) Monitor I&O
      (2) Postoperative cholecystectomy client—open cholecystectomy
         (a) Same interventions as listed above
         (b) T-tube care if present
            (i) Prevent kinking
            (ii) Keep bile drainage bag below level of abdomen

           (iii) Change dressing as needed—bile, having a very high pH, is irritating to skin

           (iv) Never irrigate tube

           (v) Do not allow traction on tube

           (vi) Measure drainage every shift

           (vii) Clamp tube when ordered during meals to determine patency of common bile duct; if client has nausea or vomiting unclamp tube—some edema is probably still present

      (c) Jackson-Pratt drainage tube—empty when half full or every shift; measure drainage; recharge after emptying

      (d) Atelectasis is a common problem postoperatively due to close proximity of incision to rib cage; client must turn, cough, and deep breathe every two hours; best achieved with adequate pain relief and use of incentive spirometer

      (e) Demerol is the drug of choice; morphine can cause spasm of the sphincter of the common bile duct and result in increased pain

  b. Home care regarding client education

    (1) Postoperative diet—clients have no dietary restrictions after discharge unless something they eat bothers them

    (2) Instructions about how to care for incision if traditional surgery, and puncture wounds if laparoscopic surgery

    (3) What findings, indicative of wound infection, should be called to the physician

10. Evaluation protocol

  a. How do I know that my interventions were effective?

    (1) Vital signs are ± 10% of baseline

    (2) Client states pain is relieved

    (3) NG is patent with minimal drainage

    (4) I&O is balanced; within ± 300 ml

    (5) T-tube is patent and draining approximately 200 ml/day of yellow-brown drainage

    (6) Skin around T-tube is intact, without breakdown

    (7) Client is turning, coughing, using incentive spirometer, and deep breathing every two hours; lung sounds are clear

      b.   What criteria will I use to change my interventions?
- (1) Vital signs not ± 10% of baseline
- (2) Client states pain is unrelieved
- (3) NG drainage has decreased or stopped
- (4) I&O is not within ± 300 ml
- (5) Skin around T-tube is red and edematous
- (6) No drainage from T-tube or drainage is other than yellowish-brown
- (7) Basilar breath sounds are diminished

      c.   How will I know that my client teaching has been effective?
- (1) Client states they are following a regular diet without gastric upset
- (2) Client states the changes in their wound that should be called to physician
- (3) Client demonstrates a wound that is clean and dry without evidence of infection

11. Older adult alert
- a. Gallbladder disease incidence increases with age and should be suspected with new onset of right upper quadrant pain
- b. Cancer of the gallbladder is a disorder of older adults. Clients must be carefully evaluated.

F. Pancreatitis
1. Definition—inflammation of the pancreas
- a. Acute—sudden onset
- b. Chronic—long-term process with a continuous course of symptoms

2. Pathophysiology
- a. Inflammation of the pancreas causes the pancreatic ducts to close off
- b. Eating stimulates the pancreas to release enzymes
- c. Enzymes become trapped in the pancreatic duct and the duct eventually ruptures
- d. Rupture of duct causes release of pancreatic enzymes into pancreas
- e. Enzymes begin to autodigest the pancreas; hemorrhage can result
- f. Necrosis of the pancreas can occur
- g. Walls are formed around this cystic fluid and debris and form pseudocysts; may lead to abscess formation

3. Etiology—biliary disease, alcohol abuse, trauma, obstruction of the pancreatic duct or duodenum

4. Assessment
   a. Ask the following questions
      (1) Are you having pain? Point to where your pain is located.
      (2) On a scale of 0 to 10 where would you rate your pain?
      (3) Have you had any nausea or vomiting?
      (4) Have you noticed that your abdomen is swollen?
      (5) Have you been running a fever?
   b. Clinical manifestations
      (1) Epigastric pain—may be severe
      (2) Hypotension, sinus tachycardia
      (3) Irretractable vomiting
      (4) Abdominal distention
      (5) Low grade fever
      (6) Steatorrhea—fatty stools; more with chronic type
   c. Abnormal laboratory findings
      (1) Serum amylase elevated
      (2) Serum lipase elevated
      (3) Calcium—low
      (4) CBC—elevated WBC
      (5) Serum glucose elevated if endocrine function affected
   d. Abnormal diagnostic tests
      (1) Abdominal ultrasound—pancreatic edema, pancreatic fluid collection
      (2) CT scan—pancreatic edema, necrosis, fluid collections, abscesses, and pseudocysts
5. Expected medical interventions
   a. Stabilization of vital signs by use of monitoring lines, with instillation of fluids commonly at high rates of 150 to 250 cc/hr and blood or blood products such as plasmanate
   b. Pain relief—Demerol drug of choice; morphine causes spasm of sphincter of Oddi
   c. Insulin for hyperglycemia
   d. Sodium bicarbonate for metabolic acidosis of pH <7.10
   e. NPO, NG tube to decrease stimulation of pancreatic enzyme release
   f. Hyperalimentation if NPO maintained for long periods
   g. Surgery for ruptured pseudocysts or hemorrhage
   h. Antibiotics are not used to treat the pancreatic inflammation; antibiotics are usually for secondary infections

6. Nursing diagnoses
   a. Pain related to inflammatory process of the pancreas
   b. Fluid volume deficit related to blood loss and fluid shifts
   c. Decreased cardiac output related to blood loss and fluid shifts
   d. Altered nutrition—less than body requirements related to nausea, vomiting
7. Client goals
   a. Client will state pain is relieved or decreased
   b. Client will maintain vital signs within ± 10% of baseline and appropriate I&O
   c. Client will demonstrate appropriate cardiac output as evidenced by BP and HR within ± 10% of normal baseline
   d. Client will maintain weight within 10% of baseline
8. Nursing interventions
   a. Acute care
      (1) Vital signs at least every two hours until ± 10% of normal or more often if not within set parameters
      (2) Pain medication as needed
      (3) Maintain IV access and monitor intravenous fluid administration
      (4) Monitor electrolyte balance and acid base balance
      (5) Maintain NPO status, maintain NG tube patency and evaluate drainage; test pH and administer antacids as per physician orders
      (6) Maintain total parenteral nutrition (TPN) as ordered (Table 7-3)
      (7) Monitor drainage tubes or sump tubes if in place; evaluate drainage and sites
   b. Home care regarding client education
      (1) Diet—low fat, high calorie, high carbohydrate
      (2) Restrictions—no alcohol, no caffeine
      (3) Alcohol rehabilitation if alcohol consumption is the source of pancreatitis
      (4) Pancreatic enzyme administration if needed
      (5) Insulin administration if continued endocrine function is impaired
      (6) Medical follow-up
9. Evaluation protocol
   a. How do I know that my interventions were effective?
      (1) Vital signs are within set parameters
      (2) Pain is controlled

Table 7-3. Total Parenteral Nutrition (TPN)

Definition

TPN is a method for nutritionally sustaining clients who cannot or should not ingest, digest, or absorb nutrients. TPN solutions consist of an individually calculated combination of amino acids, glucose, minerals, vitamins, and trace elements. Lipid emulsions are frequently added to make the feedings complete.

Administration

TPN may be delivered through either a peripheral or central vein. Peripheral delivery necessitates excellent venous access, and glucose concentrations are limited to 10%. Solutions of 15% to 35% glucose may be administered centrally. TPN is associated with significant potential risks of infection and metabolic imbalance and necessitates careful monitoring.

Nursing Interventions

Monitor insertion site; provide site care and dressing changes according to institution policy.
Administer TPN solutions through inline filters; lipids do not require filters.
Weigh client daily and maintain records.
Assess for fluid overload.
Monitor laboratory values daily.
Avoid drawing blood or administering other fluids and medications through TPN catheter.
Monitor blood glucose levels throughout therapy; provide sliding-scale insulin coverage as needed.
Encourage active exercise as tolerated to support the production of muscle rather than fat cells.
Monitor respiratory rate; excess carbohydrates increase CO_2 production and may cause tachypnea.
Instruct client to use Valsalva maneuver and clamp tube during tubing changes to prevent air emboli.
Carefully monitor infusion times and do increase drip rate to catch up if behind.

      (3) I&O is balanced; within ± 300 ml
      (4) Amylase and calcium levels are within acceptable range
      (5) NG is patent with appropriate drainage; pH maintained with antacid administration
      (6) TPN administered without complications
   b. What criteria will I use to change my interventions?
      (1) Vital signs not within ± 10% of baseline
      (2) Client's pain is unrelieved or increased

   (3) I&O, enzyme levels, and electrolytes are out of balance

   (4) Client is experiencing complications of TPN—central line infection, hyperglycemia, fluid overload

  c. How will I know that my client teaching has been effective?

   (1) Client produces a diet diary with documentation of appropriate food intake

   (2) Client discusses alcohol rehabilitation process positively

   (3) Client demonstrates appropriate insulin administration

   (4) Client demonstrates appropriate pancreatic enzyme administration

 10. Older adult alert

  a. Older clients may not have the physical stamina to survive the life-threatening nature of pancreatitis

  b. There is a decreased production of pancreatic enzymes in older clients, which may be valuable in decreasing the occurence of complications of pancreatitis

G. Cirrhosis

 1. Definition—a disorder which results in widespread fibrosis of the liver and subsequent dysfunction

 2. Pathophysiology—cirrhosis is the outcome of liver insult

  a. The liver insult will leave the liver with scar tissue and destroyed hepatocytes which are responsible for bile formation; this function will be decreased and eventually lost

  b. Blood flow through the liver is impeded by massive scar tissue, and blood will back up into the portal vein and then eventually into the veins that empty into the portal vein (mesenteric veins, pancreatic and splenic veins) and this leads to *portal hypertension*

  c. Through the process of inflammation and injury, the liver becomes inflamed and enlarged in the early stages of insult

  d. In the later stages the liver will become hard and nodular

  e. Through these changes the liver will lose its ability to perform necessary functions, and the client will suffer the consequences of hepatic insufficiency

  f. When blood cannot enter the portal vein because of high pressure, collateral circulation develops around liver to return blood flow to the superior vena cava; collateral circulation has thin walls unable to withstand the high pressures exerted on them by the portal hypertension and they then rupture—esophageal bleeding

    g. High pressure from portal vein causes increased pressure in veins dumping blood into the portal vein; veins dilate and venous pressure pushes plasma out of the vascular space and into the extravascular space; most common manifestation—ascites

    h. Liver is no longer able to detoxify ammonia; ammonia levels rise and become toxic to the brain—hepatic encephalopathy

    i. Damaged hepatocytes are unable to produce albumin; vascular fluid is normally held in the vascular space by the osmotic pull of albumin; without albumin, vascular fluid will leave the vascular space—generalized interstitial edema, anasarca

3. Etiology—alcohol ingestion, hepatitis, chemical or drug ingestion
4. Incidence—more common in the male population
5. Assessment
    a. Ask the following questions
        (1) Have you been feeling tired lately?
        (2) Have you experienced loss of appetite or nausea and vomiting?
        (3) Have you experienced any discomfort in the right upper side of your abdomen?
        (4) Have you noticed a change in your skin coloration?
    b. Clinical manifestations
        (1) Early findings—may not seek physician's care
            (a) Fatigue
            (b) Weakness
            (c) Anorexia
            (d) Nausea, vomiting, diarrhea
            (e) Epigastric or right upper quadrant abdominal discomfort
            (f) Flatulence
        (2) Progressive findings
            (a) Jaundice
            (b) Bleeding tendencies—bruising, gum bleeding
            (c) Gastrointestinal bleeding
            (d) Frequent infections
            (e) Menstrual irregularities in females
            (f) Gynecomastia, impotence in the male
            (g) Spider angioma on the skin—an elevated red dot from which thin blood vessels radiate in a star-like effect
            (h) Ascites

            (3)   Hepatic encephalopathy

                (a)   Asterixis—flapping tremor of the hands

                (b)   Drowsiness, stupor, hepatic coma

    c.   Abnormal laboratory findings

            (1)   Alanine aminotransferase (ALT) elevated

            (2)   Aspartate aminotransferase (AST) elevated

            (3)   Lactate dehydrogenase (LDH) elevated

            (4)   Prothrombin time elevated

            (5)   Partial thromboplastin time elevated

            (6)   Bilirubin (total and direct) elevated

            (7)   Serum albumin decreased

            (8)   Sodium, potassium, chloride decreased

            (9)   Hemoglobin-hematocrit decreased

    d.   Abnormal diagnostic tests

            (1)   Paracentesis—done to confirm presence of ascites; also used for evacuation of fluid to ease breathing effort

            (2)   Abdominal ultrasound—presence of ascites

            (3)   Esophagogastroduodenoscopy (EGD)—presence of esophageal varices

            (4)   Electroencephalography (EEG)—abnormal tracing in the event of encephalopathy

6. Expected medical interventions

    a.   Elimination of cause—alcohol, drugs, chemicals

    b.   High protein, high calorie diet—decrease protein in the event of encephalopathy

    c.   Sodium, fluid restriction for ascites

    d.   LeVeen shunt for reinfusion of ascites (Figure 7-5)

    e.   For bleeding esophageal varices

            (1)   NPO, NG intubation

            (2)   Room temperature saline lavage of NG tube

            (3)   IV fluid and blood replacement

            (4)   Balloon tamponade of bleeding varices with Sengstaken-Blakemore tube (Figure 7-6)

            (5)   IV vasopressin to vasoconstrict arteries and decrease bleeding

            (6)   Endoscopic injection sclerotherapy—injection of sclerosing agent into varices to cause inflammation followed by fibrosis; controls and prevents bleeding

    f.   Portacaval shunt—to decrease portal hypertension; diversion of blood from portal vein to inferior vena cava

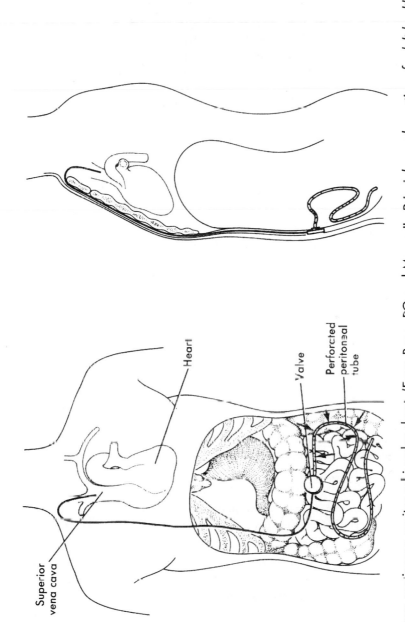

Superior
vena cava

Heart

Valve

Perforated
peritoneal
tube

Figure 7-5. LeVeen continuous peritoneal jugular shunt. (From Beare PG and Myers JL: *Principles and practice of adult health nursing*, ed 2, St Louis, 1994, Mosby.)

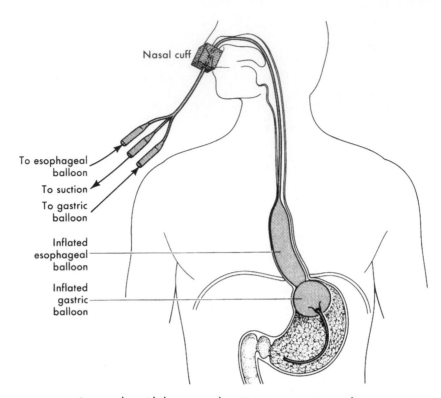

Figure 7-6. Sengstaken-Blakemore tube. (From Beare PG and Myers JL: *Principles and practice of adult health nursing*, ed 2, St Louis, 1994, Mosby.)

    g. Bowel cleansing with Lactulose and Neomycin to prevent or minimize ammonia production in the bowel and thus decrease or prevent hepatic encephalopathy

7. Nursing diagnoses
    a. Ineffective breathing pattern related to pressure on the diaphragm from enlarged liver and presence of ascites
    b. Pain related to enlarged, inflamed liver and spasms of the bile ducts
    c. Altered nutrition—less than body requirements related to nausea, anorexia, and vomiting
    d. Activity intolerance related to fatigue secondary to anemia
    e. Risk for injury (hemorrhage) related to decreased clotting factors

8. Client goals
    a. Client will maintain RR of 20 to 24 per minute without use of accessory muscles
    b. Client will state pain is decreased or improved

    c. Client will maintain baseline weight + or – 1 kg

    d. Client will increase activity by 10% each day without increase in fatigue as stated by client

    e. Client will show no evidence of bleeding or bruising

9. Nursing interventions

    a. Acute care—client regime

      (1) Rest with elimination of substances toxic to the liver such as sedatives and acetaminophen

      (2) Nutritional support for weight and energy maintenance

      (3) An increase in activity by 10% each day, i.e., walk 10 additional feet per day

      (4) Avoidance of infections and contact with others that are suffering from infection

      (5) Evaluation of all stools and urine for blood as well as any other bodily excrement

      (6) Prevention of any trauma that could cause bruising or bleeding; avoid intramuscular injections

      (7) Care of the client with bleeding esophageal varices

        (a) Vital signs every 5 to 15 minutes until within ± 10% of normal; temperature every four hours and PRN

        (b) Large bore IVs for fluid and blood administration

        (c) NG lavage with room temperature saline to clear stomach of clots and slow bleeding

        (d) Compare amount of lavage inserted to amount drained to evaluate fluid loss

      (8) Monitoring Sengstaken-Blakemore tube

        (a) Be aware of pressure in each balloon and utilize correct amount of traction if ordered

        (b) Evaluate airway frequently—displacement of tube could cause airway obstruction

        (c) Have scissors at bedside to quickly deflate balloon in the face of airway obstruction

      (9) Accurate I&O, daily weight

      (10) Abdominal girth q shift

      (11) Evaluate electrolyte balances

      (12) Monitor intake of dietary protein

    b. Home care regarding client education

      (1) Avoidance of precipitating factors; substances which could be toxic to liver or require detoxification by the liver

        (2) Diet requirements—enough protein to build tissue but not so much as to cause encephalopathy; low sodium, fluid restriction

        (3) What changes should be brought to attention of physician

10. Evaluation protocol

   a. How do I know that my interventions were effective?

      (1) Airway is patent and unobstructed

      (2) Vital signs are within ±10% of baseline

      (3) Fluid balance is adequate with I=O ±300 ml

      (4) Urine output is at least 30 ml/hr

      (5) Abdominal girth is within 1" of baseline

      (6) No evidence of trauma or bruising to skin or extremities

      (7) Urine, stool, and excrement is free of blood

      (8) No evidence of infection—WBC within acceptable parameters

      (9) Client has balanced rest and activity; OOB activity is increasing by 30 minutes per day

      (10) No substance ingested that is toxic to the liver

   b. What criteria will I use to change my interventions?

      (1) Obstructed airway

      (2) Vital signs not within ±10% of baseline

      (3) Findings indicative of infection

      (4) Findings indicative of bleeding, bruising, or trauma to the tissues

      (5) I&O out of balance

      (6) Abdominal girth increasing in size of >½" at each measurement

   c. How will I know that my client teaching has been effective?

      (1) Diet diary indicative of correct food choices

      (2) Client indicates what substances to avoid

      (3) Client is able to identify the changes in their health status that would necessitate calling the physician

11. Older adult alert

   a. Older adults have a higher occurrence of congestive heart failure and ingestion of multiple hepatotoxic drugs

   b. Concerns with clients over the age of 50 are a decrease in liver size, a decrease in storage capacity, a decreased ability to synthesize protein, and a potential decreased hepatic blood flow from a decrease in cardiac output

H. **Hepatitis**
   1. Definition—an inflammation of the liver; may be acute or chronic
   2. Pathophysiology—virus invades the liver through the portal tracts; causes inflammation of the liver
      a. Liver parenchyma cells are destroyed
      b. Destruction of hepatocytes occur
      c. Leukocytes invade liver
      d. Liver enzymes released, liver function decreased
      e. Hepatocytes are removed and replaced with scar tissue
      f. Can lead to cirrhosis or chronic hepatitis
   3. Etiology—can be caused by virus, bacteria, hepatotoxins, or drugs (Table 7-4)
   4. Incidence—over 70,000 cases per year
   5. Assessment
      a. Ask the following questions
         (1) Have you had symptoms that made you feel like you have the flu?
         (2) Have you been feeling tired and weak?
         (3) Have you been noticing a loss of appetite?
         (4) Have you noticed a change in your skin color?
         (5) Has your urine become dark in color?
         (6) Are your bowel movements a gray color?
      b. Clinical manifestations
         (1) Preicteric stage (prodromal stage)—lasts one week
            (a) Flu-like symptoms
            (b) Malaise
            (c) Weakness
            (d) Low grade fever
            (e) Cough, chills, rhinitis
            (f) Anorexia

Table 7-4. Hepatitis Etiology, Transmission, and Incubation

	Transmission	Incubation
Hepatitis A	Feces, contaminated water and food	2-6 weeks
Hepatitis B	Parenteral, sexual	4 weeks-6 months
Hepatitis C	Posttransfusion	5-10 weeks
Hepatitis D	Complication of Hepatitis B	N/A
Hepatitis E	RNA virus	2-9 weeks

        (g) Nausea, vomiting, diarrhea
        (h) Dyspepsia
        (i) Dull pain over right upper abdominal quadrant
        (j) Hepatomegaly
        (k) Lymphadenopathy
        (l) Urticaria
        (m) Weight loss
    (2) Icteric stage—lasts two to six weeks; most contagious stage
        (a) Jaundice—liver cannot metabolize bilirubin
        (b) Dark amber urine—bilirubin excreted via kidneys instead of stool
        (c) Clay-colored stools—no bilirubin in stool to induce brown color
        (d) Pruritus
        (e) Fatigue, weakness continue
        (f) Abdominal pain continues
        (g) Abnormal lab findings
    (3) Posticteric stage—lasts two to six weeks
        (a) Client remains quite fatigued
        (b) Liver size decreases as do liver enzymes
        (c) Symptoms slowly recede
  c. Abnormal laboratory findings
    (1) Direct bilirubin elevated
    (2) ALT, AST elevated
    (3) Blood glucose may be decreased
    (4) Prothrombin time may be elevated
    (5) LDH elevated
    (6) Stool positive for hepatitis A

6. Expected medical interventions
  a. Vaccination against hepatitis B in high risk clients or health care personnel
  b. Hepatitis B immune globulin for clients who have been in transmission contact with another person
  c. Immune globulin for clients traveling to areas of high levels of hepatitis A or for clients who have been exposed to hepatitis A
  d. Bedrest
  e. No substances are to be administered that are toxic to the liver such as acetaminophen or alcohol
  f. Treat findings that occur

7. Nursing diagnoses
   a. Pain related to inflammation of the liver
   b. Fatigue related to increased metabolic demands of the body
   c. Fluid volume deficit related to vomiting and diarrhea
   d. Diarrhea related to inability of liver to metabolize food appropriately
8. Client goals
   a. Client will state pain has decreased or is relieved
   b. Client will tolerate longer periods of activity without increased fatigue
   c. Client will have an I–O ±300 ml
   d. Client will have decreased episodes of diarrhea within the next 24 hours
9. Nursing interventions
   a. Acute care
      (1) Universal precautions must be maintained
      (2) Balance rest and activity to meet client needs
      (3) Turn, cough, and deep breathe, and leg exercises to prevent the complications of bedrest
      (4) Encourage the use of electric razors and soft toothbrushes to decrease risk of bleeding
      (5) Monitor nutrition—high carbohydrate, low fat diet
      (6) Antiemetic agents before meals to decrease nausea and increase nutrition
      (7) Increase fluid intake to 3000 ml/day
      (8) Avoid soap and harsh linens if client suffers from pruritus
      (9) Administer antihistamines if pruritus is severe
   b. Home care regarding client education
      (1) Not to share personal items or meal items
      (2) Sexual intercourse should be avoided during infectious period
      (3) Launder client's clothes separately
      (4) Use separate bathroom facilities, or cleanse shared bathrooms with chlorine solution daily
      (5) Abstain from alcohol for at least one year
      (6) Physicians check-ups every two to three months for at least one year
      (7) Inform health care individuals of illness for up to one year following treatment

10. Evaluation protocol
   a. How do I know that my interventions were effective?
      (1) Is client feeling more rested or less fatigued?
      (2) Is client having any difficulty breathing? Is client
          taking deep breaths every two hours? Is client
          flexing ankles at least three times an hour?
      (3) Has client noticed any blood in urine or stool, or
          blood when brushing teeth?
      (4) Is client feeling of nausea diminished?
      (5) Is client's itchy skin feeling better?
   b. What criteria will I use to change my interventions?
      (1) Fatigue is more pronounced
      (2) Client has developed atelectasis, pneumonia, or
          phlebitis
      (3) Bruising is evident or bleeding of gums
      (4) Nausea is preventing maintenance of nutrition intake
      (5) Pruritus is intractable
   c. How will I know that my client teaching has been
      effective?
      (1) Client states the use of separate bathroom and eating
          utensils and washing clothes separately
      (2) Client states the avoidance of all alcohol products
      (3) Client indicates the avoidance of sexual intercourse
          at present
      (4) Client indicates the schedule of a monthly
          appointment with the physician
      (5) Client indicates the conveyence of the illness to
          health care providers
11. Older adult alert
   a. Older adult clients will be at great risk for complications
      related to their illness and must be monitored carefully
   b. Older adults have a decreased cardiac output as well as the
      respiratory efficiency. These factors open older adults up
      to many complications during times of illness such as
      hepatitis.

I. **Inflammatory bowel disease**
   1. Definition—chronic inflammatory disorder of the small and/or
      large bowel
      a. Two disorders
         (1) Ulcerative colitis—chronic inflammatory process of
             the mucosa of the colon, usually descending, and
             rectum

(2) Crohn's disease or regional enteritis—chronic inflammatory disorder of any area of the GI tract, from mouth to anus

2. Pathophysiology—(Table 7-5)
   a. Ulcerative colitis—affects only the large bowel and only the mucosa; begins at the rectosigmoid area and moves up the descending to the transverse colon over to the right side of the colon, the ascending colon; small abscesses form in the walls of the colon and progress to purulent large ulcerations; stools will eventually be liquid and full of pus and blood from the ulcerated areas
   b. Crohn's disease—affects any area of the bowel and all layers; usually starts in the ileum and moves toward the left colon; granulomas found initially in the lymph follicles of the mucosa eventually ulcerate; lymphatics are destroyed and edema and inflammation result; fibrosis, serositis occur as well as the development of fistulas from the bowel to other areas of the bowel or adjacent structures
   c. Toxic megacolon—life-threatening complication of both disorders, though more often a complication of ulcerative colitis—destruction of circular and longitudinal muscles causes colon to dilate; walls become thin and rupture is imminent

3. Etiology—genetic, environmental, microbial, and immunological as well as psychological factors have all been implicated in these disorders

4. Incidence—more common in the 20 to 30-year-old age group; more common in the higher socioeconomic group

5. Assessment
   a. Ask the following questions
      (1) Do you ever have rectal bleeding or bloody diarrhea?
      (2) Do you ever experience abdominal cramping?
      (3) Have you been losing weight?
      (4) Do you ever feel as if you must strain to have a bowel movement? (intestinal tenesmus)
   b. Clinical manifestations—dependent on pathological findings
      (1) Ulcerative colitis—(see Table 7-5)
      (2) Crohn's disease—(see Table 7-5)
      (3) Toxic megacolon
         (a) Severe abdominal pain
         (b) Abdominal distention

Table 7-5. Comparison of Ulcerative Colitis and Crohn's Disease

	Ulcerative Colitis	Crohn's Disease
Usual area affected	Left colon, rectum	Distal ileum, right colon
Extent of involvement	Diffuse areas, contiguous	Segmental areas, noncontiguous
Inflammation	Mostly mucosal	Transmural
Mucosal appearance	Ulcerations	Cobblestone effect, granulomas
Character of stools	Blood Present No fat Frequent liquid stools	No blood present Steatorrhea Three to five semisoft stools per day
Abdominal pain	May occur, mild	Right lower quadrant pain, cramping
Abdominal mass	No	Common in right lower quadrant
Complications	Toxic megacolon Pseudopolyps Hemorrhoids Hemorrhage	Fistulas Perianal disease Strictures Abscesses Perforation
Extraintestinal manifestations	Anemia Erythema nodosum Pyoderma gangrenosa Arthritis Liver disease Iritis, conjunctivitis Stomatitis Thrombophlebitis	Anemia Malabsorption of fat and fat-soluable vitamins Arthritis Hepatobiliary disease Iritis, conjunctivitis Renal stones, obstructive uropathy
Reasons for surgery	Poor response to medical therapy Complications	Presence of complications
Response to surgery	Curative	Noncurative, high recurrence rate

From Phipps WJ, Long BC, Woods NF, Cassmeyer VL: *Medical surgical nursing concepts and clinical practice,* ed 5, St Louis, 1995, Mosby.

      (c) Fever

      (d) Leukocytosis

      (e) Tachycardia

  c. Abnormal laboratory findings

     (1) CBC—H&H may be low as well as RBCs

     (2) Stool for blood—positive during period of active bleeding

  d. Abnormal diagnostic tests

     (1) Upper GI (in Crohn's)—will show ulcerations and fistula formations, "cobblestoning of mucosa," narrowing

     (2) Barium enema—ulcerations and mucosal irregularities in both disorders

     (3) Endoscopy—inflamed mucosa, with "cobblestoning of mucosa" in Crohn's; granular appearance in ulcerative colitis

     (4) CT scan—mesenteric abnormalities, colon wall thickening

     (5) Biopsy—shows diffuse inflammation and rules out malignancy

6. Expected medical interventions

  a. IV fluids and possibly TPN during acute exacerbations

  b. Blood administration as needed

  c. Regular diet; ask client to remove those foods that exacerbate symptoms; high residue foods may cause this

  d. The four A's medication approach—Antiinflammatory, Antibacterial, Antidiarrhea, Antianxiety and immunosuppressive drugs are utilized

  e. Surgical intervention may be necessary if all medical regime has failed or if life-threatening illness has occurred

7. Nursing diagnoses

  a. Altered nutrition—less than body requirements related to increased peristalsis and poor absorption

  b. Diarrhea related to inflammatory process of the bowel

  c. Risk for fluid volume deficit related to frequent diarrhea stools

8. Client goals

  a. Client will maintain baseline weight within 1 to 2 kg

  b. Client will have decreased episodes of diarrhea by two bowel movements per day

  c. Client will demonstrate a balanced I&O within ± 300 ml

9. Nursing interventions
   a. Postoperative care
      (1) See routine postoperative care in Chapter 10, p. 315
      (2) Maintain NG suction—irrigate as per orders
      (3) Begin ostomy care—ileostomy drainage may begin almost immediately after surgery
      (4) Alkaline effluent from the ileostomy is corrosive to the skin; protect skin by using an appliance with a protective barrier such as stoma adhesive
      (5) Evaluate stoma
         (a) Immediate postop may be pale
         (b) When client warms—stoma may be red, ruddy, and be slightly edematous
         (c) Within several weeks stoma should be pink with no edema
         (d) Any change should be reported to the physician immediately
   b. Home care regarding client education
      (1) Self-care of the stoma
      (2) Changes in the stoma that must be reported to physician
         (a) Stoma colors of grey, blue, bright red
         (b) Bleeding spots on stoma
         (c) Swollen stoma
      (3) Encourage fluids but no special diet—have client remove from the diet those items that are irritating
      (4) Findings associated with fluid and electrolyte imbalance as this is a major issue with a client with an ileostomy
10. Evaluation protocol
   a. How do I know that my interventions were effective?
      (1) NG drainage decreases as bowel sounds return
      (2) Stoma remains pink and above the level of the skin
      (3) Skin surrounding the stoma remains free of breakdown
   b. What criteria will I use to change my interventions?
      (1) NG drainage continues in large amounts, >600 ml/day
      (2) Peristalsis does not return within 24 to 48 hours
      (3) Stoma color changes to a dusky pink, blue, or black
      (4) Skin ulcerates around stoma
   c. How will I know that my client teaching has been effective?

           (1) Client demonstrates all aspects of ileostomy care, including care of the appliance

           (2) Client states changes in the stoma that should be reported to the physician

           (3) Client states assessment findings associated with fluid and electrolyte imbalance that should be reported to the physician

           (4) Client indicates what foods have been removed from the diet and why

11. Older adult alert

    a. These disorders are uncommon to the older adult population

    b. If the client is an older adult and requires surgery, care of the ostomy may require more time than the younger adult would require

    c. Older clients may not be able to care for the ileostomy and care may have to be assumed by family members

J. **Diverticular disease**

  1. Definition

    a. Diverticulosis—outpouching of the wall of the colon (diverticulum)

    b. Diverticulitis—inflammation and obstruction of a diverticula

  2. Pathophysiology—fiber in the diet assists in passing feces through the colon quicker and more efficiently; due to decreased fiber content passage time is decreased, lumen pressure increases and pressure on the wall increases; impairs blood supply to the area and results in outpouching of the wall

  3. Etiology—diets low in fiber and roughage

  4. Incidence—over 30 million people are affected in the United States; largest percentage of those affected are over age 60

  5. Assessment

    a. Ask the following questions

        (1) Have you ever experienced an unusual pain in the left lower side of your abdomen?

        (2) Do you ever have alternating diarrhea and constipation?

        (3) Have you ever noticed rectal bleeding?

    b. Clinical manifestations

        (1) May be asymptomatic until diverticulitis occurs

        (2) Unusual pain in left lower quadrant of the abdomen

        (3) Alternating diarrhea and constipation

              (4) Rectal bleeding

              (5) Diverticulitis

                  (a) Crampy, left lower quadrant pain

                  (b) Abdominal distention

                  (c) Nausea, vomiting

                  (d) Low grade fever

    c. Abnormal laboratory findings

        (1) WBC—elevated

        (2) CBC—H&H may be low

    d. Abnormal diagnostic tests

        (1) Flat-plate of the abdomen—evaluates for free air under the diaphragm with perforation of bowel

        (2) Barium enema—identifies diverticular sacs with decreased lumen size

        (3) Sigmoidoscopy, colonoscopy—openings to the diverticula may be directly visualized; rule out carcinoma

6. Expected medical interventions

    a. High fiber diet, omitting seeds or kernels that can lodge in diverticula

    b. Bran therapy or Metamucil or a similar agent taken daily

    c. During acute diverticulitis—NPO, or low residue diet, IV fluid, and antibiotics

    d. Colon resection with end to end anastomosis if episodes of diverticulitis are more frequent

    e. Colon resection with diverting colostomy if bowel perforation has occurred—reanastomosis at a later date

    f. Peritonitis as a result of bowel perforation—correction of the rupture with irrigation of the peritoneum and IV antibiotic therapy

7. Nursing diagnoses

    a. Alteration in bowel elimination—constipation, diarrhea related to bowel inflammation

    b. Pain related to bowel inflammation

8. Client goals

    a. Client will state bowel movements have become soft and formed and occur once or twice a day

    b. Client will state pain is decreased or relieved

9. Nursing interventions

    a. Acute care

        (1) Diverticulitis

            (a) Maintain IV access

        (b) Maintain hydration via oral or IV fluids

        (c) Pain medication as needed by client, may take the form of antispasmodic agents

    (2) Post operative

        (a) See routine postoperative care in Chapter 10, p. 315

        (b) Maintain NG patency if present, irrigating as per orders

        (c) Evaluate stoma for color and size if present; see stoma assessment p. 246

        (d) Begin stoma care—dressings may be used initially; apply appliance when appropriate, usually within 48 hours

  b. Home care regarding client education

    (1) Diet—high fiber, Metamucil or similar agent daily

    (2) Stool softeners if needed

    (3) Assessment findings that must be called to attention of physician—abdominal distention, sudden onset of severe abdominal pain; indicative of perforation

    (4) Stoma care if stoma present

10. Evaluation protocol

  a. How do I know that my interventions were effective?

    (1) Client states pain is relieved or decreased

    (2) I&O is adequate, I=O ±300 ml; 30 ml/hr of urine output

    (3) Stoma remains pink or reddish color

    (4) Stoma output begins in two to three days

  b. What criteria will I use to change my interventions?

    (1) Pain unrelieved

    (2) I&O not balanced within ±300 ml

    (3) Stoma changes color—dusky pink, blue, black

    (4) Stoma output does not begin within three days

  c. How will I know that my client teaching has been effective?

    (1) Client produces a food diary indicative of high fiber content

    (2) Client reports taking Metamucil every day

    (3) Client states no need stool softeners

    (4) Client demonstrates care of the stoma and appliance

11. Older adult alert

  a. This is a disorder of older adults and may require frequent teaching periods regarding dietary changes. Eating habits are difficult to change.

     b. The ability to care for a stoma requires evaluation for minimal vision and manual dexterity. If the client is unable to do the care due to arthritis or vision defects, another person may have to assume the responsibility.

K. **Colorectal cancer**

   1. Definition—malignancy of the colon or the rectum

   2. Pathophysiology—tumors are graded according to cell differentiation; most favorable when cells are well differentiated; tumor spreads through the walls of the colon, through lymphatics, via the bloodstream, across the peritoneum, or via incision lines or drain; intestinal obstruction can be the result as well as wall ulceration and hemorrhage, abscess, or fistula formation

   3. Etiology—risk factors

      a. Ulcerative colitis or Crohn's disease for extended years

      b. High fat, low fiber diet

      c. Family history

      d. Polyposis—presence of polyps in the colon

   4. Incidence—second most common type of cancer; over 150,000 new cases per year in the United States; most are found in the rectum with the next most common being found in the sigmoid colon

   5. Assessment

      a. Ask the following questions

         (1) Have you noticed any rectal bleeding?

         (2) Have you had a change in your bowel movements lately?

         (3) Have you lost any weight over the last year? Were you trying to lose weight?

      b. Clinical manifestations

         (1) Rectal bleeding

         (2) Vague abdominal pain

         (3) Alternating constipation and diarrhea

         (4) Spastic pain of the colon or sphincters

         (5) Abdominal distention

         (6) Weight loss

      c. Abnormal laboratory findings

         (1) Stool for occult blood or guiac—positive

         (2) H&H—low

         (3) Carcinoembryonic antigen (CEA)—elevated indicative of intestinal tumor

    d. Abnormal diagnostic tests
       (1) Digital rectal exam—feel presence of tumor
       (2) Barium enema—depicts a constriction in colon and tumor placement
       (3) Sigmoidoscopy or colonoscopy—presence of lesion; biopsy confirms malignancy
       (4) Endorectal ultrasound—identifies involved lymph nodes

6. Expected medical interventions
    a. Surgical resection of the tumor; end to end anastomosis if possible; anterior-posterior resection if necessary with permanent colostomy
    b. Removal of involved lymph nodes
    c. Radiation therapy as an adjunct to surgery
    d. Chemotherapy if surgery not advised, or to reduce tumor before surgery

7. Nursing diagnoses
    a. Altered nutrition—less than body requirements related to anorexia
    b. Fatigue related to tumor growth and decreased nutrition
    c. Body-image disturbance related to presence of colostomy

8. Client goals
    a. Client will maintain present weight or gain ½ kg/week
    b. Client will state fatigue is reduced
    c. Client will state feeling comfortable with presence of the colostomy

9. Nursing interventions
    a. Acute care—will be identical to the client with inflammatory bowel disease and diverticular disease pp. 246, 248
    b. Home care regarding client education
       (1) Stoma care, appliance care, and where to purchase equipment
       (2) Normal diet—plenty of fluids
       (3) Colonoscopy may be repeated 6 to 12 months after surgery and then yearly
       (4) Stool for occult blood done yearly
       (5) CEA levels are drawn at regular intervals, every three to six months, for the next five years
       (6) Technique for colostomy irrigation if necessary (Figure 7-7)
          (a) Remove appliance

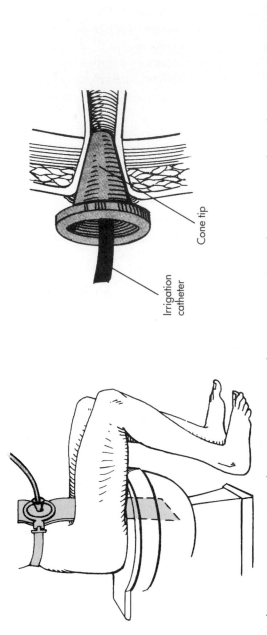

Irrigation
catheter

Cone tip

Figure 7-7. Colostomy irrigation. **A,** Colostomy irrigation with person sitting on toilet: irrigating sleeve drains into toilet. **B,** Cone irrigating tip inserted into stoma. (From AJN/Mosby Nursing board review, ed 9, St Louis, 1994, Mosby.)

          (b)   Use 1000 ml of warm water, hang bag 18 to 24″ above stoma

          (c)   Insert cone into stoma until it forms a seal to prevent irrigation fluid from coming out

          (d)   Let water run in stoma

          (e)   Remove cone and allow solution to drain

          (f)   Apply clean appliance

10. Evaluation protocol

    a. How will I know that my client teaching has been effective?

       (1) Client demonstrates effective care and irrigation of the colostomy

       (2) Client indicates the following of a regular diet without difficulty

       (3) Client exhibits an understanding of the postoperative laboratory and diagnostic regime

11. Older adult alert—these will be the same as for the client with inflammatory bowel disease and diverticular disease pp. 247, 249

REVIEW QUESTIONS

1. Clients with gastroesophageal reflux should be counseled to remove what items from their diet
   a. Pizza only
   b. Alcohol only
   c. Whatever bothers them
   d. Coffee and soda only

2. When lavaging a client's stomach tube for gastric bleeding, the nurse must calculate the correct gastric output. This is accomplished by
   a. Subtracting the output from the intake
   b. Subtracting the intake from the output
   c. Add the intake to the output
   d. Irrigate the gastric tube and remove the irrigation immediately

3. When evaluating a client's abdomen who is postoperative open cholecystectomy, the nurse notices that the continuous portable suction device is half full. It is only four hours into the shift. The best intervention at this time is to
   a. Empty the device now
   b. Wait until eight hours have passed to empty the device
   c. Wait another hour until emptying
   d. Squeeze the air out of the device but don't empty it

4. A client with pancreatitis has asked the nurse why the insulin shot is needed. The best response would be
   a. "You are producing more glucose due to your illness so we must give you extra insulin"
   b. "Your pancreas usually makes insulin, but because it is inflamed, the insulin is not made in the amounts you need"
   c. "We are giving you more glucose in your IV feeding today, so you need a little extra insulin"
   d. "You ate a little more today, so you need some extra insulin"

5. A priority assessment for clients with ascites is
   a. Abdominal girth
   b. Blood pressure
   c. Heart rate
   d. Respiratory effort

6. The nurse's understanding of the pathophysiology of cirrhosis of the liver allows the nurse to explain to the client's family why their family member is having bleeding episodes. The nurse explains that
   a. The bleeding is because of this inability to eat; it has left his body in a weakened state
   b. The liver is responsible for making substances that produce clotting of the blood. A liver that is affected by cirrhosis will not make those substances and the blood will not clot.
   c. Something in the medication we are giving him to help his liver is affecting the clotting of his blood
   d. This is a temporary problem caused by the inflammation of his liver. It will subside within a week.

7. A client with hepatitis B is complaining of severe nausea. This is interfering with his eating of meals. The best nursing intervention is to
   a. Decrease the diet to a clear liquid diet
   b. Decrease the diet to a soft diet
   c. Offer antiemetics before meals
   d. Offer antiemetics after meals

8. During the assessment of a client who has just returned from the operating room following a total colectomy and placement of an ileostomy, the nurse expects the ileostomy stoma to be what color?
   a. Pale
   b. Deep purple
   c. Red
   d. Slightly cyanotic

9. Which of the following statements by a client would alert the nurse to encourage the client to see a physician?
   a. "I have diarrhea when I drink milk"
   b. "I have a crampy right lower abdominal pain just before a bowel movement"
   c. "I keep changing back and forth between diarrhea and constipation"
   d. "I use laxatives several times a month"

10. A classic finding associated with a perforated diverticulum is
    a. Rectal bleeding
    b. Abdominal distention
    c. Severe abdominal pain
    d. Fever

ANSWERS, RATIONALES, AND TEST-TAKING TIPS

Rationales	Test-Taking Tips
1. Correct answer: c Clients can eat whatever does not cause symptoms of the reflux.	If you have no idea of the correct answer, cluster options *a, b* and *d* with the word "only." Select option *c.*
2. Correct answer: b The output should be higher than the amount instilled into the NG; i.e. 1000 ml instilled, 1300 drained out = 300 ml of gastric drainage.	The best approach to this type of question is to write a sample on the provided scratch paper. Then reread the question and each option to select option *b.*
3. Correct answer: a Drains should be emptied when half full or at the end of eight hours, whichever comes first.	Read the options carefully. Avoid allowing the destractor "now" in option *a* push you to select option *d.* THE question asks for a best action "at this time"; option *a* best answers THE question.
4. Correct answer: b An inflamed pancreas is unable to appropriately manufacture or release insulin, so it must be administered subcutaneously.	If you have no idea of the correct answer, simply match words—the client has "pancreatites"—select option *b* that has the word "pancreas" in it.
5. Correct answer: d Respiratory effort always has top priority over other assessments, especially in the client who has ascites which pushes up on the diaphragm and impedes ventilation.	Use the ABC's to guide the selection of option *d* if you have no idea of the correct answer.
6. Correct answer: b In cirrhosis the liver is no longer able to produce	If you have no idea of the correct answer, an approach is to select

clotting factors at the same pace or even at all.

the most complete statement which is option *b*.

7. Correct answer: c

Removing the nausea before a meal may allow the client to eat some of the meal.

Key words in the stem are "severe nausea." It follows that medication would be given prior to meals.

8. Correct answer: a

The stoma is initially pale, and as the client warms it becomes red. Cyanotic or purple indicates vascular compromise of the stoma.

Key words in the stem are "who just returned." The stoma color will be similar to the client's color right after surgery, pale.

9. Correct answer: c

Alternating constipation and diarrhea may be indicative of colon cancer.

The approach to this situation is to use common sense. Options *a* and *b* may be normal findings. Option *c* is considered within normal usage of laxatives. Option *c* needs further assessment.

10. Correct answer: c

Severe abdominal pain is more indicative of a ruptured diverticulum; abdominal distention could be indicative of an obstruction.

If you have no idea of the correct answer, try an approach to match the level of severity in the question and response. "Perforated" bowel can be matched with "severe abdominal pain"—both are intense findings.

The Renal System

STUDY OUTCOMES

After completing this chapter, the reader will be able to do
the following:

▼ Identify assessment findings of the client with a renal disorder.

▼ Choose the appropriate nursing diagnoses for renal disorders.

▼ Choose appropriate nursing interventions for the client with a
renal disorder.

▼ Evaluate the progress of the client with a renal disorder for
establishment of new nursing interventions based on evaluation
findings.

KEY TERMS

Azotemia	Toxic condition where there is an excess of nitrogenous waste in the blood.
Diffusion	The movement of solutes across a semipermeable membrane from an area of higher concentration to an area of lower concentration until an equal distribution is established between the two areas.
Glomerular filtration rate (GFR)	The amount of fluid that is passed through all of the nephrons in one minute.
Homeostasis	A balance or constancy in the internal functioning of the body.
Osmosis	The movement of a pure solvent such as water across a semipermeable membrane, from an area with a lower solute content to a higher solute content.
Uremia	Presence of excess urea and other waste in the blood.

CONTENT REVIEW

  I. **The renal system is responsible for excreting water soluble wastes, stimulating RBC production, and maintaining the balance of pH, plasma water, and electrolytes**

  II. **Structure and function**

    A. **Pair of organs each approximately 6 oz in weight, situated at the level of the costovertebral angle (CVA) in the retroperitoneum**

    B. **Three distinct structural areas in the kidney (Figure 8-1)**

      1. Cortex—outer layer; glomeruli, proximal and distal tubules

      2. Medulla—middle layer; 6 to 10 renal pyramids comprised of collecting ducts and tubules

      3. Pelvis—interior layer or collection area

      4. Calyces separate the pyramids of the medulla from the renal pelvis

    C. **Nephron—functional unit of the kidney; approximately 1 million per kidney (Figure 8-2)**

      1. Structure and blood flow sequence

        a. Renal corpuscle—glomerulus of renal capillaries situated in Bowman's capsule; filtration

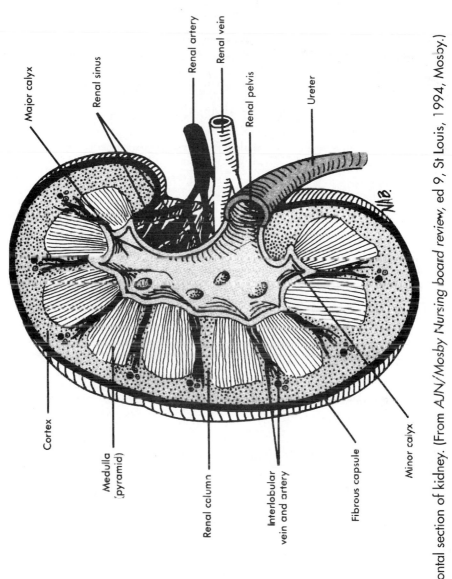

Figure 8-1. Frontal section of kidney. (From AJN/Mosby Nursing board review, ed 9, St Louis, 1994, Mosby.)

Major calyx

Renal sinus

Renal artery

Renal vein

Renal pelvis

Ureter

Cortex

Medulla (pyramid)

Renal column

Interlobular vein and artery

Fibrous capsule

Minor calyx

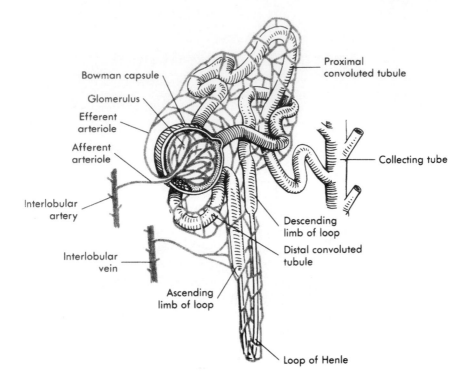

Nephron.

Part of Nephron	Function	Substance
Glomeruli	Filtration	H_2O and solute, electrolytes (Na, K, PO_4, Ca, Cl, Mg), urea, creatinine, uric acid, glucose, amino acids
Proximal tubules	Reabsorption, secretion	H_2O, electrolytes (Na, K, Mg, Ca, Cl, HCO_3), glucose, amino acids
Loop of Henle	Reabsorption	H_2O, electrolytes (Na, K)
Distal tubule	Acid-base balance, secretion	Hydrogen ions (H), Na
Collecting tubule	Concentration	H_2O

Figure 8-2. Nephron. (From *AJN/Mosby Nursing board review,* ed 9, St Louis, 1994, Mosby.)

     b. Proximal convoluted tubule—reabsorption and secretion
     c. Loop of Henle—reabsorption
     d. Distal convoluted tubule—acid-base balance and secretion
     e. Collecting ducts—concentration

D. **Functions of the kidney**
  1. Fluid and electrolyte balance
     a. Sodium—filtered by the glomeruli and reabsorbed in the tubules
     b. Chloride—follows sodium
     c. Potassium—filtered by the glomeruli and reabsorbed in the proximal tubules
     d. Water—antidiuretic hormone (ADH) concentration in the collecting duct controls reabsorption
  2. Acid-base balance
     a. Excretes organic acids
     b. Releases free hydrogen ions
     c. Conserves bicarbonate
  3. Excretion of waste products—urea and creatinine, bacterial toxins, drugs and drug metabolites
  4. Produces and secretes erythropoietin, which stimulates bone marrow to manufacture hemoglobin
  5. Production and activation of vitamin D, which is necessary for calcium metabolism
  6. Regulates arterial BP by releasing renin and activating reninangiotensin system (Figure 8-3)

III. Targeted concerns
A. Pharmacology—priority drug classifications
  1. Diuretic agents—induce the renal excretion of water, sodium, and/or potassium from the body
     a. Expected effect—reduction in circulating blood volume
     b. Commonly given drugs
        (1) Loop diuretics—act on ascending loop of Henle; Furosemide (Lasix), Bumetanide (Bumex)
        (2) Thiazide diuretics—inhibit sodium and chloride reabsorption in the distal tubule; Hydrochlorothiazide (Diuril)
        (3) Potassium-sparing diuretics—action is in the collecting tubule; Spironolactone (Aldactone)
        (4) Osmotic diuretics—pulls water from extravascular space into vascular space; Mannitol (Osmitrol)
     c. Nursing considerations
        (1) Hydration level and electrolyte balance must be monitored carefully in clients who receive diuretic drugs
        (2) Potassium supplements may be required with loop and thiazide diuretics

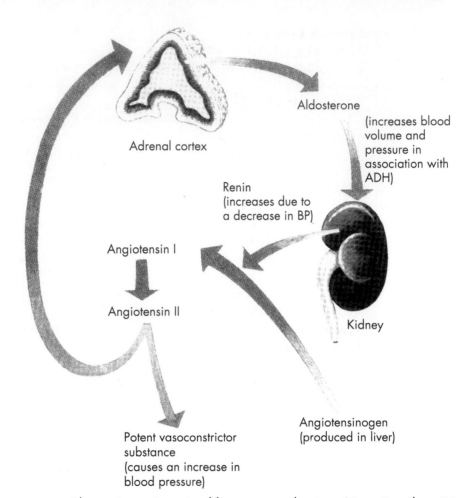

Aldosterone
(increases blood volume and pressure in association with ADH)

Adrenal cortex

Renin
(increases due to a decrease in BP)

Angiotensin I

Angiotensin II

Kidney

Potent vasoconstrictor substance
(causes an increase in blood pressure)

Angiotensinogen
(produced in liver)

Figure 8-3. The renin-angiotensin-aldosterone mechanism. (From Brundage DJ: *Renal disorders,* St Louis, 1994, Mosby.)

      (3)   With potassium-sparing diuretics, life-threatening hyperkalemia can occur if clients are not instructed that they do not require potassium supplements or high potassium foods in the diet

  2. Phosphate-binding agents—bind with phosphate in the treatment of hyperphosphatemia

    a. Expected effect—ingested phosphates bind with aluminum in the intestine, forming a complex that can be excreted in feces

    b. Commonly given drugs

      (1)   Aluminum carbonate (Basaljel)

      (2)   Aluminum hydroxide (Amphojel)

      (3)   Calcium acetate (Phos-Ex)

    c. Nursing considerations

        (1) Aluminum preparations are constipating and should be given with a stool softener

        (2) Phos-Ex should not be given in the client with high calcium levels

3. Erythrocyte-stimulating hormone—treats anemia caused by a lack of erythropoietin in chronic renal failure; promotes the production of erythrocytes

    a. Expected effect—increase in hematocrit is seen approximately two weeks after therapy has begun

    b. Commonly given drug—recombinant human erythropoietin (Epogen)

    c. Nursing considerations

        (1) May elevate BP

        (2) Do not shake the vial as it will inactivate the drug

        (3) Clinical response will not be seen for several weeks; not for immediate correction of anemia

B. **Procedures**

1. Urinalysis—identifies normal and abnormal constituents; can indicate abnormalities in the kidney function or structure; requires a clean specimen

2. Urine culture and sensitivity—identifies bacterial organisms and the antibiotics to which the organisms are sensitive; requires a sterile specimen

3. Creatinine clearance—most useful test of kidney function; 24-hour specimen

    a. Measures amount of creatinine filtered by the glomeruli

    b. A decrease in creatinine cleared indicates a drop in glomerular filtration rate

4. Kidney-ureter-bladder x-ray (KUB)—abdominal x-ray without contrast dye; standing or supine; renal structures may be seen; calculi may be visualized

5. Renal sonogram—sound waves used to project an image of the kidney and structures; calculi and renal tumors can be identified

6. Radionuclide imaging—following injection of radionuclide tracer substances, kidney can be scanned and evaluated for obstruction or insufficiency

7. Intravenous pyelogram (IVP) or excretory urogram—use of contrast dye in conjunction with radiographic x-rays allows visualization of the kidney structures and their function through sequencing x-rays

8. Nephrotomograms—x-rays taken at several angles to distinguish abnormalities in the kidneys

9. Retrograde pyelogram—catheter passed up into one or both of the ureters and contrast medium injected up into the kidney; allows for visualization of kidney structures and function when clients are not capable of concentrating or excreting urine

10. Renal arteriogram—catheter inserted into the renal artery, through the femoral artery and dye injected into the renal vasculature; used to evaluate patency of renal vascular structures

11. Renal computed tomography (CT)—computer generated plane images of kidney used to identify masses or tumors

12. Magnetic resonance imaging (MRI)—computer generated images that are created by changes in the magnetic field of the body; very useful for visualization of the kidney and abnormalities

13. Renal biopsy—needle inserted percutaneously into the kidney to obtain a sample of kidney tissue; used to evaluate hematuria, proteinuria, or nephrotic syndrome

14. Nephroscopy—endoscopic examination of the kidney; renal pelvis and calyces can be visualized; percutaneous tract established followed by the endoscope into the kidney

C. **Psychosocial**

1. Anxiety—the uncomfortable feeling associated with an unknown direct cause; renal clients may display this when symptoms begin but the cause has not yet been identified; also seen when clients are unsure of the outcome of their acute or chronic illness

2. Fear—an uncomfortable feeling associated with a real danger; the real danger may be death in many of these clients due to irreversible kidney failure

3. Social isolation—may be identified in clients who are confined due to hemodialysis or physical impairment from chronic renal impairment

4. Depression—in response to a long-standing incurable illness

5. Hopelessness—commonly seen in clients who are waiting for renal transplants

6. Dependency—may be observed in the client who is in need of renal dialysis; physical limitations may require that the client enlist aid from significant others to complete activities of daily living

D. **Health history—question sequence**
1. Please describe the problem that you have been experiencing
2. Do you have any other conditions for which you are receiving care?
3. Have you ever suffered any injury to or a problem with your kidneys?
4. Are you currently taking any prescription or nonprescription medications?
5. What is your current height and weight?
6. Has there been any change in your weight? Over what period of time?
7. Is there any history of renal disease in your family?
8. Have you experienced any pain over your sides?
9. Have you noticed any change in your pattern of urinating?
10. Have you experienced any urgency, frequency, burning?
11. Have you noticed blood or any other particles in your urine?
12. Does your urine have a strange odor or color?
13. Have you experienced any loss of appetite, nausea, vomiting, or diarrhea?
14. Have you experienced frequent urinary tract infections?

E. **Physical examination—appropriate sequence**
1. Airway, breathing, circulation—vital signs
2. Skin color, temperature, turgor, moisture
3. Inspection of upper abdomen and flank areas
4. Deep palpation of the kidneys bilaterally
5. Percussion of the kidneys posteriorly and anteriorly to outline them
6. Auscultation of the kidneys for bruits—indication of stenosis or aneurysm of the renal artery

IV. Pathophysiologic disorders

A. **Acute renal failure**
1. Definition—a sudden loss of kidney function; may be reversible
2. Pathophysiology—many theories persist as to what occurs in the kidney experiencing acute renal failure, however, there is no one accepted theory. The clinical course is
   a. Oliguric phase—client produces <400 ml/day of urine; lasts one to eight weeks; the longer it lasts the poorer the prognosis

      b.   Diuretic phase—client produces >3000 ml/day of urine; lasts several days to one week

      c.   Recovery phase—gradual return to pre-renal failure kidney function; lasts 3 to 12 months; creatine levels gradually return to normal

3. Etiology—three anatomical areas identified as location of causes

      a.   Pre-renal—poor circulating blood volume; poor cardiac output

      b.   Renal—injury or destruction to renal structures

      c.   Post-renal—obstruction of urinary tract distal to kidney

4. Assessment

      a.   Ask the following questions

          (1)   Have you noticed that you have been urinating less?

          (2)   Has your weight increased? By how much?

          (3)   Have you noticed swelling in any part of your body?

          (4)   Have you felt weak or tired?

          (5)   Have you noticed a change in the way your urine looks or smells?

      b.   Clinical manifestations

          (1)   Neurologic—altered sensorium, weakness, headache

          (2)   Respiratory—Kussmaul's respiration (deep, rapid), pneumonia

          (3)   Cardiovascular—anemia, hypertension, dysrhythmias

          (4)   Gastrointestinal—nausea, vomiting, GI bleeding

          (5)   Integumentary—generalized edema, bruising

      c.   Abnormal laboratory findings (Table 8-1)

      d.   Abnormal diagnostic tests

          (1)   EKG—dysrhythmias, T wave abnormality related to hyper- or hypokalemia

          (2)   Renal ultrasound—may indicate abnormally shaped kidney

          (3)   Renal scan—may show impaired perfusion

          (4)   Renal biopsy—indicates extent of damage to renal structures

5. Expected medical interventions

      a.   Prevention of further injury—increased fluids and osmotic diuretics to increase renal filtration

      b.   Peritoneal dialysis or hemodialysis to maintain hemostasis until renal function returns (Figure 8-4)

Table 8-1. Abnormal Laboratory Findings of Acute Renal Failure

Laboratory Tests	Oliguric Phase	Diuretic Phase	Recovery Phase
Serum sodium	Decreased	Elevated, normal, or decreased	Normal
Serum potassium	Increased	Elevated, normal, or decreased	Normal
BUN, creatinine ratio	Increased— ratio >10:1	Increased— ratio >20:1	Normal— ratio <20:1
Specific gravity	Increased	Decreased	Normal
Blood volume	Hypervolemia	Hypovolemia	Normal
Blood pressure	Hypertensive	Hypotensive	Normotensive
Serum phosphorus	High	Same	Resolving
Serum calcium	Low	Same	Resolving
Hemoglobin/ hematocrit	Anemia	Anemia	Anemia
	Hemodiluted— low	Hemoconcen- trated—high	Resolving
Serum creatinine	Elevated	Elevated	Resolving

    c. Maintenance of electrolyte balance

    d. Treatment of infections or anemia as they become apparent

 6. Nursing diagnoses

    a. Fluid volume deficit related to failed renal regulatory mechanisms (Diuretic phase)

    b. Fluid volume excess related to failed renal regulatory mechanisms (Oliguric phase)

    c. Altered nutrition—less than bodily requirements related to anorexia

    d. Potential for infection related to depressed immune response

    e. Potential for sensory-perceptual alterations related to abnormal blood chemistry

    f. Potential for impaired skin integrity related to peripheral edema

 7. Client goals

    a. Client will maintain fluid volume at appropriate levels as evidenced by CVP reading of 5 to 15 mm Hg (CVP readings may be at the higher end of normal in this client due to fluid retention that is expected until resolution of the illness)

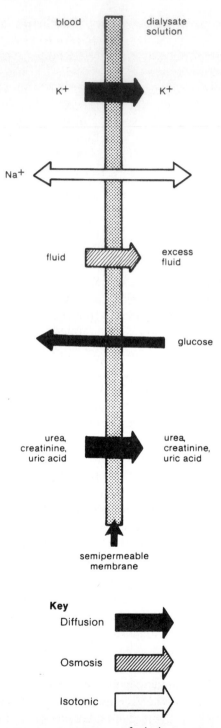

Figure 8-4. Schematic representation of dialysis. (From *AJN/Mosby Nursing board review,* ed 9, St Louis, 1994, Mosby.)

      b.   Client will have adequate caloric and protein intake daily

      c.   Client will not suffer from an infectious process as evidenced by a normal temperature and white cell count

      d.   Client will be oriented to person, time, event, and place

      e.   Client will have skin integrity remain intact as evidenced by no skin tears or open areas

8. Nursing interventions

    a.   Acute care

       (1) Assess

          (a)   Neurologic status at least every two hours

          (b)   Vital signs with postural BP every two to four hours

          (c)   Central venous pressure (CVP) readings with vital signs

          (d)   Lung sounds for fluid accumulation and heart sounds for gallops with vital signs

          (e)   Daily weights—same time, same scale, same amount of clothing

          (f)   For accuracy of I&Os

          (g)   Blood chemistries as ordered for desired changes

       (2) Care of the client receiving in-hospital peritoneal dialysis

          (a)   Use meticulous aseptic technique during procedure and dressing changes of peritoneal catheter

          (b)   Client maintained in supine position with HOB up as needed to promote ventilation

          (c)   Warm dialysate to body temperature before installation

          (d)   Instill two liters into abdomen (inflow)

          (e)   Allow dwell time of 20 to 30 minutes

          (f)   Drain fluid from peritoneum; document loss or gain of fluid during procedure (outflow)

          (g)   Outflow should be greater than inflow by 100 to 200 ml each exchange

          (h)   Turn client to ensure appropriate drainage

          (i)   Check outflow for

             (i)   Cloudiness—sign of infection

             (ii)   Red tinged—sign of bleeding

             (iii)   Brown tinged—sign of bowel perforation

          (j)   Repeat cycles for the number as ordered by physician; usually 24 in 24 hours

   (3) Evaluate nutritional likes and dislikes to encourage an appropriate nutritional status; consider the use of antiemetics before meals to ensure adequate intake

   (4) Meticulous skin care with turning every two hours, range of motion exercises, and consider use of a special mattress or bed to decrease the risk of skin breakdown; use a draw sheet for repositioning to prevent skin sheering

  b. Home care regarding client education

   (1) How to weigh client daily

   (2) The importance of keeping an accurate record of intake and output daily

   (3) Special dietary needs of the client with preparation suggestions

   (4) Medications prescribed on discharge—desired effects, side effects, effects to report to physician

9. Evaluation protocol

  a. How do I know that my interventions were effective?

   (1) Does client know who they are; where they are; what day or year it is; or what situation they are in? Neurologic status should slowly improve.

   (2) Have headaches improved?

   (3) Does client feel their strength returning?

   (4) Assess for improvement

    (a) Vital signs, CVP readings

    (b) Blood chemistries

    (c) Edema

    (d) Daily weight

    (e) I&Os

  b. What criteria will I use to change my interventions?

   (1) Neurologic status shows decreased level of consciousness

   (2) Vital signs not within ±10% of baseline

   (3) CVP readings >15 mm Hg

   (4) Peripheral edema has increased or not improved

   (5) Weight gain >2 lb/week

  c. How will I know that my client teaching has been effective?

   (1) Client or family member shows a chart of daily weights

   (2) Client tells amount of fluid taken in and urinated each day

   (3) Client shows types of food eaten each day

10. Older adult alert
    a. Older adult clients are at increased risk for developing acute renal failure as a result of unstable cardiovascular status. They have declining cardiac outputs.
    b. Fluid balance is extremely precarious in older adult clients and difficult to maintain
    c. Older adult clients have less reserve nephrons than younger adults so that there will be less to compensate for in the face of nephron damage
    d. The glomerular filtration rate begins to decline with age and is significantly decreased after the age of 50

B. **Chronic renal failure**
    1. Definition—irreversible failure of the kidneys; fatal unless client receives dialysis or a kidney transplant
    2. Pathophysiology—the affecting etiology causes a destruction of the nephrons, leading to a progressive loss of renal function; normal GFR is 125 ml/min; uremia is present when the GFR drops to 10 to 20 ml/min
    3. Etiology—the causes are endless; injuries, disease processes, drug toxicities, and infectious processes are just a few of the categories that are offenders
    4. Incidence—most common in the middle-aged adult; incidence is on the rise
    5. Assessment
        a. Ask the following questions
            (1) Do you urinate frequently? How much urine do you void when you urinate?
            (2) Do you ever have difficulty breathing?
            (3) How is your appetite?
            (4) Do you ever feel like you cannot think clearly?
            (5) Do you ever feel a burning or tingling sensation in your hands or feet?
            (6) Is your hair and skin dry?
            (7) Has there been a change in your menstrual pattern?
        b. Clinical manifestations (Table 8-2)
        c. Abnormal laboratory finding (see Table 8-2)
        d. Abnormal diagnostic tests
            (1) KUB x-ray—small, dense kidneys
            (2) Renal ultrasound—small, dense kidneys
    6. Expected medical interventions
        a. Dialysis—continuous ambulatory peritoneal dialysis (CAPD) or hemodialysis

Table 8-2. Clinical Manifestations of Chronic Renal Failure

Focus	Assessment Findings
Urine output	Oliguria <400 ml/day, anuria <100 ml/day
Metabolic	BUN & creatinine increased, no ratio; Phosphorus increased; Calcium decreased; Potassium increased, Metabolic acidosis; Sodium increase/decrease depends on body water
Neurologic, central	Decreased level of consciousness, decreased motor function, decreased cognition
Cardiovascular	Hypertension, congestive heart failure, pericarditis
Hematologic	Erythropoietin decreased (anemia); platelet function decreased (bleeding); leukocyte function decreased (infection increased); If on CAPD, hypoalbumenia
Respiratory	Kussmaul's respiration due to metabolic acidosis, pulmonary edema, pleural effusions, apnea, uremic breath from ammonia (uremic fetor)
Gastrointestinal	Anorexia, nausea, vomiting, mucosal irritation in GI tract, hematemasis, melena, diarrhea, or constipation
Neurologic, peripheral	Peripheral neuropathy, parathesias—numbness, tingling
Musculoskeletal	Soft tissue calcifications, osteodystrophy—bone defect, bone and joint pain
Dermatologic	Pruritus, dry skin (sweat glands atrophy) pallor or sallow skin color, bruising, dry-brittle hair, uremic frost (urea on skin—late sign)
Endocrine	Hypothyroidism
Reproductive	Decreased fertility, decreased libido, amenorrhea, impotence, decreased sperm and testosterone

    b. Maintaining acceptable electrolyte levels

    c. Fluid restriction

    d. Controlled protein, carbohydrate, fat, sodium, potassium, and phosphate diet if on hemodialysis; if on CAPD usually unrestricted diet with higher protein intake to replace loss of albumin

    e. Supportive drug therapy

    f. Kidney transplantation—live or cadaver

7. Nursing diagnoses

    a. Fluid volume excess related to inability of kidney to excrete water

    b. Altered nutrition—less than bodily requirements related to anorexia and inability of body to tolerate certain foods

      c. Impaired skin integrity related to tissue edema and skin structure changes

      d. Sensory-perceptual alterations related to blood chemistry abnormalities

      e. Potential for infection related to altered immune response

      f. Potential for injury related to altered sensorium and/or seizure activity

      g. Potential for body image disturbance related to need for altered elimination of nitrogenous wastes (dialysis)

8. Client goals

      a. Client will maintain an appropriate fluid balance as evidenced by a stable weight within 1 to 2 pounds

      b. Client will demonstrate an appropriate dietary intake as evidenced by food diary indicating appropriate food choices

      c. Client will maintain skin integrity as evidenced by no new skin tears and skin tears that are no longer weeping fluid

      d. Client will indicate name, location, situation, date

      e. Client will have no indication of infection as evidenced by normal temperature and WBC

      f. Client will be free of injury as evidenced by no bruising, fractures, or lacerations

      g. Client will talk about own perception of body image

9. Nursing interventions

      a. Acute care

          (1) Assess all body systems for alterations; changes in any body system are likely

          (2) Care of client—hemodialysis

              (a) Assess access site (Figure 8-5)

                 (i) Palpate for a thrill; vibration felt at site

                 (ii) Listen for a bruit—turbulent sound

                 (iii) Do not use affected extremity for BP or venipuncture; prevents bruising and bleeding

                 (iv) If external shunt, have clamps or tourniquets available for bleeding from site

                 (v) Do not allow constrictive clothing over site

                 (vi) Keep site and extremity warm

                 (vii) Check site for infection; wash site daily with antibacterial soap and water; any deodorant soap is acceptable

              (b) Prepare client for dialysis as many as three times per week; four to six hours per day

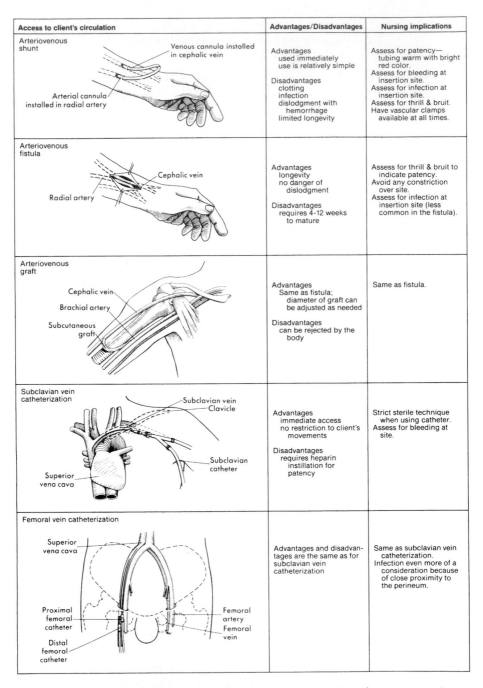

Access to client's circulation	Advantages/Disadvantages	Nursing implications
Arteriovenous shunt Venous cannula installed in cephalic vein Arterial cannula installed in radial artery	Advantages used immediately use is relatively simple Disadvantages clotting infection dislodgment with hemorrhage limited longevity	Assess for patency—tubing warm with bright red color. Assess for bleeding at insertion site. Assess for infection at insertion site. Assess for thrill & bruit. Have vascular clamps available at all times.
Arteriovenous fistula Cephalic vein Radial artery	Advantages longevity no danger of dislodgment Disadvantages requires 4-12 weeks to mature	Assess for thrill & bruit to indicate patency. Avoid any constriction over site. Assess for infection at insertion site (less common in the fistula).
Arteriovenous graft Cephalic vein Brachial artery Subcutaneous graft	Advantages Same as fistula; diameter of graft can be adjusted as needed Disadvantages can be rejected by the body	Same as fistula.
Subclavian vein catheterization Subclavian vein Clavicle Subclavian catheter Superior vena cava	Advantages immediate access no restriction to client's movements Disadvantages requires heparin instillation for patency	Strict sterile technique when using catheter. Assess for bleeding at site.
Femoral vein catheterization Superior vena cava Proximal femoral catheter Distal femoral catheter Femoral artery Femoral vein	Advantages and disadvantages are the same as for subclavian vein catheterization	Same as subclavian vein catheterization. Infection even more of a consideration because of close proximity to the perineum.

Figure 8-5. Access to client's circulation. (From *AJN/Mosby Nursing board review,* ed 9, St Louis, 1994, Mosby.)

      (c)   Evaluate temperature and BP before dialysis

      (d)   Monitor BP throughout dialysis

  (3)   Monitor vital signs for a change $>\pm10\%$ of baseline

  (4)   Daily weights

  (5)   Accurate I&Os

  (6)   Use anitemetics to control nausea and improve nutrition

  (7)   Encourage proteins of high biologic value—meat, milk, and eggs

  (8)   Institute seizure precautions if necessary

  (9)   Monitor blood chemistries—compare levels vs. physical findings

 (10)   Avoid soap for bathing to prevent drying of skin; use oil in bath water

b. Home care: regarding client education

  (1)   Continuous ambulatory peritoneal dialysis (CAPD)

      (a)   Prepare client and significant others for CAPD

         (i)   How to record daily weight and blood pressures

        (ii)   Use strict sterile technique during procedure

       (iii)   Instill two liters of room temperature dialysate using strict sterile technique

       (iv)   Keep dwell time four hours during day; eight hours at night

        (v)   Continue with usual daily activities

       (vi)   Allow outflow of fluid and discard into commode

      (vii)   Repeat with fresh solution at least four times per day

     (viii)   Have dialysate dwell overnight

      (ix)   To maintain dietary changes, increase protein to 1.5 g/kg/day, increase potassium, salt, and water intake

       (x)   Follow-up for laboratory studies and their needed frequency

      (xi)   Follow medications, schedule and report pertinent side effects

     (xii)   Report problems of which physician should be made aware

  (2)   Hemodialysis

      (a)   Teach client and significant others

         (i)   Check for infection in access site—fever, redness, swelling, pain

      (ii) They will require dialysis—three times a week, four to six hours per day

      (iii) If the client has an external AV shunt in place, have clamps or tourniquets available at all times in case of dislodgement and teach how to use

      (iv) Notify physician immediately if access site bleeds or becomes dislodged

      (v) Not to allow access site extemity to be used for BPs or venipunctures

      (vi) Not to wear constrictive clothing over access site

10. Evaluation protocol

    a. How will I know that my client interventions were effective?

      (1) Vital signs and neurologic status are stable

      (2) Weight is stable

      (3) I&Os are within normal limits for client

      (4) Electrolytes studies are within normal limits for client

      (5) Access site is free from infection and patent for dialysis use

      (6) Nutritional status is appropriate—client indicates eating suggested diet

      (7) Skin is clean and moist without tears or breakdown

      (8) Client is free of any injury

    b. What criteria will I use to change my interventions?

      (1) Vital signs not within ±10% of baseline

      (2) Neurologic status decreased

      (3) Weight gain

      (4) Abnormal electrolyte balance

      (5) Skin breakdown is evident

      (6) Bruising, lacerations, or fractures are apparent

    c. How will I know my client teaching has been effective?

      (1) Client is able to demonstrate CAPD using appropriate technique and strict sterile technique

      (2) Client selects correct food choices as indicated on a food diary

      (3) Client maintains stable weight and BP as indicated on weight and BP records

      (4) Client has appointments made for laboratory studies and catheter change

        (5)   Client has a list of adverse reactions that should be called to physician

        (6)   Client identifies protection measures that should be taken for extremity with access site

11. Older adult alert

    a. Older adult clients may have limited options for access sites for hemodialysis as a result of having long-standing cardiovascular disease

    b. Renal transplantation may not be an option for older adult clients as a result of their age. Clients over the age of 60 must be evaluated on an individual basis to identify if transplantation is a viable option.

    c. Peritoneal dialysis may not be an option for older adult clients that have had several abdominal surgeries and adhesions from the surgeries

C. **Renal calculi**

1. Definition—a stone formed and possibly lodged in the kidney; may cause obstruction of urine flow out of the kidney

2. Pathophysiology—stone components are calcium oxalate and carbonate, uric acid, cystine, and struvite; three factors lead to the production of renal calculi

    a. Urine saturation with a stone element

    b. Inhibitor deficiency or substances that would prevent stone formation

    c. A matrix formation, or the presence of a basis for the stone

3. Etiology—ingestion of calcium carbonate, vitamin D, vitamin C in large doses, and several drug therapies can predispose a client to renal calculi; abnormalities in the kidney and environmental factors can predispose a client to stone formation

4. Incidence—seen in the male population more than the female; more common in the southeastern United States; common age group is 30 to 50

5. Assessment

    a. Ask the following questions

        (1)   Do you have pain? Point to location with one finger.

        (2)   Is your pain sharp or dull?

        (3)   On a scale of 0 to 10 where would you rate your pain?

        (4)   Did your pain come on suddenly or over a period of time?

        (5)   Does your pain radiate anywhere else in your body?

        (6)   Have you experienced any nausea, vomiting, or sweating associated with this episode?

    (7) Did you try anything to make your pain better? Did it work?

    (8) Did anything make your pain worse?

  b. Clinical manifestations

    (1) Sharp, severe pain, sudden onset, deep in the lumbar region and radiating into the testicle of the male or bladder of the female if stone is lodged in renal pelvis; in contrast stones lodged in the ureter cause radiation down into the genitalia and the thigh

    (2) Pallor

    (3) Nausea, vomiting

    (4) Diaphoresis

    (5) Pain may be intermittent as the stone passes

  c. Abnormal laboratory findings—stone analysis—identifies constituents of stone

  d. Abnormal diagnostic tests

    (1) KUB x-ray—identification of stone and placement

    (2) IVP—identifies obstruction and hydronephrosis (dilation of pelvis and calyces of kidney by urine unable to drain)

6. Expected medical interventions

  a. Hydration—increased fluids to flush out stone

  b. Ambulation—to use gravity to assist removal of stone

  c. Surgery

    (1) Cystoscopy with basket to remove stone

    (2) Transcutaneous shock wave lithotripsy—client in tub of water; sonic shock waves fired at calculi resulting in disintegration of calculi

    (3) Percutaneous lithotripsy—endoscope passed through nephrostomy tract; lithotripsy used to disintegrate stone

    (4) Pyelolithotomy—removal of renal stone through flank incision (Figure 8-6)

    (5) Nephrolithotomy—stone removed from renal parenchyma through flank incision (see Figure 8-6)

    (6) Ureterolithotomy—stone removed from ureter through flank incision (see Figure 8-6)

7. Nursing diagnoses

  a. Pain related to irritation from stone

  b. Anxiety related to pain and unknown cause

  c. Knowledge deficit—dietary restrictions related to new onset and need for education

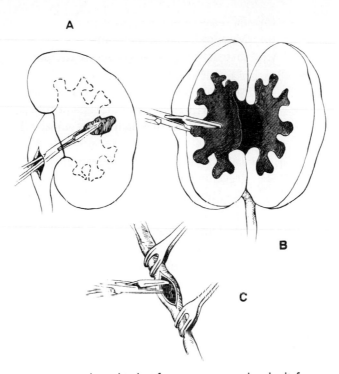

Figure 8-6. Location and methods of removing renal calculi from upper urinary tract. **A,** Pyelolithotomy, removal of stone through renal pelvis. **B,** Nephrolithotomy, removal of staghorn calculus from renal parenchyma (kidney split). **C,** Ureterolithotomy, removal of stone from ureter. (From *AJN/Mosby Nursing board review,* ed 9, St Louis, 1994, Mosby.)

8. Client goals
   a. Client will state pain is relieved following pain medication or passage of stone
   b. Client will state feeling less anxious
   c. Client will discuss postacute care
      (1) Indicate foods to avoid to prevent stone formation
      (2) Indicate the need to drink two to three liters of water per day
      (3) Plan to void at least every two hours every day for the prevention of urinary stasis and stone formation
9. Nursing interventions
   a. Acute care
      (1) Administer pain medication to control pain; narcotics usually required; assess effectiveness
      (2) Strain all urine for stones
      (3) Maintain IV access

        (4)   Increase oral intake if tolerated

        (5)   Monitor intake and output

        (6)   Instruct client to void every two hours to prevent stasis of urine

        (7)   Monitor incision for signs of infection

        (8)   Evaluate drainage from drains or tubes—DO NOT IRRIGATE TUBES unless specifically directed by physician

   b.   Home care regarding client education

      (1)   Prevention of reoccurance

          (a)   Increase daily fluid intake to 3000 ml/day; water is preferable

          (b)   Limit dietary intake dependent on stone analysis

          (c)   Void every two hours or when urge to void occurs to prevent urine stasis

          (d)   Follow-up with physician for urinalysis and laboratory studies as ordered

      (2)   Postoperative care

          (a)   Keep incision clean and dry

          (b)   Notify physician if incision becomes red, swollen, or drainage occurs

          (c)   Notify physician if experiencing urgency, frequency, or burning on urination

10. Evaluation protocol

   a.   How do I know that my interventions were effective?

      (1)   Has client pain improved or been relieved?

      (2)   Has a stone been retrieved when straining urine?

      (3)   Has client been ingesting and urinating 3000 ml/day?

      (4)   Is incision clean, dry, and free of infection?

   b.   What criteria will I use to change my interventions?

      (1)   Unrelieved pain

      (2)   Stone has not passed

      (3)   Client is urinating only 1000 ml/day with ingestion of 3000/day

      (4)   Incision is red and swollen

   c.   How will I know that my client teaching has been effective?

      (1)   Client is drinking 3000 ml/day

      (2)   Client has eliminated appropriate foods from the diet

      (3)   Client voids as soon as the urge occurs or at least every two hours

      (4)   Client has an appointment to see the physician for follow-up

11. Older adult alert—take extreme care in hydrating older adult clients with renal stones, due to risk of fluid overload with a compromised heart and diminished vascular tone. They are at greater risk for pulmonary edema.

D. Pyelonephritis
  1. Definition—bacterial infection of the renal pelvis, calyces, and parenchyma; can be acute or chronic
  2. Etiology—usually a result of an ascending urinary tract infection
  3. Pathophysiology—usually originates as lower urinary tract infection that travels up the urinary tract and infects the kidney as well; exudate accumulates in the interstitium of the kidney, and abscesses develop
  4. Assessment
    a. Ask the following questions
      (1) Do you have a fever? Do you have chills?
      (2) Do you have pain in your back?
      (3) Do you have blood in your urine?
      (4) Do you have any particles in your urine?
      (5) Do you have pain when you urinate?
      (6) Do you have frequency or urgency?
    b. Clinical manifestations
      (1) Flank pain; pain at the costovertebral angle; may be described as an aching back or a kink in the back
      (2) Fever, chills
      (3) Nausea, vomiting
      (4) Hematuria, pyuria
      (5) Foul smelling urine
      (6) May be accompanied by symptoms of cystitis—burning, frequency, and urgency
    c. Abnormal laboratory findings
      (1) Urinalysis—bacteria, pus, WBC, and casts in the urine
      (2) CBC—elevated WBC
      (3) Urine culture and sensitivity—identifies bacteria responsible for infection and which antibiotic would be effective
  5. Expected medical interventions
    a. Antiinfective agents, initially IV, followed by PO administration
    b. IV and oral fluids as tolerated
  6. Nursing diagnoses
    a. Pain related to acute inflammatory process of the kidney
    b. Altered body temperature related to inflammatory process of the kidney

7. Client goals
   a. Client will state pain is relieved
   b. Client will maintain body temperature at normal level for client or between 37° to 37.5° C
8. Nursing interventions
   a. Acute care
      (1) Administer antibiotics as ordered
      (2) Monitor culture and sensitivity results
      (3) Administer analgesics, antiemetics, and antipyretics as required by exhibited findings of client
      (4) Assess hydration status; maintain appropriate hydration
   b. Home care regarding client education
      (1) Necessity of completing all of the antibiotic
      (2) Need to make arrangements for repeat urine cultures after antibiotics completed
      (3) Instruction about the need to seek medical advice as soon as symptoms of urinary tract infection are apparent
      (4) How to prevent further episodes
         (a) Drink at least eight glasses of water per day
         (b) Void at least every two hours or as soon as urge is felt
         (c) For females, wiping from front to back
         (d) Wear cotton underwear especially under pantyhose
9. Evaluation protocol
   a. How do I know that my interventions were effective?
      (1) Has client pain improved or been relieved?
      (2) Does client feel hot?
      (3) Does client feel nauseated?
   b. What criteria will I use to change my interventions?
      (1) Flank pain persists
      (2) Fever persists
      (3) Nausea and vomiting persist
   c. How will I know that my client teaching has been effective?
      (1) Client states that all the antibiotic is completed
      (2) Client states a repeat urine culture was completed in the physician's office
      (3) Client states an intake of at least eight glasses of water a day
      (4) Client states voiding at least every two hours

10. Older adult alert
    a. In response to the normally decreased cardiac output and perfusion seen in older adult clients, blood levels of antibiotics may vary. Due to this, antibiotic therapy must be closely evaluated for effectiveness in older adult clients.
    b. The kidneys of older adult clients may be slower to respond to therapy because of the decreased perfusion

E. **Renal cancer**
  1. Definition—malignancy of the kidney
  2. Etiology—unknown
  3. Incidence—more common in the male population; renal cancer represents approximately 3% of all malignancies
  4. Pathophysiology—adenocarcinoma is most common; malignancy begins in the cortex and then progresses slowly until the parenchyma is compressed; lungs are the most common site of metastasis
  5. Assessment
    a. Ask the following questions
      (1) Do you ever have blood in your urine?
      (2) Do you ever have pain in your back?
      (3) Have you noticed a weight loss?
      (4) Do you ever feel very tired?
    b. Clinical manifestations
      (1) Intermittent gross hematuria
      (2) Flank pain
      (3) Palpable abdominal or flank mass
      (4) Weight loss
      (5) Fatigue
    c. Abnormal laboratory findings
      (1) CBC—anemia if diminished renal function or polycythemia if erythropoietin is increased
      (2) Erythrocyte sedimentation rate (ESR) elevated
      (3) Urinalysis—hematuria
    d. Abnormal diagnostic tests
      (1) KUB—lesion identified
      (2) Renal ultrasound—identifies solid mass vs. a cyst
      (3) Renal biopsy—identifies type of malignancy
  6. Expected medical interventions
    a. Nephrectomy if lymph nodes are not believed to be involved
    b. Radical nephrectomy if lymph nodes are believed to be involved
    c. Radiation therapy helpful before surgery, and after surgery to destroy any residual tumor

7. Nursing diagnoses—postoperative
   a. Pain related to effects of surgery
   b. Ineffective breathing pattern related to incisional pain
   c. Anxiety related to unknown prognosis
8. Client goals
   a. Client will state pain has been relieved or is at a tolerable level
   b. Client will maintain a respiratory rate of 16 to 20 and will take 10 deep breaths every two hours
   c. Client will state anxiety has been reduced
9. Nursing interventions
   a. Acute care
      (1) Vital signs every two to four hours, evaluating for within ±10% of baseline
      (2) Deep breathing and coughing every two hours and incentive spirometer every one hour with three to five breaths per session; difficult due to close proximity of incision to the diaphragm; pain medication must be effective and liberal
      (3) Splinting incision is also helpful when coughing and deep breathing
      (4) Assess lungs sounds at least every one to two hours for atelectasis and possible pneumothorax induced by surgery
      (5) Monitor urine output for <30 cc/hr and serum creatinine carefully for postoperative acute renal failure
      (6) Assess bowel sounds at least every two to four hours for postoperative paralytic ileus; common complication post-renal surgery
      (7) Dressing changes as needed to protect skin from drainage
   b. Home care regarding client education
      (1) How to care for incision; indications of infection in incision to report
      (2) Need to continue coughing and deep breathing and incentive spirometer exercises
      (3) Have client make appointment for follow-up care with physician
10. Evaluation protocol
    a. How do I know that my interventions were effective?
       (1) Vital signs are within ±10% of baseline
       (2) Has client pain been relieved or decreased?

       (3)   Is client having any difficulty breathing?

       (4)   Is client having any abdominal pain or bloating?

  b.   What criteria will I use to change my interventions?

       (1)   Vital signs >10% ± of baseline

       (2)   Unrelieved pain

       (3)   Shortness of breath

       (4)   Ineffective coughing and deep breathing or respiratory effort during incentive spirometer exercises

       (5)   Decreased urine output

       (6)   Absent bowel sounds

       (7)   Skin excoriation from drainage

  c.   How will I know that my client teaching has been effective?

       (1)   Client demonstrates incision care

       (2)   Client demonstrates coughing, deep breathing, and incentive spirometer exercises, with indications of how often to do the exercises

       (3)   Client states when physician follow-up visit has been scheduled and what abnormal findings to report

11. Older adult alert

  a.   Renal surgery is a major surgical procedure which may require long anesthesia time. Older adult clients must be medically cleared for this surgery with the cardiovascular status closely monitored.

  b.   Older adult clients' renal status must be evaluated carefully pre- and postoperatively, keeping in mind that one kidney is now completing all the functions of two. Renal excretion is decreased as a normal course of aging.

REVIEW QUESTIONS

1. When monitoring a client who is in the diuretic phase of acute renal failure, a central venous pressure (CVP) line would help to evaluate the
   a. Blood volume of the client
   b. Fluid volume of the client
   c. Renal perfusion capability of the client
   d. Cardiac output of the client

2. Hypertension in the client with chronic renal failure is expected as a result of
   a. The decreased urine output
   b. The decreased hemoglobin and hematocrit
   c. Increased electrolyte balance
   d. The increased fluid volume in the circulation unable to be excreted by the kidneys

3. One of the best indicators of peritonitis in the client receiving peritoneal dialysis is
   a. Fever
   b. Bloody returned dialysate
   c. Brown returned dialysate
   d. Cloudy returned dialysate

4. A concern in the older adult client presenting with kidney stones is
   a. High risk for infection
   b. Myocardial infarction
   c. Fluid overload while attempting to flush out stone
   d. Electrolyte imbalance from frequent urination

5. When caring for a client with an internal access site for hemodialysis, an important assessment to make initially would be
   a. Site color
   b. Site warmth
   c. A bruit at the site
   d. A pulse below the site

6. Near the end of completion of intermittent peritoneal dialysis on a client in acute renal failure, the nurse observes that the return from the last two runs was less than what was inserted. The best intervention to employ at this time is

a. Call the physician
b. Turn client carefully from side to side to allow drainage of all areas of the abdomen
c. Place the catheter to suction for 10 minutes
d. Irrigate the catheter with sterile saline

7. The peripheral parasthesias seen in clients with chronic renal failure are most often as a result of
a. Low potassium
b. High phosphorus
c. Low hemoglobin/hematocrit
d. Low calcium

8. The client with CAPD is permitted more protein intake than the client having intermittent peritoneal dialysis. This would be related to the fact that
a. More protein is lost through CAPD due to extended contact with the dialysate
b. Protein levels are preserved with CAPD
c. Protein levels are preserved with intermittent peritoneal dialysis
d. There is some urine formation with CAPD

9. Suggestions given to the nursing assistant for bathing a client with chronic renal failure would include to
a. Use a deodorant soap due to skin odors from urea on skin
b. Use bath oil only—soap is drying and skin is already dry due to skin changes
c. Use soap to clean and bath oil to counteract the dryness of the skin
d. Use only a bubble bath due to the cleansing nature of the bath but no skin friction

10. A client with chronic renal failure (CRF) has a blood study returned. The nurse reviews it before placing it on the chart. The hemoglobin is 7 and the hematocrit is 24. The next action would be to
a. Call the physician immediately
b. Order blood from the blood bank
c. Understand this is normal for a CRF client
d. Order a type and cross match for a blood transfusion

ANSWERS, RATIONALES, AND TEST-TAKING TIPS

Rationales	Test-Taking Tips

1. Correct answer: b

CVP is an accurate assessment of fluid volume balance in the body; it is the right atrial pressure that reflects preload.

Think venous- volume—preload. Arterial = afterload—resistance to pump against. Cluster responses *a, c,* and *d* under the focus of specific and response *b* is more general, thus the correct response. Use this approach if you don't know the correct answer.

2. Correct answer: d

The kidneys of a client in CRF are unable to remove fluid from the body. Thus fluid volume rises and results in hypertension.

Test strategy = the longest response gives the most thorough explanation. Or use the general vs. specific clustering of responses *a, b, c,* and response *d* is the most general. Or note that the key word in the stem is "hypertension" and of the responses an "increased fluid volume" would most likely raise one's blood pressure.

3. Correct answer: d

Bloody dialysate is indicative of a bleeding incident in the abdomen; brown dialysate is indicative of ruptured bowel; fever is nonspecific and too general of a response.

-itis typically means an inflammation or infection. Cloudy fluid from the body typically means infection.

4. Correct answer: c

Fluids are usually increased to attempt to flush stones out of the urinary tract system; this could cause acute heart failure in older adult clients.

Match key word in stem "stone" with response that has this word—response *c*. Responses *b* and *d* are not even considerations for high risk of stones. For the selection of response *c* remember stones are strained after saturating or hydrating the body with water.

5. Correct answer: c

A bruit felt over the access site indicates there is turbulent flow and patency of the site.

Responses *a, b,* and *d* are fine to do but are not the "initial" assessment. The flow or circulation of blood is a priority so response *c* is the best.

6. Correct answer: b

Turning the client from side to side would allow pooled fluid to exit the abdomen; the catheter should never be placed to suction, nor should it be irrigated.

Noninvasive interventions are typically more appropriate than invasive which eliminates *c* and *d.* Then, of the choices *a* or *b,* further nursing intervention is indicated before calling the physician.

7. Correct answer: d

Serum calcium runs low in the CRF client because phosphorus is high; low calcium can be exhibited by numbness or tingling around the mouth or fingers, or dizziness.

Remember the low calcium train: tingling, twitching, and tetany.

8. Correct answer: a

More protein is lost through CAPD than through peritoneal dialysis.

Use common sense—with a continuous procedure like CAPD, clients are more likely to lose protein than with an intermittent procedure.

9. Correct answer: b

Any type of soap would be drying to the skin and the skin of this client is dry already due to atrophy of sebaceous glands.

Cluster the three responses *a, c,* and *d* that have soap in them. The correct answer is *b.*

10. Correct answer: c

Due to lack of erythropoietin, which is produced by the kidney, the CRF client has a chronically low H&H.

Look at key words: "immediately" eliminates response *a*—more physical assessment data would be needed before calling the physician; "order" in responses *b* and *d* are inappropriate for the nurse to do independently.

▼ ▼ ▼ ▼ ▼ ▼ ▼ ▼ ▼   ▼ ▼ ▼

The Urinary System

STUDY OUTCOMES

After completing this chapter, the reader will be able to do
the following:

▼ Identify assessment findings of clients with alterations in
the urinary system.

▼ Choose appropriate nursing diagnoses for the urinary disorders
discussed.

▼ Implement appropriate nursing interventions for the client with
a disorder of the urinary system.

▼ Evaluate the progress of the client with a disorder of the
urinary system to establish the need for a change in nursing
interventions.

KEY TERMS

Dysuria	Painful urination.
Efflux	Movement of urine from the kidneys, through the ureter to the bladder.
Frequency	The feeling of a need to void often.
Incontinence	Uncontrolled leakage of urine from the bladder; refer to page 300 for specific definitions of incontinence.
Micturition	Urination, voiding; the process of emptying the bladder.
Reflux	Movement of urine in a backward motion from the bladder into the ureters and possibly to the kidneys.
Retention	Inability to empty the bladder completely.
Urgency	The feeling of a need to void immediately.

CONTENT REVIEW

I. **The urinary system is responsible for the transportation, storage, and elimination of urine**

II. **Structure and function**
    A. Ureters—originate at the renal pelvis and enter the bladder on the dorsal surface; purpose is to propel urine from the kidneys to the bladder; urine is actively propelled by peristalsis
    B. Bladder—situated in the pelvis; comprised of four layers
        1. Transitional epithelium—innermost layer
        2. Submucosal—supports inner layer
        3. Layer of smooth muscle bundles referred to as the detrusor muscle; urination occurs when the detrusor muscle contracts and the internal sphincter relaxes
        4. Serous layer of peritoneum—covers only in the upper surface of the bladder
    C. Urethra—allows passage of urine from the bladder to the meatus so that it can exit the body; male urethra is 18 to 20 cm in length and the female urethra is 3 to 4 cm in length; the male urethra is surrounded by the prostate gland at the proximal end and also serves to carry semen during ejaculation

III. Targeted concerns

  A. Pharmacology—priority drug classifications

    1. Antiinfective agents (Table 9-1)

    2. Urinary analgesic agent (see Table 9-1)

    3. Anticholinergics/antispasmodics/spasmolytics—relax smooth muscle in the bladder

      a. Expected effects—increases bladder capacity; used to treat instability incontinence

      b. Commonly given drugs

        (1) Flavoxate (Urispas)

        (2) Oxybutynin (Ditropan)

        (3) Propantheline (Pro-banthine)

      c. Adverse reactions—commonly occur with anticholinergic agents: drowsiness, dry mouth, blurred vision; medication is usually continued unless findings are severe

      d. Nursing considerations

        (1) Administer one hour before meals

        (2) Instruct client about the possibility of orthostatic hypotension

        (3) Warn client of possible drowsiness, and to avoid driving or using machinery until accustomed to the response

    4. Cholinergic agent—increases esophageal and ureteral peristalsis, and detrusor contraction

      a. Expected effect—increase voiding pressure and decrease bladder capacity

      b. Common agent—Bethanechol (Urecholine)

      c. Nursing considerations

        (1) PO doses should be taken on an empty stomach

        (2) Warn clients about orthostatic hypotension and how to intervene by dangling for five minutes before standing from a lying position

        (3) Warn clients that until they feel comfortable with the dizziness that may occur, they should not use heavy machinery or drive

        (4) Bladder spasms might occur and need to be reported

  B. Procedures

    1. Urinalysis—see Chapter 8 p. 265

    2. Urine culture and sensitivity—see Chapter 8 p. 265

    3. KUB X-ray—see Chapter 8 p. 265

    4. IVP—see Chapter 8 p. 265

Table 9-1. Drugs Used to Treat Urinary Tract Infection

Generic Name (Trade Name)	Action/Use	Side Effects	Nursing Implications
Urinary Analgesic			
Phenazopyridine hydrochloride (Pyridium)	Exerts an anesthetic effect on the mucosa of the urinary tract as it is excreted in the urine Used for relief of urinary tract pain	Red-orange or rust discoloration of urine	Inform that urine will be orange-colored Take drug with food Use Clinitest for urine testing
Urinary Antiseptics			
Cinoxacin (Cinobac) Methenamine hippurate (Hiprex) Nitrofurantoin (Furadantin, Macrodantin)	Act as disinfectants within the urinary tract Concentrated by the kidneys and reach therapeutic levels only within the urinary tract Used to treat UTIs	Nausea, vomiting, GI upset, diarrhea, hypersensitivity reaction, and dizziness Brown or rust discoloration of urine	Keep urine acidic; give vitamin C (6-12 g/day) or cranberry, plum, prune, or apple juice Give after meals to minimize GI upset Warn that urine may be brown- or rust-colored Monitor I&O; maintain fluid intake of 1500-2000 ml/day

Sulfonamides

Drug	Action/Use	Side Effects	Nursing Implications
Trimethoprim/Sulfamethoxazole (Bactrim, Septra) Sulfasalazine (Azulfidine) Sulfisoxazole (Gantrisin)	Bacteriostatic against gram-positive and gram-negative organisms Excreted unchanged and dissolves well in urine Used to treat UTIs, acute otitis media, inflammatory bowel disease, chronic bronchitis, parasitic infections, and for preoperative bowel sterilization	GI disorders, hypersensitivity reactions, headache, peripheral hearing loss, cystaluria, and hypoglycemia	Force fluids to 3000-4000 ml/day Keep urine alkaline Give with at least 8 oz water 1 hr before or 2 hr after meals for maximum absorption Monitor I&O Monitor clients with potential renal or hepatic impairment closely Advise clients to complete drug course Warn about potential increased effect of oral hypoglycemics and false positive Clinitest results when appropriate

Other Antiinfectives

Drug	Action/Use	Side Effects	Nursing Implications
Ciprofloxacin (Cipro)	Broad-spectrum antibiotic used for mild to moderate UTIs	GI disturbances, headache, and rash	Give 2 hr before or after administration of antacids containing magnesium Give 2 hr after meals Drink plenty of fluids

5. Retrograde pyelogram—using an endoscope, the bladder and ureters are directly visualized with the assistance of contrast dye that can be gently injected into the upper urinary tract

6. Voiding cystogram—client is catheterized and contrast material instilled into the bladder; x-rays are taken of the bladder during filling and during voiding; used to evaluate the bladder for trauma, anomalies, or reflux

7. Retrograde urethrogram—contrast material injected into the tip of the male urethra while x-rays are taken; used to evaluate urethra for strictures or structural changes

8. CT scan—provides axial images of the urinary system; helpful in locating tumors, abscesses, or masses

9. Magnetic resonance imaging (MRI)—use of a magnetic field to give an excellent image of the structures of the pelvis, but not particularly useful for urinary calculi

10. Endoscopy
    a. Ureteroscopy—visualization of the ureters using a fiberoptic scope
    b. Cystourethroscopy—visualization of the urethra, bladder, and ureters using a fiberoptic scope; any abnormalities of the structures visualized can be identified

11. Urodynamic testing—a series of tests that are used to measure the transportation, storage, and elimination of urine
    a. Cystometrogram (CMG) (most commonly used)—evaluates bladder filling, bladder capacity, and detrusor stability

12. Ultrasonography—ureters, bladder, and prostate can be visualized using high frequency sound waves; identification of tumor, urinary calculi, or masses can be accomplished

13. Biopsies—anticipate some bright red blood afterwards for about 24 to 48 hours
    a. Ureter biopsy is accomplished during endoscopy using a nylon brush to retrieve tissue for study
    b. Bladder and urethra biopsy is also accomplished during endoscopy; small forceps will pull away pieces of tissue from several areas for study

      c. Prostate biopsy is accomplished using a transrectal approach with the assistance of an ultrasonic probe; several pieces of tissue are retrieved for study

C. **Psychosocial**
1. Anxiety—that uncomfortable feeling associated with an unknown direct cause; common in the client with any alteration to urinary elimination as a result of the private nature of the matter
2. Fear—an uncomfortable feeling associated with real danger; common in the client facing any type of malignancy
3. Anger—common response when the client is facing a malignancy
4. Altered body-image—a concern for the client who must face a change in bodily functions, such as surgery that will change urinary elimination
5. Social isolation—may occur if the client has incontinence or is uncomfortable with a new body-image, such as urinary diversion
6. Depression—not uncommon in the client facing changes in life-style or body-image change
7. Embarrassment—seen in the client with a condition that is difficult to control, such as incontinence

D. **Health history—question sequence**
1. Describe the problem you are experiencing
2. How often do you urinate?
3. Do you urinate in large or small amounts each time?
4. Do you wake up at night to urinate?
5. Do you use any method to stimulate you to begin voiding?
6. Do you have difficulty beginning a stream of urine or maintaining that stream of urine?
7. Have you noticed a change in the force or shape of your urination stream?
8. Do you ever feel the need to urinate immediately?
9. Do you have difficulty controlling urination?
10. What color is your urine?
11. Is there an unusual odor associated with your urine?
12. Do you ever notice particles floating in your urine?
13. Have you experienced a large number of urinary tract infections?
14. Have you ever been hospitalized for a urinary tract problem, or had surgery for a urinary tract problem?

15. Have you experienced any nausea, vomiting, or diarrhea?
16. What prescription and nonprescription medications are you presently taking?

E. **Physical exam—appropriate sequence**
1. Airway, breathing, circulation—vital signs
2. Inspect abdominal and flank area for masses or other abnormalities
3. Palpation of the kidneys, bladder
4. Percussion of the kidneys over the posterior trunk, and bladder over the suprapubic area
5. Inspection of the perineum and urinary meatus
6. Palpation of the penis and perineum for masses or tenderness; palpation of the female perineal area for tenderness

IV. Pathophysiologic disorders

A. Incontinence
1. Definition—uncontrolled loss of urine from the bladder; two major classifications
   a. Acute—temporary incontinence associated with an acute illness or infective process
   b. Persistent (established)—continued incontinence after acute illness has subsided; five subdivisions
      (1) Stress—loss of urine during activities that increase abdominal pressure, such as coughing
      (2) Urge—incontinence following an immediate urge to void
      (3) Total—continuous leakage of urine without knowledge of the need to void
      (4) Functional—incontinence related to a client who is unable to utilize accepted elimination methods due to decreased cognition or mobility
      (5) Reflex—abnormal spinal cord reflex which causes a leakage of urine from the bladder
2. Etiology
   a. Damage or weakness of the sphincter—may be due to injury during childbirth, damage during prostatectomy, or congenital weakness
   b. Deformity of the urethra—frequent UTIs, gynecologic surgery or trauma
   c. Change in the angle between the bladder and the urethra—urethra normally lies at a 90 degree angle to the

bladder; pregnancy, surgery, or aging may decrease that angle to less than 90 degrees and allow the sphincter to open and become inefficient

d. Unstable detrusor muscle—bladder tumors, spinal cord lesions

e. Weakened abdominal and perineal muscles—obesity, childbirth, prostatectomy

3. Assessment

a. Ask the following questions

(1) Do you ever have difficulty controlling your urine?

(2) Do you wear any special pads or garments to keep you dry?

(3) How frequently do you void?

(4) How much do you void each time?

(5) Do you ever feel burning when you void?

(6) Do you drink a large amount of beverages that contain caffeine?

(7) Are you being treated by a physician for any medical problems?

(8) What color is your urine? Is there any unusual odor? Are there any particles in your urine?

(9) Is it difficult for you to get to the bathroom?

b. Clinical manifestations

(1) Stress incontinence—loss of urine during coughing, sneezing, laughing

(2) Urge incontinence—loss of urine associated with a feeling of urgency

(3) Reflex incontinence—a regular loss of urine without awareness of it occurring

(4) Total incontinence—continuous leakage of urine

(5) Functional incontinence—loss of urine before the client can reach the appropriate facility

c. Abnormal laboratory findings

(1) Urinalysis—positive for bacteria, pyuria, hematuria if incontinence is caused by UTI

(2) Urine C&S—high colony count, positive for a specific bacteria

d. Abnormal diagnostic test

(1) Urodynamics—abnormalities in the voiding patterns indicative of incontinence

(2) IVP—identifies obstruction in the urinary tract

4. Expected medical interventions
   a. Surgical—bladder suspension
   b. Artificial urinary sphincter
   c. Pharmacologic therapies—Urispas, Ditropan
   d. Therapies such as bladder training and exercises such as pelvic floor to minimize incontinence
5. Nursing diagnoses
   a. Altered patterns of urinary elimination—incontinence related to muscle weakness and decreased ability to control bladder
   b. Body-image disturbance related to inability to control urinary elimination
   c. Social isolation related to fear of inability to control urinary elimination in public
   d. Impaired skin integrity related to skin in frequent contact with urine
6. Client goals
   a. Client will demonstrate decreased incidences of incontinence over a 24-hour period
   b. Client will state feeling more comfortable with body-image as a result of being able to control incontinence
   c. Client will state having no hesitation leaving the home as a result of having more control of incontinence
   d. Client will indicate perineal skin is intact and free of breakdown
7. Nursing interventions
   a. Pelvic floor exercises also termed pubococcygeal muscle exercises or Kegel exercises; instruct client to
      (1) Tighten muscles in perineum—as if trying to stop the flow of urine
      (2) Hold tight muscles for 6 to 10 seconds
      (3) Repeat tightening 4 to 6 times
      (4) Repeat total exercise 3 to 4 times per day
   b. Bladder training; instruct client to
      (1) Void hourly throughout the day
      (2) Increase interval to two hours between voiding
      (3) Increase interval to three hours between voiding
   c. Incontinence garments
   d. External urinary drainage devices available for men and women

e. Skin care
   (1) Skin cleansed as necessary
   (2) Protective skin creams or ointments
   (3) Change damp underwear garments as soon as possible
f. Client education related to specific medical regime

8. Evaluation protocol
   a. How do I know that my interventions were effective?
      (1) Has client noticed decrease in incontinent episodes?
      (2) Has client felt comfortable in leaving the home and spending more time becoming involved outside of the home?
      (3) Is client having any difficulty in skin breakdown or redness?
   b. What criteria will I use to change my interventions?
      (1) Increased episodes of incontinence
      (2) Client refusing to leave the home for any reason
      (3) Skin breakdown in the perineal area
   c. How will I know that my client teaching has been effective?
      (1) Client demonstrates effective technique for care of devices to be utilized
      (2) Client states correct regime for medication administration
      (3) Client states correct individually developed bladder training or pelvic exercises sequence

9. Older adult alert
   a. As a normal course of aging there is a decrease in the amount of urine clients can hold in the bladder and a decrease in the muscle strength of the detrusor muscle and muscles of the pelvis. This predisposes older adults to urinary incontinence.
   b. Nurses need to be careful not to assume, however, that incontinence is a normal aging process. Instead, evaluation as to the cause of incontinence as it occurs is needed, and then implementation of an appropriate course of action.
   c. An important reminder is that many of the medications older adults take can also predispose them to incontinence

B. Urinary tract infection
   1. Definition—cystitis is an inflammation of the wall of the bladder; urinary tract infection (UTI) is an infection at any point along the urinary tract

2. Pathophysiology—as pathogens invade the urinary tract the bladder mucosa is affected and the wall will lose its efficiency for contraction; clients may complain of frequent voiding but still have the feeling their bladder is not empty; as the inflammation spreads across the bladder wall, clients complain of painful urination or dysuria and hematuria, or blood in the urine may be seen

3. Etiology—most common cause is bacterial, although other organisms can induce this disorder; the majority of UTIs occur because of contamination from the gastrointestinal tract; close proximity of the urethra to the rectum in the female is the most commonly identified cause of urinary tract infection; infections can descend or ascend from origin of the infection and thus infect other internal structures if not treated properly

4. Assessment
   a. Ask the following questions
      (1) Do you have pain when you urinate?
      (2) Does it burn when you urinate?
      (3) Do you feel like you must urinate frequently?
      (4) Do you feel like you must run to the bathroom to urinate quickly?
      (5) Does your urine smell unusual?
      (6) Is there blood or other particles in your urine?
      (7) Have you been running a fever?
   b. Clinical manifestations
      (1) Frequency
      (2) Urgency
      (3) Dysuria, burning
      (4) Suprapubic pain
      (5) Foul smelling urine
      (6) Hematuria, pyuria
      (7) Fever
   c. Abnormal laboratory findings
      (1) Urinalysis—positive for pathogen, blood, and possibly pus; RBCs and WBCs present
      (2) Urine culture and sensitivity—colony count >100,000; pathogen identified, sensitivity identifies appropriate antibiotic therapy
   d. Abnormal diagnostic tests
      (1) Cystoscopy—identifies inflamed bladder wall

(2) Urodynamics—identifies voiding abnormalities with associated etiology; usually done if clients have frequent UTIs

5. Expected medical interventions
   a. Urinary analgesic for pain—Pyridium
   b. Antiinfective therapy dictated by the culture and sensitivity result
   c. Education for prevention

6. Nursing diagnoses
   a. Pain related to urinary tract inflammation
   b. Altered patterns of urinary elimination—urgency, frequency related to urinary tract inflammation
   c. Knowledge deficit—care of and prevention of UTI related to client teaching not yet completed

7. Client goals
   a. Client will state pain is relieved or reduced in level on a scale of 1 to 10
   b. Client will state frequency and urgency have subsided
   c. Client will state care procedure related to diagnosis and how to prevent the disorder in the future

8. Nursing interventions
   a. Acute care
      (1) Increased fluid intake up to 3000 ml/day to flush out urinary tract
      (2) Void at least every two hours
      (3) Drink fluids free of caffeine and citrus because of the aggravating effect on the bladder
      (4) Sitz baths for perineal pain
   b. Home care regarding client education
      (1) Continue all interventions listed under acute care
      (2) Instruct on the importance of finishing all of the antibiotic
      (3) Discourage use of bubble bath and any bathing products with perfume, such as soap, powder, or bath gels
      (4) Wiping the perineum from front to back ONLY
      (5) Wearing only cotton underwear—allows absorption of vaginal and/or urinary excretions as opposed to nylon which will not absorb but hold excretions close to urinary meatus; wet nylon is a good medium for bacterial growth

        (6) Voiding as soon as feasible after sexual intercourse— allows a flushing of the urethra following mechanical friction which may introduce bacteria

9. Evaluation protocol
   a. How do I know that my interventions were effective?
      (1) Does client still have pain when urinating?
      (2) Does client still have the urge to void immediately or void frequently?
      (3) Has client's urine returned to a normal color with normal odor?
      (4) How much fluid and what type of fluid is client drinking each day?
   b. What criteria will I use to change my interventions?
      (1) Pain, frequency, urgency continues
      (2) Hematuria, pyuria continues
      (3) Client begins to experience bladder spasms
      (4) Temperature stays elevated or gets higher
   c. How will I know that my client teaching has been effective?
      (1) Client is voiding every two hours or at the first urge to void
      (2) Client urinates within one hour or sooner after sexual intercourse
      (3) Client is wearing only cotton underwear or cotton underwear under pantyhose
      (4) Client is careful to wipe only from front to back
      (5) Client has changed the brand of soap/powder to one without perfume

10. Older adult alert
    a. Urinary tract infections in older adults may be asymptomatic
    b. In older adult clients the only manifestations of UTI may be anorexia, malaise, and low-grade fever
    c. Incontinence in older adults, especially those that are confused, may also be an indication that a UTI exists

C. **Bladder cancer**
   1. Definition—malignancy of the bladder
   2. Pathophysiology—most bladder tumors begin as papillomatous growths and at some point begin to invade the wall of the bladder; staging of the cancer is determined by the depth of infiltration into the bladder wall; metastasis is generally to local lymph nodes, liver, lungs, and bones
   3. Etiology—cigarette smoking has a high correlation with bladder cancer; use of the drug phenacetin has been implicated;

exposure to aniline dyes (made from poisonous liquid extracted from the indigo plant, or made synthetically), rubber, and textiles are also implicated

4. Incidence—more common in the male population; accounts for approximately 2% of all deaths from cancer in the United States
5. Assessment
   a. Ask the following questions
      (1) Do you experience pain when you urinate?
      (2) Do you ever see blood in your urine?
      (3) Do you feel as if you must void frequently?
      (4) Do you have an urge to void immediately at times?
   b. Clinical manifestations
      (1) Painless hematuria
      (2) Dysuria, burning
      (3) Frequency
      (4) Urgency
      (5) Pyuria
   c. Abnormal laboratory findings
      (1) Urinalysis—microscopic or gross hematuria
      (2) Urine cytology—malignant cells identified in voided specimen
   d. Abnormal diagnostic tests
      (1) Cystoscopy with biopsy—definitive diagnostic measure; positive for malignant cells
      (2) CT scan may be helpful with staging
6. Expected medical interventions
   a. Noninvasive tumors
      (1) Transurethral resection of tumors
      (2) Laser fulguration (burning away) of tumors
      (3) Intravesical chemotherapy
   b. Invasive tumors
      (1) Partial or radical cystectomy
      (2) Urinary diversion (Figures 9-1 and 9-2)
         (a) Ileal conduit—piece of ileum is dissected away, closed at one end, ureters implanted on top and other end of ileum is pulled out to the abdomen; stoma devised; appliance required
         (b) Kock's pouch—a continent ileal reservoir; ureters implanted on a 2 ft piece of the terminal ileum; left attached to its blood supply; ileum is formed into a reservoir with a nipple that is pulled out to the abdominal wall; reservoir is

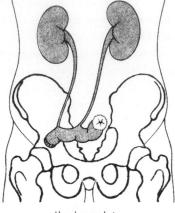

Ileal conduit

Figure 9-1. Ileal conduit. (From Beare PG and Myers JL: *Principles and practice of adult health nursing,* ed 2, St Louis, 1994, Mosby.)

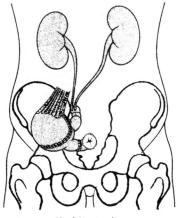

Kock's pouch

Figure 9-2. Kock's pouch. (From Beare PG and Myers JL: *Principles and practice of adult health nursing,* ed 2, St Louis, 1994, Mosby.)

            catheterized every three to four hours; no
            appliance required

    (3) Adjunct chemotherapy and/or radiation therapy
  7. Nursing diagnoses
    a. Anxiety, fear related to diagnosis and unknown outcome
    b. Pain related to the effects of surgery

    c. Body-image disturbance related to change in the manner of urinary elimination

    d. Sexual dysfunction related to nerve impairment secondary to bladder surgery

    e. High risk for impaired skin integrity related to urine contact with skin from stoma

8. Client goals

    a. Client will state anxiety and/or fear has decreased in intensity

    b. Client will state pain has decreased on a scale of 0 to 10 or has been relieved

    c. Client will indicate by behavior and verbalization an acceptance of the change in body-image and structure

    d. Client will indicate by verbalization an acceptance for alternative methods of sexual expression

    e. Client will have no skin breakdown around the stoma

9. Nursing interventions

    a. Acute care

        (1) Preoperative education

            (a) Routine operative instructions

                (i) Turn, cough, and deep breathe every two hours; incentive spirometer every one to two hours

                (ii) Leg muscle exercises every hour while in bed; dorsi and plantar flex ankles

            (b) Procedure, type of stoma and device

            (c) Introduction to general care of the stoma and device if utilized

            (d) Possibility of NG tube

            (e) Visit from stomal therapist before surgery

            (f) Changes in sexual functioning and the possibility of impotence postoperatively

            (g) Bowel prep before surgery

        (2) Postoperative care

            (a) Vital signs

            (b) Careful I&O with strict attention to urinary output

            (c) Increased fluid intake as tolerated by the cardiovascular system

            (d) Carefully monitor for bleeding, evaluate dressing and drainage from drains—drainage devices such as Jackson-Pratts should be drained when half full or every eight hours, whichever occurs first; document amount and color of drainage

        (e) Pain assessment

        (f) Monitor stoma for bleeding and drainage

        (g) NG tube output

        (h) Specific instructions from stomal therapist as to care of stoma and devices

        (i) Sexual counseling and a visit from a member of an ostomy support group would be appropriate as the client progresses postoperatively

   b. Home care regarding client education

     (1) Incontinent urinary diversion care—the stoma and device or continent urinary diversion care

     (2) Need to be aware of findings associated with UTI and, upon occurrence, to call physician

     (3) Use of straight drainage and gravity devices at night to prevent reflux into ureters with an incontinent diversion

     (4) Need for follow-up care with physician and for chemotherapy or radiation therapy

10. Evaluation protocol

   a. How do I know that my interventions were effective?

     (1) Can client demonstrate exercises such as incentive spirometer use every two hours after surgery?

     (2) Does client know what kind of stoma or device that will be utilized?

     (3) Has client's pain decreased or been relieved?

   b. What criteria will I use to change my interventions?

     (1) Vital signs are not within ±10% of baseline; bleeding from operative site

     (2) Pain is not relieved or decreased

     (3) Client is not aware of postoperative regime

     (4) Client is unclear as why there is a stoma postoperatively

   c. How will I know that my client teaching has been effective?

     (1) Client states using a gravity drainage bag at night to prevent a kidney infection

     (2) Client states effective visits with a therapist for sexual counseling or attending a support group

     (3) Client states having an appointment to see physician in two weeks

(4) Client demonstrates correct procedure for emptying a continent diversion and for applying a device on an incontinent diversion

11. Older adult alert
   a. The older adult population is the age group most likely to suffer from this disorder, so careful attention must be paid to symptoms suggestive of cancer of the bladder
   b. Older adult clients' dexterity must be evaluated to determine capability of performing appropriate stomal care. Arthritis may cause some difficulty in preparing and applying the pouches. Because of impaired vision, older adults may need home visits from a nurse to do ostomy care.

REVIEW QUESTIONS

1. The nurse is caring for an older adult client who has become confused over the past three hours and is now incontinent when the client had previously been continent. The nurse suspects
   a. Stress incontinence
   b. CVA
   c. Urinary tract infection
   d. Bowel obstruction

2. A client requests instructions for irrigation of the ileal conduit. The nurse's most appropriate response would be
   a. Irrigation is done daily with 100 ml of water
   b. Technique is much like giving an enema
   c. Irrigation is done with 1000 ml of warm water
   d. Irrigation is usually not done on an ileal conduit since the output is a continuous liquid; irrigation can be done if mucous plugs are suspected

3. When teaching a female client how to prevent her frequent urinary tract infections, it would be a priority to include instruction to
   a. Void immediately after intercourse
   b. Void every four hours
   c. Wipe, after toileting, from vagina to urinary meatus
   d. Wear only nylon underwear, especially under pantyhose

4. The definitive diagnostic test for a urinary tract infection is
   a. Urinalysis
   b. Intravenous pyelogram
   c. Kidneys, ureters, bladder x-ray
   d. Urine culture

5. When planning care for a client who is taking Bactrim for a urinary tract infection, the nurse is careful to instruct the client to include
   a. Apple juice with all meals
   b. Administration of medications with meals
   c. An increased fluid intake to at least 3000 ml/day
   d. Careful monitoring of intake only

ANSWERS, RATIONALES, AND TEST-TAKING TIPS

Rationales	Test-Taking Tips

1. Correct answer: c

In an older adult client who has been continent and is now incontinent, and also is confused, you must consider urinary tract infection.

The question is asking about the urinary tract, therefore responses *a* and *c* are the best choices. Of these two, response *c* is the best. The clue given is that there is an acute change of client status and infection typically can cause such an acute change. In addition, there is no data in the stem to support response *a*.

2. Correct answer: d

Instructions would have to be centered around the fact that the output from an ileal conduit is liquid and will not require irrigation unless there is an increase of mucus production and mucous plugs with an evident decreased or cloudy urine output. Mucus comes from the mucosa of the piece of ileum that is used as a reservoir.

Cluster out responses *a* and *c* because they are quite specific. Common sense gives a clue that the lumen of the ileal conduit is much smaller than lumens of openings to give an enema and could not be correct. Note that a key word in the stem is that the client is asking for "guidelines" not steps in a procedure.

3. Correct answer: a

Clients should be urged to void immediately or within an hour after sexual intercourse to flush the urethra of any bacteria that may have been introduced through the friction of intercourse. Wiping should be from front to back or from urethra to rectum. Women should void every 2 hours and wear only cotton underwear due to its absorbency.

Do not let the word "immediately" distract you from the correct answer. The other responses are obviously incorrect. Be aware of your bias from personal behaviors that might lead you not to select *a* as the correct response. A key word in the stem is "prevent."

4. **Correct answer: d**

A urine culture will tell what organism is the cause of infection in the urine. A urinalysis would show WBCs but not specify the type of organism.

The key word "definitive" means with great certainty. Responses *b* and *c* reflect what anatomical deviations or if stones are found in the urinary system.

5. **Correct answer: c**

Urine should be made alkaline since sulfonamides are most effective in alkaline urine; so apple juice would not be appropriate. Bactrim should be taken on an empty stomach. Intake and output should be monitored. Fluids should be increased to at least 3000 ml/day.

Sulfonamides are included in that group of medications along with tetracycline and carafate that are taken on an empty stomach.

▼ ▼ ▼ ▼ ▼ ▼ ▼ ▼ ▼ ▼   ▼ ▼ ▼

The Reproductive System

STUDY OUTCOMES

After completing this chapter, the reader will be able to do the following:

▼ Describe the structure and function of the organs of the reproductive system.

▼ Identify assessment findings associated with disorders of the reproductive system.

▼ Choose appropriate nursing diagnoses for the reproductive disorders discussed.

▼ Implement appropriate nursing interventions for the client with disorders of the reproductive system.

▼ Evaluate the progress of the client with a reproductive disorder for the establishment of new nursing interventions based on evaluation findings.

KEY TERMS

Amenorrhea	Absence of menstruation.
Dysmenorrhea	Painful menstruation.
Epididymitis	Acute or chronic inflammation of the epididymis from venereal disease, UTI, prostatitis, or prostatectomy.
Menorrhagia	Abnormally heavy menstruation.
Metrorrhagia	Uterine bleeding not associated with menstruation.
Nocturia	Awakened at night by the urge to urinate, usually several times during the night.

CONTENT REVIEW

I. Definition

A. The female reproductive system is responsible for
1. Production of ova
2. Provision for the means to fertilization, growth, and maturation of the embryo that will grow from a fertilized ovum
3. Provision of milk for nutrition of the newborn

B. The male reproductive system is responsible for
1. Production of sperm
2. Instillation of sperm into the female vagina so that fertilization can take place

II. Structure and function

A. Female
1. Ovaries—primary sex organs; two oval glands located on either side of the fallopian tubes; responsible for production of the hormones estrogen and progesterone
2. Uterus—supports and nourishes a growing fetus; pear-shaped organ located in the pelvis
3. Fallopian tubes—hollow tubes situated between the ovaries and uterus; propels ova from ovaries to uterus
4. Vagina—an internal canal that accepts penile penetration during sexual intercourse; serves as birth canal during childbirth
5. Breasts—mammary glands; found on each side of the chest between the second and sixth rib; responsible for milk production to nourish infants

B. Male
  1. Testes—two oval glands located in the scrotum, behind the penis in the perineal area; responsible for secretion of testosterone
  2. Prostate gland—found just below the bladder, surrounding the urethra; secretes fluid emitted with sperm during ejaculation that will ensure sperm motility
  3. Penis—external reproductive and urinary organ; responsible for urinary elimination and reproduction; ejaculates sperm into the female vagina during sexual intercourse for the purpose of fertilization of an ovum and subsequent reproduction

III. Targeted concerns

A. Pharmacology—priority drug classifications
  1. Estrogens—hormones given through oral or dermal route
     a. Expected effects
        (1) Prostate cancer—causes tumor cells to atrophy
        (2) Menopause-induced vaginitis—can reduce symptoms of dryness
        (3) Prevents osteoporosis in menopausal women
        (4) Replacement therapy
     b. Commonly given drugs
        (1) Estradiol valerate (Delestrogen)
        (2) Ethinyl estradiol (Estinyl)
        (3) Diethylstilbestrol (DES)
     c. Nursing considerations
        (1) Warn clients about the possibility of dizziness
        (2) Clients should brush with a soft toothbrush and floss regularly due to the gingival irritation that can occur while on estrogen therapy
        (3) Clients should not smoke while on estrogen therapy because of the vasoconstrictive effects of smoking and thromboemboletic effects of estrogen
  2. Antiandrogenic agents—block the action of androgens, or the production of androgens
     a. Expected effects—used for palliative treatment of prostate cancer and to treat benign prostatic hypertrophy; prevent stimulation and growth of tissue
     b. Commonly given drugs
        (1) Flutamide (Eulexin)
        (2) Goserelin (Zoladex)
        (3) Leuprolide (Lupron)

    (4) Megestrol acetate (Megrace)

    (5) Finestaride (Proscar)

   c. Nursing considerations

    (1) Instruct client about feeling hot flashes

    (2) Inform physician immediately if client has difficulty urinating

    (3) Instruct client that bone pain may increase initially but will subside; use analgesics to assist with pain relief

  3. Alpha-adrenergic blockers—produce alpha 1 and alpha 2 blockade

   a. Expected effect—relaxation of bladder outlet to decrease symptoms of benign prostatic hypertrophy bladder outlet obstruction

   b. Commonly given drugs

    (1) Terazosin (Hytrin)

    (2) Prazosin (Minipress)

   c. Nursing considerations

    (1) Caution about orthostatic hypotension

    (2) Remind client about feeling fatigue for a period of time

  4. Androgens—hormones administered to replace a lack of testosterone

   a. Expected effects—will increase testosterone levels and promote male characteristics; used in breast cancer in postmenopausal women

   b. Commonly given drugs

    (1) Fluoxymesterone (Halotestin)

    (2) Testosterone (Histerone)

   c. Nursing considerations

    (1) Evaluate carefully for hypercalcemia

    (2) Monitor for edema

B. Procedures

  1. Papanicolaou test (Pap test)—microscopic examination of cells of the cervix

  2. Biopsies—removal of tissue for examination of cells for malignancy or other abnormalities

   a. Endometrial—tissue from walls of the uterus; aspiration method

   b. Cervical—tissue from cervix; punch biopsy method; cervical conization—cone of tissue removed from cervix if no specific lesion is identified

      c. Breast—tissue from breast lesion; open method or needle biopsy method

      d. Prostate—tissue from the prostate gland; needle biopsy using a transrectal or perineal approach

  3. Fiberoptic examinations

      a. Colposcopy—direct visualization of vagina and cervix

      b. Culdoscopy—direct visualization of peritoneal cavity via an incision into the cul de sac of the vagina

      c. Laparoscopy—direct visualization of pelvic contents via an incision made in the abdomen

      d. Hysteroscopy—direct visualization of cervical canal and internal uterus; scope inserted through cervix and into uterus

  4. Hysterosalpingography—contrast medium injected into uterus and fallopian tubes via a tube placed in the cervix to determine patency of fallopian tubes and uterine abnormalities

  5. Mammography—radiologic examination of breasts for abnormalities and lesions

  6. Ultrasonography—sound waves used to emit images of the examined areas; abdominal cavity, pelvic cavity, breasts, prostate (transrectal), and the scrotum, which is the preferred method for evaluation of scrotal abnormalities

  7. Prostate specific antigen (PSA)—elevated serum levels can be indicative of prostate cancer or inflammation

  8. Testicular scintigraphy—nuclear medicine scan of the testicles; requires injection of radioactive contrast medium; helpful in identifying testicular torsion

C. **Psychosocial**

  1. Reproductive disorders can be associated with a change in the client's self-concept, body image, personal identity, and role at home

  2. Sexuality and sexual functioning can be altered by a reproductive disorder

  3. When working with a client with a reproductive disorder, extreme sensitivity must be utilized

  4. Fear/anxiety—the uncomfortable feeling associated with a real or unknown threat; commonly seen in clients with a reproductive disorder as a result of the changing effect the illness has on their lives

  5. Embarrassment—related to the gynecologic and perineal exams

6. Denial—commonly seen as a defense mechanism to protect from the need to seek medical assistance and intrusive perineal exams; also to protect against the fear of change in body image and self-concept

D. **Health history—question sequence**
1. What has been bothering you? What problem are you seeking help for from the physician?
2. Are you or have you been treated in the past for any illnesses?
3. Do you have a history of disorders of the reproductive system?
4. Is there a family history of disorders of the reproductive system?
5. Have you ever had surgery involving the reproductive system?
6. Are you presently taking any prescription or nonprescription medications?
7. Do you suffer from any allergies to any medications, foods, or substances?
8. Have you experienced any breast tenderness, lumps, or nipple discharge? (Ask both females and males the previous question.) Are any of these findings associated with your menstrual cycle?
9. What type of contraceptives are you using? (Ask both male and female clients.)
10. Tell me about your menstrual cycles
11. Tell me about your pregnancies

E. **Physical exam—appropriate sequence**
1. Airway, breathing, circulation—vital signs
2. Selected assessments (Table 10-1)

Table 10-1. Physical Exam Assessments for Reproductive System

Male	Female
Inspect breasts, palpate breasts for lumps	Same
Inspect abdomen, palpate abdomen for masses, tenderness	Same
Auscultate abdomen for bowel sounds	Same
Inspect pubic hair, skin, penis for abnormalities, scrotum for abnormalities	Inspect pubic hair, skin, labia majora and minora, urethra meatus
Palpate penis and scrotum for lumps and tenderness	Palpate perineal area for lumps and tenderness

IV. Pathophysiologic disorders

A. Benign prostatic hypertrophy (BPH)

1. Definition—enlargement of the prostate gland to the point of urethral obstruction with resultant urinary dysfunction

2. Pathophysiology—circulating androgens decrease in the elderly male and may contribute to the incidence of BPH; as the prostate enlarges, the urethra is compromised and the male feels the need to exert more pressure to void; eventually there may be total occlusion of the urethra, resulting in urinary retention

3. Etiology—unknown or unclear

4. Incidence—one in every four men will require medical intervention for BPH; incidence increases after the age of 50

5. Assessment

   a. Ask the following questions

      (1) Have you noticed a decrease in the stream of your urine?

      (2) Have you felt as if your bladder was not empty when you were finished voiding?

      (3) Have you felt as if you must void frequently?

      (4) Do you waken at night with a need to void?

      (5) Have you had a normal appetite?

      (6) Have you noticed a weight loss or gain?

   b. Clinical manifestations

      (1) Change in urinary elimination pattern; decrease in force of urinary stream; normal stream assessed for

         (a) Force—enough to clear feet and reach toilet within several inches of penis

         (b) Caliber—stream diameter approximately equal to a pencil lead

         (c) Constancy—relatively constant stream

         (d) Trimness—stream constant and not spraying to the sides

      (2) Urgency frequent, yet difficulty starting and stopping stream

      (3) Nocturia

      (4) Urge incontinence

      (5) Inability to empty bladder (retention)

      (6) Frequent urinary tract infections

      (7) Urinary calculi

(8) Signs of renal insufficiency due to obstruction—nausea, vomiting, weight loss, edema with weight gain, oliguria, or polyuria

c. Abnormal laboratory findings
  (1) Urinalysis—RBCs and WBCs indicative of infection
  (2) Urine culture—positive for specific pathogen; indicative of urinary infection
  (3) Creatinine/BUN—elevated if renal insufficiency is apparent

d. Abnormal diagnostic tests
  (1) Urodynamics—voiding abnormalities
  (2) Prostatic ultrasound—enlargement of gland; can differentiate between benign and malignant glands
  (3) Cystoscopy—visualization of urethra and bladder for decreased urethra size and bladder changes consistent with an obstructive disorder

6. Expected medical interventions
  a. Indwelling catheterization allows for urinary drainage in the face of retention; may need to be long-term or repeated
  b. Pharmacologic interventions—antiandrogen agents, alpha adrenergic blocking drugs to decrease size of gland
  c. Surgical interventions—approach is dependant on the size of gland and condition of client (Figure 10-1)
    (1) Transurethral prostatectomy
    (2) Suprapubic prostatectomy
    (3) Retropubic prostatectomy
    (4) Transurethral incision of the prostate
    (5) Microwave/hyperthermia of the prostate
    (6) Transurethral laser incision of the prostate
    (7) Transurethral balloon dilation (Figure 10-2)

7. Nursing diagnoses
  a. Altered patterns of urinary elimination related to obstruction of flow through urethra
  b. Urinary retention related to obstruction of urethra
  c. Urge incontinence related to obstruction of urethra
  d. Risk for infection related to retention of urine in bladder after voiding

8. Client goals
  a. Client will return to previous urinary elimination pattern
  b. Client will state bladder is emptying completely

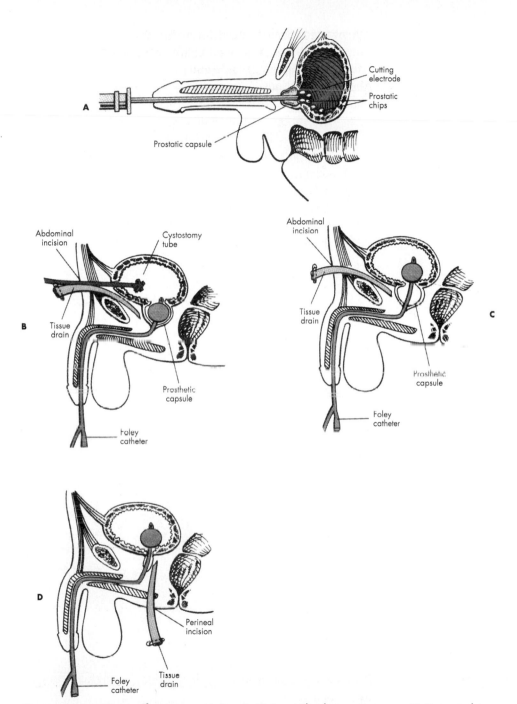

Figure 10-1. Types of prostatectomies. **A,** Transurethral prostatectomy. **B,** Suprapubic prostatectomy. **C,** Retropubic prostatectomy. **D,** Radical perineal prostatectomy. (From *AJN/Mosby Nursing board review,* ed 9, St Louis, 1994, Mosby.)

c. Client will report incidence of urge incontinence gone
d. Client will no longer exhibit factors associated with UTI (fever, burning, urgency, frequency)
9. Nursing interventions
a. Acute care
(1) Encourage 2000 to 3000 ml/day fluid intake to prevent UTI, but limit fluid intake 3 to 4 hours before bed to decrease nocturia
(2) Client may require intermittent catheterization or an indwelling catheter; not uncommon to have a slight resistance from enlarged prostate to catheter insertion; do not force catheter; physician may have to use special catheter

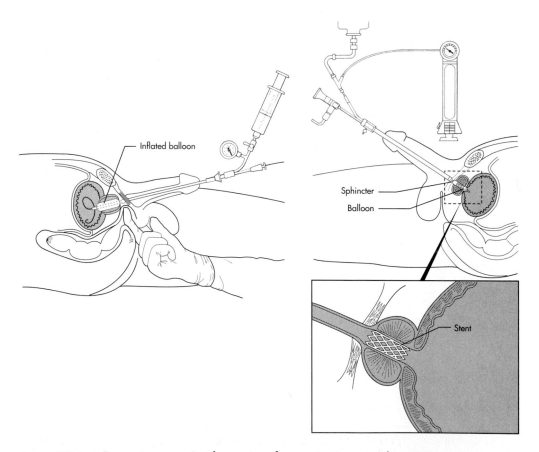

Figure 10-2. Prostatic stent. **A,** Placement of stent. **B,** Stent in place increases prostatic urethral lumen. (From Gray: *Genitourinary disorders—Mosby clinical nursing series,* St Louis, 1994, Mosby.)

(3) Assess client carefully after inserting indwelling catheter and draining bladder for shock can occur as a result of rapid blood flow into previously stretched and poorly perfused blood vessels of bladder; drain no more than 1000 cc at a time

(4) Postoperative care—TURP client

    (a) Maintain patency of three-way indwelling urinary catheter (Foley)—continuous bladder irrigation (CBI) with normal saline to maintain urine that is pink and without clots; eventually urine returns to a clear yellow color within 24 to 48 hours (Figure 10-3)

    (b) Maintain traction on the Foley for 24 hours to decrease postoperative bleeding (Figure 10-4); in

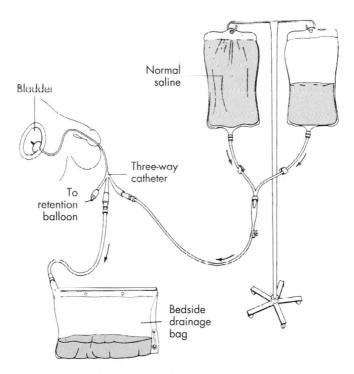

Figure 10-3. Continuous irrigation of the bladder requires a three-way Foley catheter that allows simultaneous infusion and drainage of an irrigating solution (normal saline) through the bladder. The solution is infused rapidly into the bladder, and the bedside drainage bag is assessed for evidence of excessive bleeding and then drained every 1 to 2 hours. (From Gray: *Genitourinary disorders—Mosby's clinical nursing series,* St Louis, 1994, Mosby.)

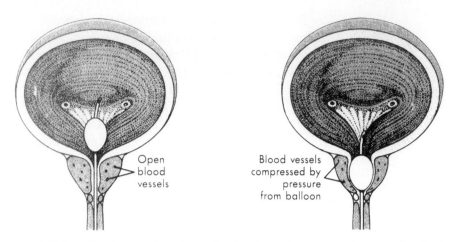

Open blood vessels

Blood vessels compressed by pressure from balloon

Figure 10-4. Gentle traction is maintained against prostatic vascular bed to prevent excessive bleeding following transurethral resection. (From Beare PG and Myers JL: *Principles and practice of adult health nursing,* ed 2, St Louis, 1994, Mosby.)

surgery the Foley will be firmly taped to leg with traction applied by physician before taping

(c) Increase continuous bladder irrigation rate if any signs of increased bleeding or clots; if increased rate does not diminish bleeding or clots, monitor vital signs, validate urinary system is patent, and notify physician

(d) Assess client carefully for TUR syndrome— caused by absorption of normal saline irrigation solution and results in electrolyte imbalance, which leads to bradycardia, hypertension, confusion, vomiting, headache, and tremors

(e) Assess intake and output carefully to ensure that irrigation is draining from the bladder and urine output is adequate

(f) CBI is normally stopped after 24 hours and Foley is removed within 72 hours

(g) Instruct client that dysuria is common after catheter removal; urine will slowly return to normal yellow color in 7 to 10 days after surgery; monitor color of urine carefully for onset of new bleeding and report to physician

   (h) Bladder spasms are common; may be caused by clot obstruction of urinary flow; Belladonna and Opium (B&O) suppositories are helpful

   (i) Pubococcygeal exercises (Kegel) should be started 48 hours after surgery to decrease postoperative dribbling; instruct client to

     (i) Tighten perineal muscles as if trying to stop urine flow

     (ii) Hold tightened muscles for 6 to 10 seconds

     (iii) Repeat exercise four to six times

     (iv) Complete total exercise three to four times per day

 b. Home care regarding client education

  (1) Encourage increase of fluid intake at home 2000 to 3000 ml/day to decrease risk of UTI

  (2) Instruct that after a prostatectomy the client will have retrograde ejaculation that will decrease his fertility yet not affect erection

  (3) Resume sexual activity in 6 to 8 weeks

  (4) Instruct about pubococcygeal exercises (Kegel) for any client with dribbling or incontinence

  (5) Advise that small flecks of burgundy colored "scabs" or clots may be shed 7 to 10 days after catheter removal and then should clear within 24 to 48 hours after onset

10. Evaluation protocol

 a. How do I know that my interventions were effective?

  (1) Is client experiencing any pain?

  (2) Does client know where he is, and the date?

  (3) Assess

   (a) Vital signs within 10% of baseline

   (b) Pink urine, no clots

   (c) Fluid in drainage bag exceeds amount of irrigation—difference is true urine output

 b. What criteria will I use to change my interventions?

  (1) Vital signs not within 10% of baseline

  (2) Bloody urine with clots

  (3) Increase in bladder spasms

  (4) Drainage bag output less than irrigation intake

    c. How will I know that my client teaching has been effective?
      (1) Client states fluid intake is approximately 1500 ml/day
      (2) Client reports pubococcygeal exercises are improving continence
      (3) Client states they will not have sexual intercourse for 6 to 8 weeks after surgery

11. Older adult alert
    a. It may be difficult to identify TUR syndrome in older adults, because symptoms may be confused with anesthesia changes or confusion changes that could be considered normal in older adults
    b. Continue to reassure clients that incontinence can be controlled with continued exercise and does not have to be a part of their lives forever

B. Prostate cancer
1. Definition—malignancy of the prostate gland
2. Etiology—exact cause unknown; prevailing theories include genetic tendency, multiple sexual partners, high fat consumption, chemical exposure, history of gonorrhea —virus
3. Incidence—most common type of cancer in the male population; Black population has the highest incidence
4. Assessment
    a. Ask the following questions
      (1) Do you have any rectal pressure?
      (2) Do you have any pain? Where?
      (3) Have you experienced painful ejaculation?
    b. Clinical manifestations
      (1) May be asymptomatic unless BPH is also present
      (2) May have no symptoms until symptoms of metastasis occur—hip or back pain
      (3) Rectal pressure may occur
      (4) Painful ejaculation may occur
    c. Abnormal laboratory findings
      (1) Acid phosphatase elevated
      (2) Alkaline phosphatase elevated
      (3) Prostatic specific antigen (PSA) elevated
    d. Abnormal diagnostic tests
      (1) Digital rectal exam—hard nodule
      (2) Transrectal ultrasound—best test for early detection; identifies tumors twice as often as rectal exams
      (3) Radionuclide imaging—bone metastasis

5. Expected medical interventions
   a. Radiation therapy with external beam and/or irradiated seeds
   b. Radical prostatectomy via retropubic or perineal approach (see Figure 10-1, pp. 323)
   c. Exogenous hormones
   d. Bilateral orchiectomy to remove androgens required by tumor to grow
   e. TURP is palliative
6. Nursing diagnoses
   a. Altered patterns of urinary elimination related to urethral obstruction
   b. Sexual dysfunction related to surgical disruption of nerves necessary for erection or related to hormonal administration
   c. Stress incontinence related to effects of prostate surgery
   d. Chronic pain related to bone metastasis
   e. Anxiety/fear related to beliefs about diagnosis of cancer
7. Client goals
   a. Client will report normal urinary elimination pattern
   b. Client will state use of alternative methods of sexual expression
   c. Client will reduce incontinence to two episodes per day
   d. Client will state pain is at a tolerable level
   e. Client will state a decrease in anxiety/fear
8. Nursing interventions
   a. Acute care
      (1) Preoperative—radical prostatectomy
         (a) Teaching regarding turning, coughing, deep breathing, incentive spirometer every 2 hours
         (b) Leg exercises every 1 to 2 hours while in bed
         (c) Urethral catheter in place for 10 to 24 days
         (d) Bowel preparation—usually enemas until clear; Go-Lytely induces rapid cleansing of bowel; followed by Neomycin for sterilization of bowel
         (e) Reinforce teaching regarding the possibility of postoperative impotence and infertility
      (2) Postoperative—radical prostatectomy
         (a) Vital signs
         (b) Monitor indwelling urinary catheter for bloody drainage and patency
         (c) Dressing for bleeding, drainage

              (d)   Pain medication as needed

              (e)   No foreign objects in rectum for at least 5 days or until the anastomosis between the bladder and urethra heals

        (3)   Radiotherapy therapy

              (a)   Diarrhea may occur so client must increase fluid intake to prevent dehydration

              (b)   Avoid fatty foods

        (4)   Hormonal therapy

              (a)   Discuss strategies for client and significant other to cope with impotence and fertility if that is of concern

              (b)   Take hormones with food to prevent nausea

              (c)   Thromboembolism is a risk and client must be instructed about symptoms of which physicians should be notified

    b. Home care regarding client education

        (1)   Available information for alternatives for sexual expression if dysfunction has not disappeared after 12 months

        (2)   Urinary dysfunction that has not disappeared after 12 months should be brought to the attention of the urologist; medications may help in the interim

        (3)   Chronic pain (Table 10-2)

              (a)   Eliminate activities that exacerbate pain; effective way to treat chronic pain is to prevent it if possible

              (b)   Identify realistic goals for client and have significant other assist with reorganizing activities so goals can be met

Table 10-2. Characteristics of Acute and Chronic Pain

Acute	Chronic*
Short duration	Lasts more than several months (usually 5 to 6)
Usually well-defined cause	May or may not be well defined
Decreases with healing	Begins gradually and persists
Reversible	Exhausting and useless
Mild to severe	Mild to severe
May be accompanied by anxiety	May be accompanied by depression and fatigue

*Chronic malignant, chronic nonmalignant, and chronic intermittent pain.

        (c) Work with physician to find acceptable pain medication that is effective

        (d) Refer client to support group or community agency

9. Evaluation protocol

  a. How do I know that my interventions were effective?

    (1) Has client's pain decreased or been relieved?

    (2) Does client remember how long the catheter will stay in place?

    (3) Has client increased fluid intake?

    (4) Objective assessment

      (a) Vital signs stable within 10% of baseline

      (b) Urinary drainage pink without clots

      (c) Dressing dry and intact

  b. What criteria will I use to change my interventions?

    (1) Unrelieved pain

    (2) Client unaware time catheter will be indwelling

    (3) Vital signs unstable, or not within 10% of baseline

    (4) Urine bloody with clots

  c. How will I know that my client teaching has been effective?

    (1) Client states the finding of alternative methods of sexual expression with significant other

    (2) Client indicates regular performing of pubococcygeal exercises as ordered and incontinence is decreasing in incidence

    (3) Client states chronic pain is tolerable and activities are adjusted as needed

10. Older adult alert

  a. Older adults are the population most likely affected by this illness; careful screening must be encouraged in this age group

  b. Bone metastasis is very likely in clients with prostate carcinoma. Older adults should be evaluated for ambulatory stability as a result of the risk of falling and fractures.

  c. Homes of older adult clients must be evaluated for potential causes of falls, such as the use of throw rugs in the home, poor lighting, uneven steps

C. **Testicular cancer**

1. Definition—malignancy of the testes

2. Pathophysiology—testicular cancer arises from two components of the testes: germ cells that line the seminiferous tubules and those that originate from nongerm cells

3. Etiology—unknown; factors that may contribute are testicular atrophy, failure of testes to descend, and scrotal trauma

4. Incidence—second most common cancer in the male population; manifests between the ages of 20 and 35 years of age

5. Assessment
   a. Ask the following questions
      (1) Have you noticed an increase in the size of your scrotum?
      (2) Have you noticed a full or heavy sensation in your scrotum?
      (3) Have you noticed an increase in the size of your breasts?
   b. Clinical manifestations
      (1) Testicular enlargement, unilateral or bilateral
      (2) A feeling of scrotal fullness, heaviness
      (3) Gynecomastia—enlarged, painful breasts
      (4) Hardness of testes or lumps on palpation; normally testes feel spongy on palpation
   c. Abnormal laboratory findings
      (1) Serum alpha-fetoprotein (AFP) elevated
      (2) Serum beta human chorionic gonadotropin elevated
      (3) Serum LDH elevated
   d. Abnormal diagnostic tests
      (1) Testicular ultrasound—positive for tumor
      (2) Abdominal CT scan—nodal metastasis

6. Expected medical interventions
   a. Orchiectomy and lymph node dissection if lymph nodes are involved; prosthetic testes may be implanted
   b. Radiotherapy and chemotherapy if a tumor of the retroperitoneum is identified

7. Nursing diagnoses
   a. Pain related to stretching of scrotal sac and nerve pressure secondary to testicular tumor, or pain related to effects of surgery
   b. Body-image disturbance related to changes in sexuality secondary to surgery
   c. Sexual dysfunction related to effects of surgery
   d. Anxiety related to beliefs about diagnosis of cancer

8. Client goals
   a. Client will state pain is relieved or decreased
   b. Client will state feeling comfortable with bodily changes

      c. Client will state finding other ways of sexual expression

      d. Client will state anxiety is under control

9. Nursing interventions

    a. Acute care

      (1) Postoperative

        (a) Evaluate vital signs every 1 to 4 hours as client progresses postoperatively

        (b) Check dressing over scrotal wound or over abdomen if there is lymph node dissection with every set of vital signs

        (c) Evaluate urine output; call physician for <30 ml/hr

        (d) Maintain scrotal support to decrease edema

        (e) Pain medication as needed

    b. Home care regarding client education

      (1) Remind client of correct technique for monthly self-testicular exam for remaining testicle

      (2) Information about what would be seen in the face of wound infection

      (3) If chemotherapy or radiation therapy is used, the client may have decreased sperm counts; following therapy, counts may return to normal; alternative fertilization techniques can be considered

      (4) Referral to support group or community agency

10. Evaluation protocol

    a. How do I know that my interventions were effective?

      (1) Client states pain is decreased or relieved

      (2) Vital signs are stable within ±10% baseline

      (3) Urine output is at an acceptable level

    b. What criteria will I use to change my interventions?

      (1) Pain is unrelieved or increased

      (2) Unstable vital signs not within ± 10% baseline

      (3) Inadequate urine output

    c. How will I know that my client teaching has been effective?

      (1) Client demonstrates correct technique for self-testicular exam

      (2) Client describes what a wound infection would look like

      (3) Client describes alternate techniques for fertilization to be used if needed

11. Older adult alert

    a. Testicular cancer is rare in the older adult. If suspicious symptoms occur, evaluation should be completed.

Unfortunately when testicular tumors do occur in the older adult they are almost always malignant.

b. Scrotal enlargement in the older adult is more often due to hydrocele, spermatocele, varicocele, or hernia

D. **Cancer of the cervix**

1. Definition—a malignancy of the cervix
2. Pathophysiology—usually squamous cell type; spreads by direct extension or through the lymphatic system; metastasis to the liver, bones, and mediastinal nodes
3. Etiology—a major risk factor is intercourse at an early age; also multiple sexual partners, sexually transmitted diseases, pregnancies at an early age, and smoking
4. Incidence—seen more commonly in women of low socioeconomic status
5. Assessment
   a. Ask the following questions
      (1) Have you noticed any unusual bleeding from the vaginal canal?
      (2) Do you ever notice bleeding after intercourse?
      (3) Have you noticed pain in your back, legs, or groin?
      (4) Have you had difficulty voiding?
   b. Clinical manifestations
      (1) Abnormal vaginal bleeding
      (2) Bleeding after intercourse
      (3) Unusual vaginal odor or brownish discharge in between periods
      (4) Pain in the back, legs, or groin
      (5) Difficulty voiding
   c. Abnormal laboratory findings
      (1) CBC—anemia
      (2) Pap smear—abnormal cells of the cervix
   d. Abnormal diagnostic tests
      (1) Colposcopy—visualization of tumor or cells
      (2) CT scan of the abdomen—identification of tumor and the size
      (3) MRI scan of the abdomen—identification of tumor size and location
6. Expected medical interventions
   a. Treatment will depend on the stage of the cancer
   b. In the early stage, cryosurgery, electrocautery, laser surgery, and conization can be utilized for cancer

    c. Hysterectomy is used for those clients not wishing to have more children

    d. For more extensive cancers, radical hysterectomy with pelvic lymphadenectomy

    e. Ovaries will be removed if determined to be necessary at the time of surgery

    f. External radiation and intracavitary radiation can be used at some stages

    g. Pelvic exenteration used if radiation therapy has failed, includes removal of perineum, pelvic floor, levator muscles, all reproductive organs, lymph nodes, rectum, distal sigmoid colon, distal ureters; colostomy and urinary conduit are created

7. Nursing diagnoses

    a. Anxiety/fear related to beliefs about diagnosis of cancer

    b. Pain related to effects of surgery or to effects of the cervical tumor

    c. Fatigue related to anemia, anorexia

    d. Impaired skin integrity related to abnormal vaginal discharge

8. Client goals

    a. Client will state fear or anxiety is decreased to a manageable level

    b. Client will state pain has deceased or is gone

    c. Client will state fatigue is diminishing

    d. Client will exhibit a perineal area that is clear and free of breakdown

9. Nursing interventions

    a. Acute care

        (1) Postoperative care (interventions for every client having surgery)

            (a) Vital signs (normal routine: every 15 min × 4, every 30 min × 4, every hour × 4, every 2 hours × 4, then every 4 hours)

            (b) Dressing checked with every check of vital signs

            (c) Maintain IV rate as per physician order

            (d) Monitor urine output for a minimum of 30 ml/hr

            (e) Monitor NG drainage if present, amount, and color; irrigate PRN q 2 to 4 hours with 30 ml normal saline

            (f) Monitor pain and medicate as needed; if using a patient controlled analgesia (PCA) pump,

evaluate effectiveness of medication as
well as respiratory rate for depression; if
using a continuous epidural infusion pump,
evaluate respiratory rate every hour with
vital signs and urine output and lower
extremities for sensation, strength, and
movement

    (g) Turn, cough, deep breathe, and incentive
spirometer every 2 hours

    (h) Leg exercises every 1 to 2 hours

    (i) Ambulate as soon as ordered by physician

b. Home care regarding client education

    (1) Encouragment to keep follow-up appointments with
physician

    (2) Information on how to balance rest and activity until
strength has returned

    (3) Need for increased fluid intake at home to prevent
urinary stasis—at least 2000 to 3000 ml/day

    (4) Referral to support groups and sexual counseling to
improve self-image

10. Evaluation protocol

a. How do I know that my interventions were effective?

    (1) Vital signs within 10% of baseline

    (2) Dressing is dry and intact

    (3) Urine output is at optimal level with I=0 ±300 ml

    (4) Client states pain is decreased or relieved

    (5) Client is turning, coughing, and deep breathing,
using incentive spirometer, and ambulating without
difficulty

b. What criteria will I use to change my interventions?

    (1) Vital signs not within 10% of baseline

    (2) Bleeding noted on dressings

    (3) Decreased urine output; intake differs from output
by ±300 ml

    (4) Pain is increased or not relieved

    (5) Client is reluctant to turn, cough, and deep breathe
or ambulate, and lung sounds are decreased in the
bases

c. How will I know that my client teaching has been effective?

    (1) Client attends appointment with physician
for follow-up

    (2) Client reports drinking 2000 ml/day of fluid

         (3)   Client reports taking a 30 minute nap in the morning and afternoon, which results in the feeling of being stronger

         (4)   Client has contacted the American Cancer Society to locate a support group

  11.   Older adult alert

      a. The fatigue associated with the anemia in this disorder will be poorly tolerated by the older adult client because of the decreased stamina. Nursing interventions may require alterations, i.e., change in activities of daily living to include rest periods between activites, and moving the client to an area of the house where there are no steps.

      b. If extensive surgery is required for an older adult client, careful medical workup will have to be completed before surgery to determine the client's ability to withstand the surgery

E. Endometrial cancer

  1.   Definition—malignancy of the endometrium of the uterus

  2.   Pathophysiology—most are adenocarcinomas; metastasis is usually to the pelvic and periaortic nodes

  3.   Etiology—many risk factors are acknowledged: obesity, nulliparity, late menopause, use of estrogen therapy

  4.   Incidence—found most frequently in postmenopausal women; early diagnosis has significantly decreased the mortality rate

  5.   Assessment

      a. Ask the following questions

         (1)   Since menopause has started and you have stopped having periods, have you had any vaginal bleeding?

         (2)   Have you noticed any unusual pain?

      b. Clinical manifestations

         (1)   Postmenopausal bleeding

         (2)   Pain in the lumbar area, hypogastric area, or pelvic area

      c. Abnormal laboratory findings—Pap may show malignant cells

      d. Abnormal diagnostic tests—endometrial biopsy shows malignancy

  6.   Expected medical interventions

      a. Total abdominal hysterectomy with bilateral salpingo-oophorectomy; pelvic and periaortic lymph node biopsies

      b. Preoperative intracavitary radiation (Figure 10-5)

      c. Postoperative external radiation

      d. Chemotherapy

  7. Nursing diagnoses

      a. Pain related to pressure from tumor or related to effects of surgery

      b. Fear/anxiety related to beliefs about diagnosis of cancer

      c. Body-image disturbance related to need for gynecologic surgery and/or need for surgery on a sexual organ

  8. Client goals

      a. Client will state pain is decreased or relieved

      b. Client will state fear/anxiety is decreased and manageable

      c. Client will identify two ways to cope with changes in sexuality

  9. Nursing interventions

      a. Acute care

          (1) See postoperative care guidelines under Nursing Interventions of the client with cervical cancer p. 335

          (2) Care of client with intracavitary radiation—(see Figure 10-5)

              (a) Must be in private room

              (b) Nurse keeps toward head of bed during care to reduce exposure to radiation

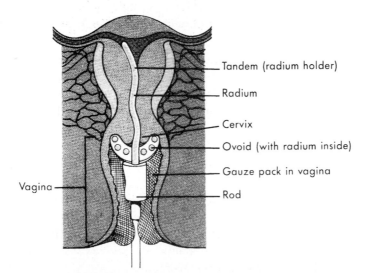

Figure 10-5. Intracavity irradiation of cervix for treatment of cervical cancer. (From Beare PG and Myers JL: *Principles and practice of adult health nursing,* ed 2, St Louis, 1994, Mosby.)

           (c) Visitors limited to 30 minutes

           (d) No children or pregnant women allowed in room

           (e) Client on absolute bedrest

           (f) May logroll and have head of bed elevated no > 45 degrees

           (g) Encourage deep breathing, coughing, incentive spirometer, and leg exercises at least every 2 hours

           (h) Urinary catheter in place and patent

           (i) Assess for temperature elevation, nausea, and vomiting; may be indicative of uterine perforation or infection

           (j) Report profuse vaginal drainage to physician immediately

           (k) Sexual activity can resume 1 week after therapy

           (l) Vaginal lubricant may be needed due to dryness of vagina from effects of therapy

           (m) Vaginal dilator may be required due to scarring from therapy

    b. Home care regarding client education

       (1) Postoperative teaching—diet, fluid, activity, and physician follow-up

       (2) Postintracavitary radiation

           (a) Fatigue is common; take frequent rest periods of 30 minutes every 2 hours

           (b) Diarrhea is a common postprocedural occurrence; follow a low-fiber diet to decrease symptoms

           (c) Report excessive nausea, vomiting, diarrhea, difficulty urinating, prolonged back or abdominal pain

           (d) Showers are preferred to tub baths because of the expected increase in vaginal discharge

10. Evaluation protocol

    a. How do I know that my interventions were effective?

       (1) Client has not developed complications of bed rest while undergoing intracavitary radiation (DVT, atelectasis)

       (2) Postoperative client demonstrates vital signs that are within 10% of baseline, with no bleeding

       (3) Postoperative pain is controlled

b. What criteria will I use to change my interventions?
    (1) Client develops DVT or atelectasis
    (2) Postoperative client has unstable vital signs or bleeding
    (3) Postoperative pain is increased or not relieved
c. How will I know that my client teaching has been effective?
    (1) Client is resting in the morning and afternoon, and has increased stamina and overall activity
    (2) Client has kept the follow-up appointments
    (3) Client uses a water-soluble lubricant for intercourse

11. Older adult alert
    a. This is a disorder most commonly seen in the older adult client. Careful assessment of the female client for findings associated with this illness is imperative.
    b. An older adult client who must have intracavitary radiation is at very high risk for complications, such as deep vein thrombosis, atelectasis, and pneumonia associated with bed rest. This client must be monitored carefully.
    c. An older adult client undergoing intracavitary radiation must also be monitored carefully for the development of fistulas

F. Ovarian cancer
    1. Definition—malignancy of the ovary
    2. Pathophysiology—risk factors are ovarian dysfunction and infertility; most are epithelial tumors; metastasis is through seeding and implantation; common sites are peritoneum, omentum, and bowel
    3. Etiology—unknown; however, there does seem to be a familial tendency for the disorder
    4. Incidence—seen in all age groups; most common in the white population
    5. Assessment
        a. Ask the following questions
            (1) Have you experienced abdominal or pelvic pain?
            (2) Have you been experiencing unusual vaginal bleeding?
            (3) Have you had any gastrointestinal complaints?
            (4) Have you noticed any changes in urinary function or any unusual symptoms with urination?
        b. Clinical manifestations
            (1) Manifestations are most often seen in advanced cases, making early treatment very difficult
            (2) Ascites

        (3) Pelvic or abdominal pain

        (4) Abnormal uterine bleeding

        (5) Persistent gastrointestinal complaints

        (6) Urinary complaints

  c. Abnormal laboratory findings—cancer antigen 125 (CA-125) elevated

  d. Abnormal diagnostic tests

        (1) Bimanual exam—palpation of the ovaries in postmenopausal women is abnormal; any ovarian mass should be considered suspicious

        (2) Ultrasonography—identification of a mass, or enlarged ovaries

6. Expected medical interventions

  a. Total abdominal hysterectomy with bilateral salpingo-oophorectomy and omentectomy as soon as diagnostic workup is completed

  b. Radiation and chemotherapy may follow surgery; intraperitoneal and systemic chemotherapy may be done

7. Care of this client will be very much the same as the client with endometrial cancer and cervical cancer; please refer to those nursing interventions and evaluations

G. **Breast cancer**

1. Definition—malignancy of the female or male breast

2. Etiology—familial tendency; history of fibrocystic disease; hormonal influence

3. Incidence—breast cancer is now the second leading cause of cancer deaths in women; it is rare in men

4. Assessment

  a. Ask the following questions

        (1) Has your mother or a sister ever been diagnosed with breast cancer?

        (2) Do you routinely do self-breast exam? When in relation to your periods?

        (3) Do you have mammographies? How often?

        (4) Did you find this lump during self-breast exam?

  b. Clinical manifestations

        (1) Single lump or thickening on one breast—earliest finding

        (2) Painless lump

        (3) Lump is irregular and nonmobile

        (4) Nipple discharge

        (5) Skin dimpling on the breast

               (6)   Change in breast shape

               (7)   Skin ulcerations (late finding)

      c. Abnormal diagnostic tests

               (1)   Mammography—defined mass with size and shape

               (2)   Biopsy—identification of malignant or benign cells

5. Expected medical interventions

    a. Lumpectomy—removal of tumor with surrounding healthy tissue

    b. Mastectomy

             (1)   Subcutaneous—removal of breast tissue; leaving skin and nipple intact

             (2)   Modified radical—breast and axillary lymph nodes removed

             (3)   Radical—breast, pectoral muscles, and axillary nodes removed

             (4)   Simple—breast removed

             (5)   Quadrantectomy—quadrant of breast is removed that houses the lesion

             (6)   Breast reconstruction is done with initial surgery in many cases

    c. Radiation therapy—internal implants or external radiation

    d. Chemotherapy

6. Nursing Diagnosis

    a. Body-image disturbance related to surgical changes in the breast

    b. Impaired skin integrity related to the effects of radiation therapy

    c. Impaired physical mobility related to acute pain following surgery extending into the axilla

    d. Pain related to pressure from tumor or to effects of surgery

    e. Fear/anxiety related to beliefs about the diagnosis of cancer

    f. Altered nutrition—less than body needs related to anorexia, nausea, and vomiting caused by chemotherapy

7. Client goals

    a. Client will state feeling comfortable with the new body image that is going to occur

    b. Client will maintain clean, dry, intact skin in association with radiation therapy

    c. Client will be able to have full, active range of motion of affected arm

        d. Client will indicate pain is decreased or gone

        e. Client will state fear or anxiety has decreased to a manageable level

        f. Client will maintain present body weight or not lose >½ lb/wk

8. Nursing interventions

    a. Acute care

        (1) Postoperative care

            (a) Usual postoperative care is maintained

            (b) Drains, continuous portable suction devices, usually present—empty when half full or every 8 hours, whichever occurs first

            (c) Elevate and abduct affected arm above level of heart when sitting or lying

            (d) Begin arm exercises as soon as client is awake enough to cooperate

                (i) Wall-walking with finger tips—up wall so arm extends above head

                (ii) Squeezing a ball

            (e) After drains are removed begin full range of motion exercises to the affected arm

            (f) Give pain medication as needed to ensure appropriate exercise regime

        (2) Have Reach for Recovery see client while in the hospital—this is usually a volunteer group from the American Cancer Society, commonly made up of women who have experienced breast cancer and can assist the client in postoperative adjustment as well as offer a temporary prosthesis to wear home

    b. Home care regarding client education

        (1) Needed care required of arm on surgical side

            (a) Avoid burn, insect bites, cuts, scrapes, and scratches if there was a loss of lymph nodes in the axilla; the greater the number of nodes removed the greater the risk for infection

            (b) Avoid procedures on the arm; such as blood pressures, injections, or blood drawing from affected arm

            (c) Need to carry heavy objects in nonaffected arm; usually at three weeks light parcels of <5 lb are allowed to be carried, and driving is permitted

            (d) Wear a medic alert bracelet to inform caregivers of disorder

9. Evaluation protocol
   a. How will I know that my interventions were effective?
      (1) Client indicates pain is decreased or tolerable
      (2) Affected arm does not become edematous
      (3) Client is able to perform assisted active range of motion exercises effectively
   b. What criteria will I use to change my interventions?
      (1) Affected arm becomes edematous
      (2) Client's pain is increased or unrelieved
      (3) Client is unable to perform assisted active range of motion exercises
   c. How will I know that my client teaching has been effective?
      (1) Client wears medical alert bracelet
      (2) Client carries packages on unaffected side
      (3) Client protects affected arm from trauma or from exposure to infection
10. Older adult alert—treatment plan for the older adult client may be modified to only hormonal manipulation and/or radiation therapy if the client cannot tolerate surgery

REVIEW QUESTIONS

1. While caring for a client who had a transurethral resection of the prostate (TURP), the nurse understands that the urinary catheter is pulled tight and taped to the leg to
   a. Prevent bladder spasms
   b. Encourage compression of the prostate and further dilate the urethra
   c. Decrease the incidence of postoperative bleeding
   d. Prevent edema in the prostate

2. A client asks why his bladder must be continuously irrigated. The best reply by the nurse is
   a. "The irrigation keeps your urine clear"
   b. "The irrigation clears any clots and blood out of your bladder"
   c. "The continuous saline drip decreases swelling in the area of the surgery"
   d. "The normal saline increases your urine output"

3. An important teaching need of the postoperative TURP client is
   a. Wound care
   b. Catheter care
   c. Pubococcygeal exercises
   d. Fluid restriction

4. When assessing a client with prostate cancer who has suffered with metastasis to the bones for over 4 months, the nurse would expect to see what kind of assessment findings indicative of pain?
   a. Facial grimacing
   b. No physical symptoms
   c. Clenched fists
   d. Fetal position

5. A clinical manifestation associated with testicular cancer is
   a. Anemia
   b. Impotence
   c. Scrotal pain
   d. Gynecomastia

6. A common problem reported by clients following intracavitary radiation therapy is
   a. Difficulty swallowing
   b. Diarrhea
   c. Hair loss
   d. Hearing loss

7. A friend asks a nurse about her risk of having ovarian cancer, since she just lost her mother to ovarian cancer. The nurse's best response would be
   a. The cause of ovarian cancer is unknown, so that risk is also unclear
   b. Ovarian cancer is so difficult to identify in the early stages that physicians are unsure of what risks might be associated with the illness
   c. There is a familial tendency for ovarian cancer; so having a complete gynecologic examination would be wise
   d. There is no known link to family heredity in ovarian cancer

8. The nurse knows that a client has grasped the concept of arm exercises following a modified radical mastectomy when the client says she will
   a. Wear her sling all the time until her incision is healed
   b. Perform wall-walking exercises with her fingertips above her head every 2 to 4 hours following pain medication
   c. Exercise only her wrist until she is at home
   d. Limit her exercising to only her bath, and only those parts that she can reach

9. The nurse explains to a client that the reason the client must not have injections, blood pressures, or venipunctures in the affected arm following a modified radical mastectomy is
   a. The lymph glands have been removed from the axilla. Lymph drainage from the arm is seriously impeded and may make the arm extremely edematous with nonabsorption of any medication if any of those procedures would occur
   b. There is an incision in the axilla that must heal before any of those procedures can be performed due to possible impaired healing of the incision
   c. Pressure from the tourniquet for venipuncture and increased fluid load from injections can impede healing of the mastectomy scar
   d. Blood pooling from the surgery makes veins impossible to find on the affected arm and injections impossible to absorb

10. When positioning a client immediately postoperatively, following a lumpectomy, the nurse would use which position?
    a. Supine with affected arm elevated on a pillow, above the level of the heart
    b. Side-lying, nonsurgical side only with affected arm elevated above the level of the heart
    c. Low fowlers with affected arm elevated on two pillows, above the level of the heart
    d. Whatever position is comfortable for the client

ANSWERS, RATIONALES, AND TEST-TAKING TIPS

Rationales	Test-Taking Tips

1. Correct answer: c

The urinary catheter is pulled tight for traction to put direct pressure on the surgical site of the prostate. This decreases bleeding. The large 30 cc balloon causes bladder spasms. Remember that the prostate is one of the more vascular areas of the body; a TURP removal is by pieces so a small piece could be retained and then bleed post-op.

The key word in the stem is "tight"; associate this with the prevention of bleeding. The key word in responses *b* and *d* is "prostate"; it has been removed; thus these are incorrect responses.

2. Correct answer: b

Continuous bladder irrigation is initiated after a TURP to flush blood and clots out of the bladder and ensure free draining urine. Answer *a* is not as clear or specific as answer *b*.

The question asks about irrigation; therefore the responses can be narrowed to responses *a* or *b*. The concept of irrigation means "to remove." Responses *c* and *d* are incorrect statements; the irrigation increases output— not urine output!

3. Correct answer: c

The postoperative TURP client must be taught how to perform pubococcygeal exercises so that urinary control can be achieved as quickly as possible after catheter removal.

Key word is "TURP"— transurethral means "through urethra"; no wound is present. The catheter is removed in 2 to 3 days— clients don't need to know about catheter care. In renal or urinary systems fluids are given to flush; the only exception not to give fluids is in renal or heart "failure."

4. **Correct answer: b**

   A client who has suffered pain for that length of time typically will not show physical evidence of pain. The physical evidence will be controlled by the client.

   The time element is important here—chronic pain is best assessed by client complaints and not physical findings; think of a "chronic complainer."

5. **Correct answer: d**

   Gynecomastia quite frequently accompanies the diagnosis of testicular cancer since tumors may produce hormones or result in a decrease in normal hormone production. Anemia can be a result of cancer therapy. Impotence would more likely result from surgery or the change in mental thoughts of the client.

   Associate that tumors may produce or inhibit hormonal production and the only response with indication of a hormonal finding is *d*. Pain is generally not present; rather a complaint of feelings of heaviness or fullness in the scrotal sac is most common.

6. **Correct answer: b**

   Diarrhea is a postintracavitary radiation therapy problem that must be treated to prevent dehydration.

   Key word in the stem is "common." Think anatomy—this radiation is for the uterus and the only response that is anatomically close in response is diarrhea—the bowel. Another approach is to cluster responses *a, c,* and *d* to be anatomically at the top of the body and diarrhea is at the middle of the body; since it stands alone it is the correct response.

7. **Correct answer: c**

   There is a familial tendency for ovarian cancer.

   Cluster the common themes in the responses *a, b,* and *d*—key words: "unknown," "difficult to identify . . . unsure" and "no known link." Response *c* is left and it gives specific information.

8. **Correct answer: b**

   Wall-walking exercises using fingertips, walking fingers above the head are appropriate exercises for this client. Every 2 to 4 hours would be appropriate, following PRN pain medication.

   Response *b* has the most specific information as a response. Cluster the other responses since they have those absolute words in them—response *a* "all the time," responses *c* and *d* "only." Responses with absolutes are usually incorrect choices.

9. **Correct answer: a**

   Removal of the lymph glands from the axilla will prevent lymph drainage from the affected arm. Blood pressure readings, venipunctures, or injections will further prevent lymph drainage out of the arm.

   Remember modified radical = removal of lymph nodes and breast tissue. Match this fact with the key word "removed" in response *a*.

10. **Correct answer: d**

    Lumpectomy does not involve removal of lymph nodes from the axilla, so arm positioning is not crucial. Position of comfort is best.

    Cluster the responses *a, b, c* under the category of very specific information. Response *d* must be correct since it is very general information. Also remember "lumpectomy = lymph still intact."

The Endocrine System

STUDY OUTCOMES

After completing this chapter, the reader will be able to do the following:

▼ Describe the complex structure and function of the endocrine system.

▼ Assess a client with a disorder of one of the endocrine glands using the appropriate technique and sequence.

▼ Identify with implementation of appropriate nursing diagnoses for the client with an endocrine disorder.

▼ Evaluate the outcomes of the client with an endocrine disorder for the purpose of change in the interventions currently in use.

KEY TERMS

Diurnal	A pattern of rise and fall of hormone levels in the blood, within a 24-hour time period.
Endocrine glands	Secrete their hormones directly into the blood stream or lymph system.
Exocrine glands	Secrete their hormones through a duct into the GI tract.
Hormone	Chemical agent secreted by the endocrine glands into the blood, responsible for eliciting a response from a target organ or structure.
Negative feedback	A method the body uses to bring the hormone to an appropriate level, but not to allow it to rise to an unacceptable level (Figure 11-1).
Target gland	Glands affected by the action of a hormone from another gland.

CONTENT REVIEW

I. **The endocrine system in association with the nervous system is responsible for controlling homeostasis in the body**

II. **Structure and function (Table 11-1 and Figure 11-2)**

III. **Targeted concerns**
   A. Pharmacology—priority drug classifications
      1. Hormones—synthetic or naturally occurring substances used to treat hypoactive states of the various endocrine organs
         a. Expected effect—replacement of insufficient hormones
         b. Commonly given drugs
            (1) Insulin (Table 11-2, p. 358)
            (2) Glucagon
            (3) Adrenocorticotropic
               (a) Corticotropin (ACTH)
               (b) Cosyntropin (Cortrosyn)
            (4) Androgens
               (a) Testosterone (Histerone)
               (b) Danazol (Danocrine)
            (5) Antidiuretic (ADH)
               (a) Desmopressin (DDAVP)
               (b) Vasopressin (Pitressin)

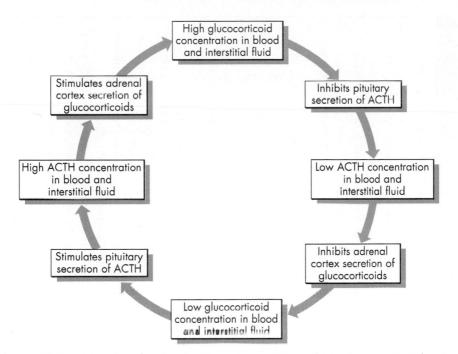

Figure 11-1. Negative feedback. (From Beare PG and Myers JL: *Principles and practice of adult health nursing,* ed 2, St Louis, 1994, Mosby.)

   (6) Estrogens
      (a) Diethylstilbestrol (DES)
      (b) Conjugated estrogens (Premarin)
   (7) Oxytocic—Oxytocin (Pitocin)
   (8) Progestin
      (a) Medroxyprogesterone (Provera)
      (b) Progesterone (Gestrol)
   (9) Thyroid
      (a) Levothyroxine (Synthroid)
      (b) Thyroid (Thyrar)
 c. Nursing considerations
   (1) Client must understand dosage schedule
   (2) Follow-up exams must be emphasized to determine effectiveness of therapy
   (3) Client must be aware of adverse reactions to report to physician
   (4) Dosage cannot be abruptly stopped; need to be tapered
   (5) Brand of medication should be consistent; avoid alternation between brand name and generic medication

Table 11-1. Hormones

Gland	Hormone	Action
Hypothalamus	Releasing hormones	Stimulates release of hormones from pituitary gland
	Inhibiting hormones	Inhibits release of hormones from pituitary gland
Pituitary, anterior lobe	Growth hormone (GH)	Acts directly on bones and other tissues to stimulate growth
	Prolactin (PRL)	Stimulates development of mammary tissue and lactation
	Thyrotropic hormone (TSH)	Stimulates thyroid gland
	Adrenocorticotropic hormone (ACTH)	Stimulates adrenal cortex
	Melanocyte-stimulating hormone (MSH)	Stimulates darkening of the skin
	Luteinizing hormone (LH)	Initiates ovulation and formation of corpus luteum
	Follicle-stimulating hormone (FSH)	Women: stimulates ovarian development of graafian follicle Men: maintains spermatogenesis
Pituitary, posterior lobe	Antidiuretic hormone (ADH, also called vasopresson) (produced in hypothalamus and stored in pituitary)	Facilitates reabsorption of H_2O in the kidneys, vasoconstriction in arterioles
	Oxytocin (also produced in hypothalamus)	Initiates expression of breast milk; stimulates uterine contractions at delivery
Thyroid	Triiodothyronine (T_3) Thyroxine (T_4)	Control body metabolism and influence physical and mental growth; nervous system activity; protein, fat, carbohydrate metabolism; reproduction
	Calcitonin	Lowers serum calcium levels; inhibits bone resorption
Parathyroid	Parathormone (PTH)	Regulates calcium and phosphorus metabolism

Gland	Hormone/Function	Function
Pancreas	Endocrine function Insulin (from beta cells)	Enables glucose to freely enter cells; helps muscle and tissue oxidation of glucose; promotes storage of glycogen
	Glucagon (from alpha cells)	Increases gluconeogenesis in liver
	Exocrine function (digestive enzymes) Amylase Trypsin Lipase	Aids carbohydrate digestion Aids protein digestion Aids fat digestion
Adrenal cortex	Aldosterone: mineralocorticoid	Facilitates reabsorption of NA^+ and elimination of K^+
	Androgens	Responsible for development of secondary sex characteristics
	Cortisol (hydrocortisone): glucocorticoid	Major effect is the conversion of protein to carbohydrate from which the resulting amino acids are converted in the liver to glucose and glycogen; thus, it regulates serum glucose by increasing rate of gluconeogenesis; suppresses the inflammatory and immune response; increases fat mobilization; supports adaption during stressful situations
Adrenal medulla	Epinephrine Norepinephrine	Initiates stress response, ↑ HR, RR, Causes severe vasoconstriction
Ovaries	Estrogen	Responsible for secondary sex characteristics, mammary duct system, growth of graafian follicle in women
	Progesterone	Prepares corpus luteum; maintains pregnancy
Testes	Testosterone	Responsible for secondary sex characteristics, normal reproductive function in men

Modified from *AJN/Mosby Nursing boards review*, ed 9, S: Louis, 1994, Mosby.

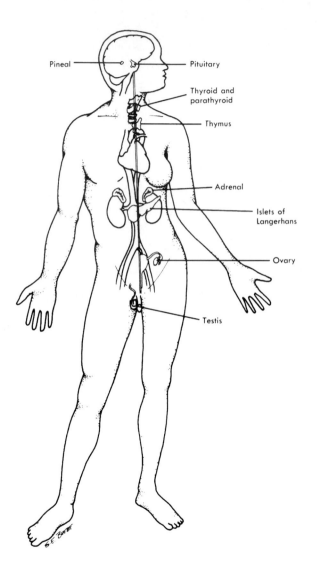

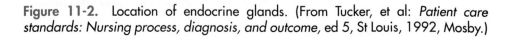

Figure 11-2. Location of endocrine glands. (From Tucker, et al: *Patient care standards: Nursing process, diagnosis, and outcome,* ed 5, St Louis, 1992, Mosby.)

2. Glucocorticoids—used as replacement therapy when client is lacking in glucocorticoids; also used in connection with many other disorders for the immunosuppressive and antiinflammatory action
   a. Expected effects—replacement of hormones; immunosuppression and antiinflammatory
   b. Commonly given drugs
       (1) Cortisone (Cortone)
       (2) Hydrocortisone (Solu-Cortef)
       (3) Methylprednisolone (Medrol)
       (4) Prednisolone (Predalone)
       (5) Prednisone (Deltasone)
       (6) Dexamethasone (Decadron)
       (7) Beclomethasone (Vanceril)
   c. Nursing considerations
       (1) Medication must be taken with meals to prevent gastric ulcers
       (2) Client must never skip a dose or stop taking medication—adrenal crisis may be the result: severe hypotension, sinus tachycardia, and tachypnea
       (3) Instruct client to report any sudden weight gain—black-tarry stools, edema, infections or increased thirst
       (4) Wear a medic-alert bracelet indicating that the medication is taken
   d. Common side effects
       (1) Hyperglycemia
       (2) Weight gain, moon face from sodium and fluid retention, edema
       (3) Mood swings
       (4) Increased frequency of infections or colds
       (5) High risk of hypokalemia
3. Hypoglycemic agents (Table 11-2)
   a. Expected effect—to modulate serum glucose levels
   b. Commonly given drugs
   c. Nursing considerations
   d. Common side effect—hypoglycemia
4. Antithyroid agents—used to treat hyperthyroidism; inhibit formation of thyroid hormone
   a. Expected effect—decrease symptoms of hyperthyroidism
   b. Commonly given drugs
       (1) Potassium iodide (Thro-Block)
       (2) Lugols's solution

Table 11-2. Hypoglycemic Medications

Medication	Onset Hours	Peak Hours	Duration Hours
Rapid Acting Insulins:			
Regular	0.5-1	2-4	6-8
Iletin, zinc suspension	0.5-1	2-8	8-16
Humulin R	0.5-1	1-3	3-5
Semilente	1-3	2-8	12-16
Intermediate Acting Insulins:			
Isophane insulin suspension (NPH)	1-2	6-12	18-26
Insulin zinc suspension (Lente)	1-3	6-12	18-26
Humulin N	1-2	8-12	26-30
Long Acting Insulins:			
Protamine zinc (PZI)	4-6	18-24	28-36
Insulin zinc suspension extented (Ultralente)	4-6	16-24	36
Humulin U	4-6	16-24	24-30
Insulin Mixture			
70% NPH 30% Regular	0.5	2-12	18-24
Oral Hypoglycemic Agents: *First Generation*			
Tolbutamide (Orinase)	1	4-6	6-12
Tolazamide (Tolinase)	1	1-6	12-24
Acetohexamide (Dymelor)	1	3-6	12-24
Chlorpropamide (Diabinese)	1	3-6	24
Oral Hypoglycemic Agents: *Second Generation*			
Glyburide (Micronase, Diabeta)	0.75-1	1.5-3	24
Glipizide (Glucotrol)	0.25-0.5	1-2	24

Nursing Considerations

Assess client carefully for hypoglycemic reactions, especially when starting a new medication or changing dosages

Check for sulfa allergies before administering oral hypoglycemic agents

Regular insulin is the only insulin that can be administered intravenously

Tablets may be crushed if client has difficulty swallowing pills

Make sure client has insulin on board at all times. Check peak and duration times for insulins given to client

Regular insulin should be given 30 minutes before a meal

Blood glucose monitoring should be done 30 minutes to one hour before giving ordered insulin

                (3) SSKI (supersaturated potassium iodide)

                (4) Methimazole (Tapazole)

                (5) Propylthiouracil (PTU)—takes about 3 months to be effective

      c. Nursing considerations

                (1) Warn client to not miss doses—may trigger hyperthyroidism

                (2) Ask client to confer with physician about eliminating foods high in iodine; iodine is needed to manufacture thyroid hormone, however, these clients have too much hormone so by decreasing iodine intake there may be a drop in the amount of thyroid hormone created

                (3) Teach findings of hypothyroidism since medication may destroy too much of the gland

B. Procedures

1. Serum and urinary measurement of hormones will be vital to diagnosing a disorder

2. Radioactive iodine uptake (RAIU)—radioactive iodine administered, then thyroid scanned for uptake of radioactive iodine

3. Thyroid ultrasonography—evaluation of thyroid using ultrasonic sound waves for detection of fluid or tissue-filled tumors

4. Thyroid biopsy—tissue sample evaluated for benign or malignant tissue type

5. Serum calcium and phosphorus are evaluated in suspected parathyroid disorders

6. Skeletal x-rays identify loss of calcium in bones of a client with a parathyroid disorder

7. CT scan of adrenal glands—helpful in identifying tumors and gland enlargement

8. Adrenal arteriogram—identification of tumors

9. Dexamethasone suppression test—confirms Cushing's syndrome; client given high or low doses of dexamethasone and 24-hour urine evaluation for response to the medication

10. Urine and plasma catecholamines—helpful in identifying pheochromocytoma

11. Fasting blood sugar (FBS)—helpful in detecting diabetes mellitus

12. Two-hour postprandial glucose test—level of glucose in body 2 hours after a meal; screens for diabetes mellitus

13. Glucose tolerance test (GTT)—the definitive test for diabetes mellitus
14. Glycosylated hemoglobin (Ghb/Hb A1c)—measurement of time-averaged values of blood glucose over the preceding 2 to 4 months; assay of Hb A1c; can be drawn without regard to meals or insulin therapy

C. **Psychosocial**
1. Anxiety—uncomfortable feeling associated with unknown direct cause; may be difficult for clients to verbalize their anxiety but they can tell you they are uneasy about the outcome of their disorder
2. Fear—uncomfortable feeling associated with a direct cause, such as change in lifestyle, body changes, or death
3. Social isolation may occur if clients have a significant change in their body or disease symptoms make it more comfortable for them to stay home
4. There are many dietary restrictions associated with disorders of the endocrine system, so eating outside their own home is difficult and may be anxiety provoking
5. Lifestyle changes are abundant especially in the client with diabetes mellitus; health maintenance must be very intense and the client must learn how to maintain correct medication administration and dietary intake

D. **Health history—question sequence**
1. Would you please describe the problem you have been experiencing?
2. Do you tire easily?
3. Do you find that you must sleep or take rest periods more than you used to?
4. Do you wake up frequently at night? Do you sleep restlessly?
5. Does cold or heat bother you?
6. Have you noticed weight gain or loss? Over what period of time?
7. Have you noticed a loss of hair? Where? How long has this been occurring?
8. Have you noticed puffiness in your face, eyes or hands? Do you notice this when you wake up or is it all the time?
9. Do you ever have heart palpitations?
10. What do you take for constipation or diarrhea? How often must you take these medications?
11. Do you ever feel very thirsty or void large amounts of urine?
12. Do you ever feel nervous or jittery for days rather than hours?
13. Do your muscles ever feel weak or painful?

E. **Physical exam—appropriate sequence**
   1. Airway, breathing, circulation—vital signs
   2. Height and weight
   3. Inspect skin for integrity, turgor, lesions
   4. Inspect hair and nails for distribution, quantity and quality; nails for thickness and clubbing
   5. Inspect head and face for exophthalmos and edema
   6. Inspect neck for any asymmetry especially in the thyroid area
   7. Palpate the thyroid for abnormalities
   8. Inspect the chest for any heaves or thrusts in the area of the heart; and gynecomastia in males
   9. Palpate the anterior chest for thrills and for position of the apical impulse
   10. Auscultate heart sounds
   11. Inspect extremities—note any tremors, asymmetry, or disproportion to the trunk
   12. Inspect abdomen for striae or scars
   13. Auscultate for bowel sounds
   14. Palpate abdomen for areas that are painful
   15. Inspect genital area for abnormal pubic hair distribution and abnormal genitalia

IV. Pathophysiologic disorders
A. **Hyperthyroidism (thyrotoxicosis)**
   1. Definition—a metabolic imbalance that is a result of an excess of thyroid hormone; Grave's disease is a form of hyperthyroidism with four components: enlarged thyroid (goiter), increased thyroid production, exophthalmos (eyes bulging out of the sockets), and skin changes
   2. Etiology—autoimmune process from an as yet unidentified cause; possibly viral; there is a familial tendency
   3. Incidence—more common in females; occurs more frequently between the ages of 20 and 40
   4. Pathophysiology—thyroid gland is stimulated by circulating immunoglobulins to oversecrete thyroid hormone
   5. Assessment
      a. Ask the following questions
         (1) Have you noticed an enlargement of your neck or difficulty swallowing?
         (2) Have you been losing weight lately?
         (3) Have you experienced diarrhea?
         (4) Do you find you are unable to tolerate any heat?

        (5) Do you tire easily?

        (6) Do you ever have difficulty sleeping?

        (7) Have you noticed a dryness of your eyes or difficulty focusing your eyes?

        (8) Have you experienced heart palpitations?

b. Clinical manifestations

        (1) Tires easily

        (2) Fine tremors

        (3) Tachycardia, palpitations

        (4) Hypertension

        (5) Heat intolerance

        (6) Thin, brittle hair

        (7) Thickness of the skin and subcutaneous tissue, especially over tibia

        (8) Exophthalmos—bulging of the eyes from the sockets

c. Abnormal laboratory findings

        (1) T_4—thyroxine total—elevated

        (2) T_3, T_3-RIA elevated

        (3) Thyroid stimulating hormone (TSH) assay decreased

d. Abnormal diagnostic tests

        (1) Thyroid scan—abnormal uptake of radioactive iodine

        (2) Thyroid ultrasonography—differentiates a cyst (fluid filled) from a tumor (tissue growth)

        (3) Thyroid biopsy—identifies thyroid tissue as malignant or benign

6. Expected medical intervention

a. Antithyroid drugs to bring the client to a euthyroid state before more therapy

b. Administration of beta blocker Inderal to decrease sympathetic symptoms associated with hyperthyroidism

c. Radioactive sodium [131]I—substance is quickly picked up by the thyroid and substance destroys thyroid tissue; within 6 to 12 weeks the thyroid will become euthyroid; major complication is hypothyroidism as the radiation dosage is difficult to prescribe accurately

d. Thyroidectomy or partial thyroidectomy with preservation of parathyroid glands

7. Nursing diagnoses

a. Altered body nutrition—less than bodily requirements related to increased metabolic rate

b. Diarrhea related to increased peristalsis

c. Potential for fluid volume deficit related to diarrhea

      d. Risk for injury—corneal ulceration related to inability of client to close eyelids

8. Client goals

      a. Client will not lose any additional weight; begin to gain ¼ lb/wk

      b. Client will have only four liquid stools per day, with frequency decreasing by one episode of diarrhea per day then have normal consistency stools after the fifth day

      c. Client will show a balanced I&O and have acceptable skin turgor, moist mucous membranes

      d. Client will maintain moist appearing cornea with no evidence of corneal ulceration

9. Nursing interventions

      a. Acute care

          (1) Quiet, restful environment

          (2) Balance rest and activity carefully

          (3) Diet high in calories, protein, and carbohydrates

          (4) Daily weights, strict I&O

          (5) Postthyroidectomy care

              (a) Semifowlers position with no high fowlers to prevent strain on incision and neck

              (b) Dressing evaluated for tightness or bleeding

              (c) Check back of neck for bleeding; blood may trickle down neck folds and pool behind neck

              (d) Tracheostomy set at bedside at all times

              (e) Evaluate for hoarseness that is worsening, indicative of laryngeal nerve damage; ability to talk in a whisper may be normal for 3 to 5 days after surgery

              (f) Assess for tetany due to accidental removal of parathyroid glands

                 (i) Tingling around mouth and in fingers is first indication

                (ii) Muscle spasms and twitching

               (iii) Positive Chvostek's sign and Trousseau's sign (Figure 11-3)

               (iv) Palpitations

              (g) Encourage client to support head and neck when moving

              (h) Have calcium gluconate available because of possibility of tetany from accidental removal of parathyroid glands

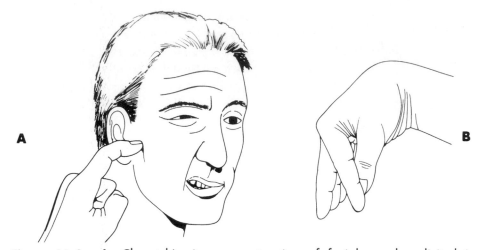

Figure 11-3. **A,** Chvostek's sign: a contraction of facial muscles elicited in response to a light tap over facial nerve in front of ear. **B,** Trousseau's sign: a carpopedal spasm induced by inflating a blood pressure cuff above systolic pressure. (From Beare PG and Myers JL: *Principles and practice of adult health nursing,* ed 2, St Louis, 1994, Mosby.)

    (6) Assess and intervene in client with thyrotoxic crises
       (a) Fever, tachycardia, flushing, sweating, dysrhythmias, shock, delirium, or coma
       (b) Administer Inderal by slow IV infusion to control sympathetic response
       (c) Intravenous Propylthiouracil to prevent further release of hormone
       (d) Possible steroid administration to support stress response
  b. Home care regarding client education
    (1) Radioactive sodium ^{131}I therapy
       (a) Isotope is administered via a tasteless, colorless liquid; a single dose
       (b) NPO after midnight
       (c) First 24 hours client should not be in contact with infants, children, or pregnant women
       (d) Increase fluids to 2000 to 3000 ml/day for several days
       (e) Flush toilet several times after each use for 2 to 3 days to decrease exposure to family members
    (2) Care of client with exophthalmus
       (a) Restrict sodium
       (b) Elevate head of bed

(c) Eye drops for moistness

(d) Sunglasses for photophobia

(3) Client must be evaluated 6 months after therapy for the need for replacement thyroid therapy, such as T_3, T_4

(4) Teach client findings associated with hypofunction of thyroid

(a) Constant fatigue

(b) Sustained constipation

10. Evaluation protocol

a. How do I know that my interventions were effective?

(1) Is client having any difficulty in breathing or swallowing?

(2) Has the client complained of a hoarse voice?

(3) Does client feel any tingling around the lips or fingers?

(4) Is client able to get some rest? Is room temperature conducive to sleeping?

b. What criteria will I use to change my interventions?

(1) Client experiencing difficulty breathing or swallowing

(2) Bleeding on the dressing or pooling of blood behind neck

(3) Evidence of thyrotoxic crisis

(4) Tingling around mouth or fingers

(5) Environment uncomfortable for client

c. How will I know that my client teaching has been effective?

(1) Client demonstrates appropriate eye care for exophthalmos

(2) Client states appropriate precautions to be taken in the home after radioisotope therapy is begun

11. Older adult alert

a. Many older adult clients are misdiagnosed because they may not present with classic findings. Their complaints many times fit nicely into a cardiac picture and will not stimulate the physician to perform thyroid testing.

b. Treatment of choice for the older adult client with hyperthyroidism is radioactive iodine

B. **Hypothyroidism**

1. Definition—decreased metabolism related to decrease in thyroid hormone

a. Myxedema is a complication of hypothyroidism; a generalized hypometabolic state

b. Myxedema coma is a life-threatening hypometabolic state

2. Pathophysiology—iodine is required for the thyroid gland to synthesize and secrete its hormone; if diet is insufficient in iodine the thyroid gland will enlarge in an attempt to compensate for the deficiency; when the pituitary gland identifies an insufficient thyroid hormone, it will increase secretion of the thyroid stimulating hormone (TSH); this is responsible for the enlarging thyroid gland, also known as a goiter

3. Etiology—most common cause is Hashimoto's Thyroiditis—an autoimmune disorder that leads to deterioration of the thyroid gland; other etiologies are iodine deficiency, congenital defects, or ineffective hormone synthesis

4. Incidence—more common in the female population; occurs most frequently between the ages of 30 and 60

5. Assessment
   a. Ask the following questions
      (1) Do you find that the cold really bothers you?
      (2) Have you found that you have been gaining weight without a change of diet or exercise?
      (3) Is your hair and skin very dry or oily?
      (4) Do you have trouble remembering things?
      (5) Do you tire easily?
   b. Clinical manifestations
      (1) Lethargy
      (2) Sinus bradycardia
      (3) Cold sensitivity
      (4) Weight gain
      (5) Constipation
      (6) Dry skin
      (7) Brittle hair
      (8) Forgetfulness
      (9) Depression
   c. Abnormal laboratory findings
      (1) TSH increased, pituitary is attempting to stimulate thyroid to produce more hormone
      (2) T_3 and T_4 decreased because thyroid gland is not producing them
      (3) H&H decreased due to the decreased metabolic rate, which affects RBC production
      (4) Cholesterol, triglycerides elevated due to decreased metabolic rate and results in disorders of lipid metabolism
      (5) Blood glucose decreased

      d. Abnormal diagnostic tests—radioactive iodide uptake (RAIU) decreased

6. Expected medical interventions
      a. Replacement drug therapy—most commonly used drug: Levothyroxine (Synthroid); lifetime maintenance dose
      b. Myxedema coma—resuscitative measures; synthroid IV, glucose, and corticosteroids
      c. Diet high in iodine easily accomplished with iodized salt

7. Nursing diagnoses
      a. Altered nutrition—more than bodily requirements related to decreased body metabolism
      b. Activity intolerance related to decreased metabolic rate
      c. Constipation related to decreased peristalsis secondary to decreased metabolic rate
      d. Hypothermia related to decreased metabolic rate

8. Client goals
      a. Client will have balanced nutrition to metabolic demands as evidenced by weight within 2 to 4 lb of baseline
      b. Client will increase activity by 10 minutes each day
      c. Client will have a bowel movement of soft consistency each day
      d. Client will maintain a temperature between 36.8° and 37° C

9. Nursing interventions
      a. Acute care
        (1) Assess vital signs every 2 to 4 hours
        (2) Assess lung sounds and heart sounds every 2 to 4 hours; be alert for heart failure: crackles, S_3
        (3) Maintain warm environment to meet client needs
        (4) Balance rest and activity as required by client needs
        (5) Meticulous skin care, paying attention to moisturize the skin and prevent skin tears
        (6) Request an order for a stool softener to alleviate constipation; increasing fluids or activity may not be as effective in hypothyroidism
        (7) Daily weight to identify fluid retention; report loss or gain of >2 lb/wk
      b. Home care regarding client education
        (1) Medication regime is lifelong as is follow-up care
        (2) Need to take medications at same time each day and on an empty stomach
        (3) Need to take pulse biweekly and reporting a pulse >100 at rest

(4) Symptoms to report to physician include chest pain, SOB, palpitations, insomnia, or feeling jittery

(5) Diet should be high in fiber and bulk, but low in calories, fat, and cholesterol

(6) Need for increased fluid intake to at least 2000 ml/day

(7) Biweekly weights on same days and times of day

(8) Moisturizers to counteract dry skin

10. Evaluation protocol
  a. How do I know that my interventions were effective?
    (1) Does client feel short of breath?
    (2) Has client noticed any palpitations?
    (3) Is client warm enough?
    (4) Is client feeling overly tired with usual activities?
  b. What criteria will I use to change my interventions?
    (1) Chest pain, shortness of breath
    (2) S_3/S_4 heart sounds, pulmonary crackles
    (3) Client still feels cold
    (4) Client feels exhausted even after minimal activity
    (5) New skin tears or breakdown areas noted
  c. How will I know that my client teaching has been effective?
    (1) Client demonstrates correct technique for taking pulse and weight
    (2) Client gives correct time span for taking pulse and weight
    (3) Client repeats correct adverse reactions to be reported to physician
    (4) Client shows a food diary that indicates correct food and fluid choices
    (5) Client reports using a moisturizer especially after bathing; no skin breakdown is evident

11. Older adult alert
  a. Hypothyroidism should be considered by a physician when ruling out a wide variety of illnesses
  b. The older adult client who is placed on drug therapy for hypothyroidism is at risk for developing ischemic heart disease because of the sudden increase in the metabolic rate. The client must be monitored carefully for cardiac complaints.
  c. A subclinical hypothyroidism is not uncommon in postmenopausal women and should be evaluated appropriately if complaints are suggestive of hypoactive thyroid

C. **Hyperparathyroidism**
  1. Definition—oversecretion of parathyroid hormone
  2. Pathophysiology—parathyroid hormone in its oversecreted state will function at an accelerated rate; increased loss of calcium from the bone leads to bone resorption, increased renal retention of calcium, and increased gastrointestinal absorption of calcium; this excess calcium is responsible for the clinical manifestations of the disease
  3. Etiology—benign adenoma in the majority of cases
  4. Incidence—more common in the female population especially after age 50; one of the most frequently identified endocrine disorder
  5. Assessment
     a. Ask the following questions
        (1) Have you experienced weakness or fatigue?
        (2) Have you noticed that you feel drowsy or sleepy a great deal of the time?
        (3) Is your appetite normal?
        (4) Have you been experiencing constipation?
        (5) Have you been urinating a great deal of urine?
        (6) Have you experienced pain in your bones?
     b. Clinical manifestations (Table 11-3)
     c. Abnormal laboratory findings—serum calcium elevated × 3
     d. Abnormal diagnostic test—parathyroid hormone radioimmunoassay test elevated (most specific)
  6. Expected medical interventions (see Table 11-3)
  7. Nursing diagnoses
     a. Constipation related to decline in peristalsis
     b. Risk for injury—pathologic fractures related to resorption of calcium from bones
     c. Activity intolerance related to fatigue
  8. Client goals
     a. Client will have a soft, formed stool at least every other day
     b. Client will not demonstrate any findings of pathologic fractures or renal calculi
     c. Client will increase activity level by 10 minutes each day
  9. Nursing interventions
     a. Acute care—client will be hospitalized for surgical removal of the parathyroid glands; see Care of the Client following a thyroidectomy, p. 363
     b. Home care regarding client education
        (1) Balance activity and rest; be aware that too much bed rest is not helpful in moving calcium back into the bones

Table 11-3. Parathyroid Gland Disorders

Disorder	Description	Symptoms	Client Management
Hyperparathyroidism	Disorder of calcium, phosphate, and bone metabolism characterized by hypersecretion of parathyroid hormone (PTH) from increased gland mass. May be caused by benign adenomas or secondary responses to hypocalcemic states. Incidence rises sharply after age 50.	Usually detected on routine chemistry profiles since most clients are asymptomatic. If present, symptoms are related to excess calcium and include hypertension, renal stones, muscle weakness, GI distress, constipation, and bone pain.	Surgical removal of affected gland; low-calcium diet, fluids, and calcium-blocking agents
Hypoparathyroidism	May be produced by a variety of disease states associated with impaired secretion of parathyroid hormone (PTH). Rare disorders and autoimmune involvement is likely.	Symptoms are variable and primarily related to the severity and rapidity of the deficiency. Calcium deficiency is a primary aspect with muscle tetany, abdominal cramping. Cardiac depression and seizures may occur.	Medications to replace calcium and vitamin D and control phosphate levels

From *AJN/Mosby Nursing boards review*, ed 9, St Louis, 1994, Mosby.

           (2)   Low calcium diet—limit dairy products

           (3)   Need to increase fluid intake to 2000 to 3000 cc to prevent renal calculi

           (4)   Need to increase fiber and bulk in diet

10. Evaluation protocol—How will I know that my client teaching has been effective?

    a.   Client indicates naps are taken in the morning and afternoon

    b.   Client shows a food diary indicating a low-calcium, high-fiber, high-fluid diet

    c.   Client reports normal pattern of bowel elimination without use of evacuation aids

11. Older adult alert—this disorder is commonly dismissed as the effects of aging in the older adult client. Be alert to significant findings that could lead you to be suspicious of hyperthyroidism.

D. **Hypoparathyroidism**

1. Definition—undersecretion of the parathyroid hormone

2. Pathophysiology—parathyroid hormone normally acts to increase bone resorption and maintain an appropriate balance between calcium and phosphate; a decrease in this hormone will lead to a decrease in serum calcium and decreased renal excretion of phosphate; hypocalcemia, hyperphosphatemia, and the resulting alkalosis will lead to an extreme in neuromuscular excitement and eventually tetany if not treated. Make the connection between low calcium and tetany.

3. Etiology—most common cause is accidental removal of the parathyroid glands during thyroidectomy or damage to the glands during the thyroidectomy

4. Incidence—more common in the female population

5. Assessment

    a.   Ask the following questions

           (1)   Have you noticed any numbness or tingling around your mouth or in your fingertips?

           (2)   Have you experienced any abdominal cramping?

    b.   Clinical manifestations (see Table 11-3)

           (1)   Numbness or tingling around mouth or fingertips

           (2)   Cardiac dysrhythmias

           (3)   Positive Chvostek's and Trousseau's sign (see Figure 11-3, p. 364)

    c.   Abnormal laboratory findings

           (1)   Serum calcium decreased

(2) Serum phosphate elevated

(3) Urinary calcium low or absent

6. Expected medical interventions (see Table 11-3, p. 370)—tetany is considered a medical emergency: laryngeal spasms may occur and subsequent respiratory obstruction, which will require immediate intervention to maintain a patent airway; must be treated with intravenous calcium immediately to return calcium to normal levels; calcium gluconate is the drug of choice

7. Nursing diagnosis—high risk for injury related to seizures or tetany caused by hypocalcemia

8. Client goal—Client will have no injury from the seizure activity or from the effects of tetany

9. Nursing interventions

   a. Acute care—monitor for the emergence of tetany

      (1) Evaluate airway and breathing frequently

      (2) Monitor the client for numbness or tingling around the mouth and fingertips—first sign

      (3) Evaluate for Chvostek's and Trousseau's signs

      (4) Have IV calcium gluconate readily available

      (5) Place client on cardiac monitor if calcium gluconate administration is required

   b. Home care regarding client education

      (1) Oral calcium and concurrent vitamin D administration to enhance absorption through the intestines

      (2) Diet high in calcium and low in phosphorus

      (3) Use of phosphate binder (Amphojel) before meals

      (4) Physician follow-up to monitor calcium levels

10. Evaluation protocol

   a. How do I know that my interventions were effective?

      (1) Vital signs are within 10% of baseline

      (2) Client is free of assessment findings that would indicate tetany, such as numbness or tingling around lips

      (3) Imminent tetany is treated promptly to prevent respiratory difficulty

   b. What criteria will I use to change my interventions?

      (1) Vital signs are not within expected parameters

      (2) Assessment findings that indicate tetany, such as numbness and tingling around mouth and in fingertips

      (3) Client experiences respiratory distress

    c. How will I know that my client teaching has been effective?
       (1) Client shows a food diary indicating appropriate food and beverage choices
       (2) Client indicates making a follow-up appointment with physician and identifying the importance of continuing the follow-up visits
       (3) Client states that Amphogel is taken before each meal
  11. Older adult alert—the nurse must emphasize to the older adult client that this disorder requires lifelong care and follow-up with a physician

E. **Adrenal insufficiency (Addison's disease)**
  1. Definition—insufficient release of hormones from the adrenal cortex (remember cortex . . . corticosteroids)
  2. Pathophysiology—adrenal insufficiency results in a decrease in the mineralocorticoids (Aldosterone), glucocorticoids (Cortisol), and the androgens; see Figure 11-4 for more information regarding the effects of the deficiency

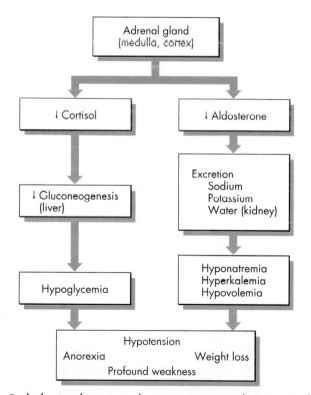

Figure 11-4. Pathologic alterations that accompany adrenocortical insufficiency. (From Beare PG and Myers JL: *Principles and practice of adult health nursing,* ed 2, St Louis, 1994, Mosby.)

3. Etiology—a common cause is autoimmune adrenalitis; can be caused primarily as a dysfunction of the adrenal gland or as a deficiency of ACTH; can also be seen in the client removed from exogenous steroid use after long-term therapy

4. Incidence—this is a rare illness that affects men and women equally

5. Assessment
   a. Ask the following questions
      (1) Have you been feeling increasingly fatigued lately?
      (2) Have you noticed weight loss recently?
      (3) Has your abdomen bothered you lately?
      (4) Have you experienced any nausea, vomiting, diarrhea, or constipation?
      (5) Have you experienced any dizzy spells?
   b. Clinical manifestations
      (1) Progressive weakness
      (2) Abdominal complaints—pain, anorexia
      (3) Nausea, vomiting, diarrhea, constipation
      (4) Amber coloration of the skin
      (5) Postural hypotension
      (6) Decreased pubic and axillary hair in the female population
   c. Abnormal laboratory findings
      (1) Electrolytes—sodium is low, potassium and calcium are increased
      (2) ACTH stimulation test—most reliable: baseline cortisol drawn; ACTH administered intravenously; 45 minutes later another cortisol level is drawn; result is abnormally low
      (3) Fasting Blood Sugar FBS—low
      (4) Melanocyte Stimulating Hormone MSH—elevated; results in bronzed skin, hyperpigmentation

6. Expected medical intervention
   a. Lifelong glucocorticoid and mineralocorticoid administration
   b. Acute Addisonian crisis, which causes vascular collapse, is treated with
      (1) Rapid infusion of saline and 5% dextrose
      (2) Intravenous dexamethasone
      (3) Hemodynamic monitoring

7. Nursing diagnoses
   a. Activity intolerance related to decreased glucose available for metabolism, secondary to decreased cortisol levels

      b.   Risk for injury—falls, related to decreased cardiac output

      c.   Risk for fluid volume deficit related to decrease in aldosterone production

8. Client goals

      a.   Client will increase activity by 10 minutes each day without expression of excessive fatigue

      b.   Client will not suffer any falls or injuries

      c.   Client will maintain a balanced I&O: I = O within 300 ml/day

9. Nursing interventions

      a.   Acute care—Addisonian crisis

         (1)   Evaluate airway, breathing, and circulation every 10 to 15 minutes until stable

         (2)   Institute IV access

         (3)   Institute cardiac monitoring to observe for cardiac dysrhythmias

         (4)   Monitor serum electrolytes

      b.   Home care regarding client education

         (1)   Lifelong replacement of glucocorticoids and mineralocorticoids

         (2)   Increasing glucocorticoid dosage during minor illnesses or stressful life events or situations; as directed by physician

         (3)   Medication supply is always a priority, need to ensure that there is always a sufficient supply, even for extended travel

         (4)   Use of medical alert bracelet or necklace

         (5)   Use of injectable cortisone for emergencies

10. Evaluation protocol

      a.   How do I know that my interventions were effective?

         (1)   Vital signs within 10% of baseline

         (2)   I = O within 300 ml

         (3)   Electrolytes are within acceptable limits

      b.   What criteria will I use to change my interventions?

         (1)   Vital signs >10% of baseline

         (2)   Output is not equal to intake within 300 ml

         (3)   Electrolytes are not within acceptable levels

      c.   How will I know that my client teaching has been effective?

         (1)   Client states that these medications must be taken for life

          (2)   Client states that illness or extreme stress will increase the need for medications and that the medications must be increased with the advice of the physician

          (3)   Client demonstrates correct use of a self-injector for an acute crisis

   11. Older adult alert

      a.   This is not a disease seen in the older adult population as a rule

      b.   When this disorder is seen in older adults, health care practitioners need to remember older adults' complaints may be more pronounced because they may already have a decreased adrenal function as a normal course of aging

      c.   The older adult client may also be more sensitive to the side effects of the corticosteroids because some of the symptoms may already be apparent as a normal course of aging, such as hypertension

F. **Adrenal hyperfunction (Cushing's syndrome)**

   1. Definition—increased secretion of glucocorticoids from the adrenal cortex or as a result of exogenous steroid administration

   2. Pathophysiology—increased glucocorticoid production has an effect on every system in the body (Table 11-4)

   3. Etiology

      a.   ACTH producing pituitary or hypothalamus lesion

      b.   Extrapituitary malignancies producing ACTH

      c.   Adrenal adenomas

      d.   Adrenal carcinoma

      e.   Exogenous steroid administration

      f.   Alcohol induced

   4. Incidence—more common in the female population; common in the 20 to 40 age group

   5. Assessment

      a.   Ask the following questions

          (1)   Have you noticed a change in the shape of your face?

          (2)   Have you noticed stretch marks on your abdomen?

          (3)   Has your hair begun to thin?

          (4)   Do you notice that it takes a long time for cuts to heal?

      b.   Clinical manifestations (see Table 11-4)

      c.   Abnormal laboratory tests

          (1)   Urinary 17-hydroxysteroids elevated

          (2)   Plasma cortisol levels elevated throughout the day with a loss of normal diurnal rhythm, which is high

Table 11-4. Cushing's Syndrome: Pathophysiologic Changes and Clinical Manifestations

Pathophysiologic Changes	Clinical Manifestations
Increased cortisol levels	Depression, apathy, mood changes, psychosis, cataracts
Sodium and water retention, potassium excretion	High blood pressure, hypokalemia, increased urinary potasium, metabolic alkalosis, edema
Increased androgen production	Acne, hirsutism, virilization, hyperpigmentation, amenorrhea, menstrual changes
Immunosuppression	Poor wound healing, leukocytosis, decreased lymphocyte and eosinophil production, increased erythropoiesis
Body fat redistribution	Moon face, truncal obesity, "buffalo hump"
Increased protein catabolism and collagen loss	Skin and hair thinning, abdominal striae, muscle weakness, atrophy
Capillary fragility	Easy bruising
Gastric hyperacidity	Peptic ulcer formation
Increased calcium loss	Increased urinary calcium, osteoporosis, backache, pathologic fractures
Increased gluconeogenesis	Hyperglycemia

From Beare PG and Myers JL: *Principles and practice of adult health nursing,* ed 2, St Louis, 1994, Mosby.

        levels in the morning, with levels falling in the evening and becoming the lowest near midnight
- (3) Urinary-free cortisol elevated
- d. Abnormal diagnostic tests
  - (1) Adrenal CT scan—identifies adrenal tumor
  - (2) X rays—used to identify tumors in other areas of the body that could be causing the disorder
6. Expected medical interventions
  - a. Surgery to remove adrenal tumors
  - b. Radiation therapy for pituitary tumors or tumors in other areas of the body
  - c. Drug therapy to suppress the release of ACTH or the synthesis of the corticosteroids
  - d. Monitor use of exogenous steroids

7. Nursing diagnoses
    a. Activity intolerance related to weakness and fatigue
    b. Risk for fluid volume excess related to increased corticosteroid production
    c. Risk for infection related to increased production of corticosteroids causing a suppressed immune system
    d. Body-image disturbance related to changes in fat deposits and hair distribution secondary to increased glucocorticoid production
8. Client goals
    a. Client will tolerate activity, 10 minutes more each day without stated excessive fatigue
    b. Client will have I = O within 300 ml
    c. Client will be free from infection as evidenced by normal white cell count and differential within accepted parameters
    d. Client will state feeling comfortable with bodily changes
9. Nursing interventions
    a. Acute care—postoperative; see Care of the Postoperative Client, Chapter 9, p. 309
    b. Home care regarding client education
        (1) Need for lifelong steroid replacement if treatment has left client in state of adrenal insufficiency
        (2) Daily weight monitoring and report gain or loss of 2 lb/wk
        (3) Maintaining a low-sodium/high-potassium diet
        (4) How to protect self from infection; careful hand washing
        (5) Need for more steroids during times of stress or illness, if client therapy requires lifelong steroid replacement
        (6) Need to take steroids with food or milk
        (7) Risks associated with stopping the steroid preparation abruptly
10. Evaluation protocol
    a. How do I know that my interventions were effective? See Evaluation Protocol for adrenal insufficiency, p. 375.
    b. What criteria will I use to change my interventions? See Evaluation Protocol for adrenal insufficiency, p. 375.
    c. How will I know that my client teaching has been effective?
        (1) Client indicates correct drug administration regime and precautions about not stopping medication abruptly

(2) Client states risks of infection due to increased steroid production or administration

(3) Client demonstrates correct method for daily weight

(4) Client shows a food diary with appropriate food and beverage choices

11. Older adult alert—the older adult client may present with excessive numbers of assessment factors because many older adults already manifest these symptoms due to the normal changes of aging

G. **Diabetes mellitus**

1. Definition—a metabolic disorder affecting a wide variety of systems but most commonly affected is glucose metabolism

   a. Diabetic ketoacidosis—life-threatening disorder caused by an ineffective level of insulin and resulting hyperglycemia; average of 600 mg/dL

   b. Hyperosmolar hyperglycemic nonketotic syndrome (HHNK)—a life-threatening disorder associated with an extremely high blood glucose, average 1100 mg/dL; dehydration and coma

   c. Hypoglycemia—low blood glucose, average <50 mg/dL

2. Pathophysiology

   a. Type 1 or insulin dependent diabetes mellitus (IDDM)—a deficiency of insulin noted as well as an increase in counterinsulin hormones: glucagon, epinephrine, cortisol, and growth hormone

      (1) Decreased insulin causes a decreased utilization of serum glucose by the cells, allowing the serum and urine glucose to rise

      (2) Lack of glucose for cellular nutrition forces the body to mobilize fat and protein stores for metabolism

      (3) This results in ketone buildup in the blood and urine

      (4) Glucose is hypertonic and will pull fluid out of the extracellular space, resulting in increased urine output, thirst, and sodium and potassium losses

   b. Type 2 or noninsulin dependent diabetes mellitus (NIDDM)—insulin levels may be low, normal, or elevated; several factors felt to contribute to the pathophysiology: slower response of insulin release, decreased number of insulin receptors, reduced responsiveness to glucose by the beta cells in the pancreas; a major factor in the advent of NIDDM is obesity

3. Etiology—several theories are presently being evaluated, including autoimmune, viral, environmental, and genetic etiologies
4. Incidence—over 12 million Americans are afflicted; over 500,000 new cases are reported each year; the majority of clients diagnosed are noninsulin dependent
5. Assessment
   a. Ask the following questions
      (1) Have you noticed that you are urinating more than usual?
      (2) Have you been very thirsty lately?
      (3) Have you been losing weight, even when eating the same amount of food or more?
      (4) Do you ever feel very tired and weak?
   b. Clinical manifestations
      (1) Polyphagia—increased appetite due to increased hunger
      (2) Polyuria—increased urination
      (3) Polydipsia—increased thirst
      (4) Weight loss
      (5) Fatigue
      (6) Weakness
      (7) Type 2 client may not show above symptoms but may be initially diagnosed with complications
      (8) DKA, HHNK (Tables 11-5 and 11-6)
   c. Abnormal laboratory findings
      (1) Blood glucose elevated
      (2) Fasting blood glucose elevated
      (3) Postprandial blood glucose elevated
      (4) Glucose tolerance test elevated with a longer time period for return to normal; this is the definitive test to diagnose diabetes
      (5) Urine ketones elevated
6. Expected medical interventions
   a. Treatment must be individualized
   b. Insulin administration
   c. Oral hypoglycemic agents
   d. Diet therapy—American Diabetic Association diet, calorie intake individualized
   e. Exercise—recommended six to seven times per week at approximately the same time each day
   f. Hypoglycemia (see Table 11-5)

Table 11-5. Differentiating Hypoglycemia from Ketoacidosis (Hyperglycemia)

	Hypoglycemia (Insulin Reaction)	Ketoacidosis (Diabetic Coma)
Causes	Delayed or missed meals, excess insulin, excess exercise (glucose less than 50 mg/dL)	Inadequate insulin, too much food, infection, injury, physical or emotional stress (glucose greater than 350 mg/dL)
Clinical Findings	Anxiety, irritability, weakness, sweating, hunger, tremor, nausea, headache (severe: confusion, unconsciousness); moist, cool skin; "feels shakey"	Thirst, increased urination, weakness, nausea, abdominal pain (classic: acetone breath odor, Kussmaul's respirations, decreased consciousness), hot, dry skin
Treatment	5 to 15 g of carbohydrate as: 4 to 8 oz soft drink (regular, not diet) 4 oz orange juice 6 to 8 Life Savers 1 to 1½ Tbs honey 1 to 2 Tbs jam Administer glucagon I.M. or S.Q. (0.5 to 1.0 mg) if unable to swallow Give some complex carbohydrate from meal plan within 1 hour after initial treatment	Correct volume depletion with IV fluids, 0.9% NS initially Administer regular insulin by infusion Replace electrolytes as volume is restored Monitor vital signs, I&O, blood glucose, and level of consciousness

Modified from *AJN/Mosby Nursing boards review*, ed 9, St Louis, 1994, Mosby.

    g. Ketoacidosis (see Table 11-5)
    h. HHNK (see Table 11-6)
  7. Nursing diagnoses
    a. Risk for infection related to impaired leukocyte function and high glucose content in tissues
    b. Potential for injury or trauma related to inability to feel pain secondary to peripheral nerve degeneration
    c. Risk for impaired peripheral tissue integrity related to microcirculatory and macrocirculatory changes

Table 11-6. Hyperglycemic Hyperosmolar Nonketotic Coma (HHNK)

A life-threatening condition characterized by severe elevation of blood glucose, dehydration and stupor or coma. It occurs primarly in elderly Type II or previously undiagnosed diabetics. It has a 15 to 20% mortality rate.

Pathophysiology:
The crisis is frequently caused by an infection or stressor which causes an outpouring of steroids and raises the blood glucose. Enough insulin is produced to prevent ketosis but hyperglycemia and dehydration become life-threatening, especially if the client cannot take oral fluids.

Clinical Findings:
Severe dehydration
Hypothermia, hypotension
Severe weakness and lethargy
Depressed mental status to coma
Blood glucose greater than 600 mg/dL; usually around 1100mg/dL
Elevated serum sodium
Serum osmolality above 350 mOsm/kg
Ketones—negative

Treatment:
IV fluid replacement, 0.9% NS initially
Low-dose IV insulin
Careful monitoring for complications (e.g.,CHF, pulmonary edema, electrolyte imbalance, seizures)

Modified from *AJN/Mosby Nursing boards review,* ed 9, St Louis, 1994, Mosby.

    d. Knowledge deficit—medication and dietary regime related to need for additional teaching

8. Client goals
   a. Client will show no evidence of infection as evidenced by normal WBC, afebrile
   b. Client will show no evidence of burns, abrasions, or cuts to extremities and will carefully assess extremities for injury several times per day
   c. Client will have appropriate tissue integrity as evidenced by intact skin without ulcerations
   d. Client will demonstrate knowledge and skills necessary to follow appropriate diet and take insulin or hypoglycemic agents as ordered

9. Nursing interventions
   a. Acute care

    (1) Ketoacidosis (serum glucose >600 mg/dL and ketones present) and HHNK (serum glucose >1100 mg/dL and ketones absent)

        (a) Maintain airway, breathing, and circulation; monitor lung sounds frequently especially the bases for the advent of CHF

        (b) Evaluate neurologic status frequently for changes

        (c) Maintain IV access and prepare to administer fluids in large quantities; 8 to 12 liters not uncommon in the first 24 hours of care; fluid of choice is 0.9% saline followed by 0.45% saline

        (d) Evaluate serum glucose levels as ordered or indicated; administer insulin bolus IV initially followed by insulin drip or SC injections as blood glucose levels decrease to a more acceptable range

        (e) Monitor urine output—anticipate large urine outputs until blood glucose has returned to baseline

        (f) Evaluate electrolyte levels as ordered—potassium and phosphorus abnormalities may not be seen immediately in the serum levels; potassium and phosphorus will be replaced as indicated by results of serum levels as pH is corrected

    (2) Hypoglycemia (insulin shock)—serum glucose <50 mg/dL

        (a) If client can tolerate PO fluids, administer approximately 15 grams of carbohydrate such as soda, sugar, candy, or orange juice

        (b) If unconscious, glucagon can be administered SQ or IM

        (c) Physician may order an IV started and 50% dextrose administered

        (d) Frequent blood sugar evaluations to ensure a return to the client's baseline

  b. Home care regarding client education

    (1) Medication administration

        (a) Insulin currently used, kept at room temperature; other vials refrigerated

        (b) Insulin must be at room temperature before administration

    (c) Roll insulin, do not shake

    (d) Correct technique for drawing insulin from the vial

    (e) If two insulins mixed, place short-acting in syringe first, followed by longer-acting—*clear to cloudy*; (tell client to associate bath water—first clear then cloudy)

    (f) Rotate sites (Figure 11-5), so all sites are used within a week

    (g) Inject at a 45 to 90 degree angle; depends on the amount of subcutaneous tissue

    (h) Do not rub site after administration, press lightly

    (i) Do not smoke for 30 minutes after administration—smoking causes vasoconstriction, which reduces absorption

Injection record								
SITE		1	2	3	4	5	6	7
Right arm	A							
Right abdomen	B							
Right thigh	C							
Left thigh	D							
Left abdomen	E							
Left arm	F							
Left buttock	G							
Right buttock	H							

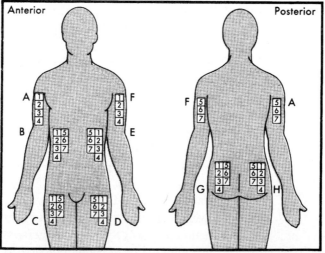

Figure 11-5. Injection record. (From Beare PG and Myers JL: *Principles and practice of adult health nursing,* ed 2, St Louis, 1994, Mosby.)

(j) Teach another person living with or near client how to inject medication, in the event the client is unable to inject own medication

(2) Glucose/ketone monitoring

  (a) Urine testing used to evaluate for ketones—test before meals and at bedtime if required; document in percentages

  (b) Teach proper needle stick technique for blood glucose monitoring

    (i) Use correct timing as per manufacturer's requirements

    (ii) Use earlobes and side of fingertips

  (c) Notify physician if levels are higher or lower than physician recommends

(3) Diet therapy

  (a) Instruct client to follow the individualized meal plan

  (b) Carefully follow the exchange list of the diet

  (c) Do not skip meals

  (d) How to modify for illness

    (i) Drink fluids hourly to replace fluids that are lost

    (ii) Make sure there is an intake of simple sugars that could be digested easily

(4) Exercise requirements

  (a) All exercise must be carefully planned; suggest 6 to 7 days a week, the same time each day to facilitate glucose control

  (b) Exercise enhances effects of insulin so it may cause hypoglycemia

  (c) Blood glucose monitoring before and after exercise

  (d) Eat at least 1 hour before exercise and make sure insulin has been taken

  (e) Carry a quick-acting carbohydrate in case of a hypoglycemic reaction

  (f) Always have medical alert bracelet or necklace on in case of hypoglycemic reaction

(5) Relationship between diet, exercise, and medication administration

(6) How to identify when ketoacidosis and hypoglycemia occur and what interventions to take (see Table 11-5, p. 381)

    (7) Diabetic foot care
        (a) Inspect feet daily for dryness, cracks, or ingrown toenails
        (b) Thoroughly cleanse and dry feet and in between toes daily
        (c) Place skin moisturizer on feet to prevent cracking
        (d) Never walk around barefoot
        (e) Always wear socks with shoes
        (f) Allow only a podiatrist to care for corns, callouses, and toenails
        (g) Must be aggressive in treating any breakdown in the foot to prevent any local and subsequent bone infection
    (8) Changes that must occur in the face of illness or surgery
        (a) Must continue to take medication
        (b) More insulin will be required
        (c) Increase frequency of blood glucose monitoring
        (d) If unable to eat, take in increased fluids, simple carbohydrates
    (9) Health care maintenance
        (a) Careful daily hygiene is imperative
        (b) Frequent checkups with dentist
        (c) At least yearly evaluation by an ophthalmologist
10. Evaluation protocol
    a. How do I know that my interventions were effective?
        (1) Client exhibits patent airway, acceptable breathing pattern, and circulation
        (2) Client maintains appropriate neurologic status—client is awake, oriented × 3
        (3) Client exhibits urine output ≥30 ml/hr and I = O within 300 ml
        (4) Client exhibits decreasing or increasing blood glucose levels with a return to client baseline
        (5) Client exhibits normal electrolyte balance
    b. What criteria will I use to change my interventions?
        (1) Unstable airway, breathing, or circulation
        (2) Decreased or decreasing neurologic status
        (3) Unbalanced I&O
        (4) Blood glucose levels that are resistant to therapy without a return to or near baseline levels
        (5) Abnormal electrolyte balance

c. How will I know that my client teaching has been effective?
   (1) Client demonstrates correct technique and timetable for administration of medication
   (2) Client produces a food diary that exhibits correct dietary management
   (3) Client demonstrates correct technique for blood glucose monitoring
   (4) Client produces a plan for exercise indicating that exercise will occur following a meal and after insulin administration, the same time each day
   (5) Client correctly identifies factors to watch for that could indicate ketoacidosis or hypoglycemia is about to occur, with interventions to be used
   (6) Client demonstrates proper foot care
   (7) Client states changes that must be made in the face of illness, surgery, or any other stressful life event or situation
   (8) Client states the frequency of appointments with the dentist and ophthalmologist for examinations
   (9) Client shows a medical alert bracelet
   (10) Client states what conditions need to be reported to the physician

11. Older adult alert
    a. Noninsulin dependent diabetes mellitus is more common in the older adult client
    b. The older adult client is at great risk for complications associated with diabetes that would require hospitalization
    c. The symptoms commonly associated with diabetes mellitus may be masked by other illnesses in the older adult client. An example is polyuria, which may manifest itself as incontinence.
    d. Many older adult clients have unusual or erratic eating that must be considered when planning their diet
    e. Keep in mind there may be decreased visual acuity or manual dexterity in older adult clients that may decrease their ability to prepare insulin
    f. Proper foot care may not be possible due to decreased mobility and visual acuity in the older adult

REVIEW QUESTIONS

1. A client is admitted to the hospital with a tentative diagnosis of Grave's disease. The nurse would expect to assess for which clinical manifestation
   a. Hypotension
   b. Bradycardia
   c. Client sleeps when undisturbed
   d. Client complaining of the room being cold

2. When caring for a client who has received radioactive iodine therapy for hyperthyroidism, the interventions must include
   a. Keeping the client in a private room
   b. The nurse wearing gowns and gloves when having direct contact with the client
   c. The client using disposable eating utensils
   d. Asking the client to flush the toilet several times after each use

3. In a client with hypothyroidism the nurse would expect to see what group of laboratory values?
   a. $\uparrow T_3$, $\uparrow T_4$, $\uparrow$TSH
   b. $\downarrow T_3$, $\downarrow T_4$, $\downarrow$TSH
   c. $\downarrow T_3$, $\downarrow T_4$, $\uparrow$TSH
   d. $\uparrow T_3$, $\uparrow T_4$, $\downarrow$TSH

4. A complication likely to occur in a client with hyperparathyroidism is
   a. Urinary calculi
   b. Fluid overload
   c. Skin breakdown
   d. Diarrhea

5. An assessment that would be appropriate for a client believed to be entering into the beginning stages of tetany would be
   a. Allen's test
   b. Pulmonary function test
   c. Reflex evaluation
   d. Evaluation for Trousseau's sign

6. A client having surgery, who is taking corticosteroids for Addison's disease, will require
   a. A smaller dose the day of surgery due to the effects of anesthesia
   b. A much larger dose due to the increased need as a result of the stress of surgery
   c. Smaller doses given over several days
   d. A larger dose followed by withholding the usual dose for one day

7. Addisonian crisis is an acute lack of corticosteroids and requires which initial nursing assessment skill?
   a. Evaluation of arterial monitoring system
   b. Dysrhythmia detection
   c. Evaluation of BP
   d. Evaluation of pulmonary function testing

8. In the client with Cushing's syndrome, it is imperative that evaluation occurs of cortisol levels. Expected normal plasma cortisol level is at its highest
   a. At midnight
   b. At noon
   c. At meal time
   d. Upon wakening

9. The exercise regime suggested for the client with diabetes mellitus is
   a. 3 times per week at the same time each day
   b. 4 times per week
   c. 6 to 7 times per week
   d. 6 to 7 times per week at the same time each day

10. The purpose for administration of a low-dose intravenous insulin in the face of hyperosmolar nonketotic coma is to
    a. Prevent severe hypotension
    b. Encourage the passage of glucose into the cells slowly to prevent lysis of cells
    c. Return blood glucose to an acceptable level for the client slowly, thus preventing profound shock
    d. Return electrolyte imbalance to normal for the client and prevent a rapid change in the electrolyte balance

ANSWERS, RATIONALES, AND TEST-TAKING TIPS

Rationales	Test-Taking Tips

1. **Correct answer: c**

   A client with Grave's disease or hyperthyroidism exhibits hypertension, tachycardia, heat intolerance, and fatigue. This is from a hypermetabolic state.

   Responses *a, b,* and *d* can be clustered under the problem of hypofunction of the thyroid. Select option *c.*

2. **Correct answer: d**

   Gowns, gloves, and a private room are not necessary for this client. The only concern is elimination by flushing the toilet several times after each use to dilute radiation that may be excreted in urine or feces.

   Cluster the responses *a, b,* and *c* under the interventions for isolation of a client. Select option *d.*

3. **Correct answer: c**

   The T_3 and T_4 would be low, due to the inability of the thyroid to produce the hormone. The pituitary hormone TSH, thyroid stimulating hormone, would be high, attempting to stimulate the thyroid to produce more hormone.

   The key word in the stem is "hypothyroidism." Therefore read down vertically through the first item in these series. Immediately the responses can be narrowed to *b* and *c.* Use common sense to think that T_3 and T_4 will be low but the TSH, thyroid stimulating hormone, will be up since it will try to get the thyroid to produce more hormones.

4. **Correct answer: a**

   Urinary calculi are not uncommon in the client with hyperparathyroidism due to the demineralization of the bones from the increased levels of PTH. Recall that the balance of calcium and phosphorus can be thought

   Recall that the parathyroid deals with the balance of two minerals, calcium, and phosphorus. Then associate that the only response given that might deal with mineral accumulation since the question is asking about hyperfunction would be the formation of kidney stones.

of as a seesaw—when calcium is up phosphorus will be down. And in parathyroid problems the calcium follows the direction of the imbalance—

hyper = ⬈ CA, ⬊ phosphorus
hypo = the opposite.

Response *a* is correct. Diarrhea would be associated with a loss.

5. Correct answer: d

Allen's test is to evaluate blood flow through the ulnar artery. Pulmonary function testing is for lung volumes; reflex evaluation would not give you enough information in this client. Trousseau's sign— carpal pedal spasm when a blood pressure cuff is inflated for at least 1 minute on the arm—if positive with these findings is indicative of impending tetany.

Responses *b* and *c* are too general to be answers to a question about a specific assessment. Remember that *A* in Allen's test is a clue that it assesses *A*rterial circulation to the hand. *T*etany is indicated by *T*rousseau's sign.

6. Correct answer: b

The stress of surgery increases the client's need for corticosteroids and thus the client needs more corticosteroids before or during surgery. Remember the *s* for *s*teroids: need to be given *s*teadily with more given in *s*tress and can't be *s*topped *s*uddenly.

Common sense about stress is that when stressed, more hormones are needed in the entire body; thus, the responses can be narrowed to either *b* or *d*. If one reads too quickly, the key words "withholding the usual dose" will be missed. These words make this response incorrect since steroids should never be stopped abruptly.

7. Correct answer: c

A severe lack of corticosteroids, or Addisonian crisis will cause cardiovascular collapse, a drop in BP, and cardiac dysrhythmias.

The key word is "initial." The nurse would assess options *a, b,* and *c.* However, initially the BP would be the most expedient since arterial monitoring and dysrhythmia detection require more sophisticated equipment and a physician order. Option *d* is not appropriate in Addisonian crisis.

8. Correct answer: d

Cortisol is highest in the morning due to the fact that there has been little use of cortisol while sleeping.

Associate the levels of cortisol with most people's energy level throughout the day. Highest in the morning and lowest in the afternoon or early evening.

9. Correct answer: d

Exercise in the diabetic client must be consistent, the same time each day and at least 6 to 7 days per week.

The cardiac client is advised to exercise three times a week. The diabetic needs to exercise about every day to facilitate the best control of the serum glucose with minimal fluctuations.

10. Correct answer: c

It is preferable to bring the glucose levels down slowly to prevent profound shock. The beginning of response *b* is correct; however the second part is incorrect.

Note the important clues in the stem: insulin given in high glucose situation. Recall basic information that insulin lowers glucose levels. Select response *c*.

The Musculoskeletal System

STUDY OUTCOMES

After completing this chapter, the reader will be able to do the following:

▼ Identify major anatomic components and functions of the musculoskeletal system.

▼ Identify assessment findings of clients with alterations of the musculoskeletal system.

▼ Choose appropriate nursing diagnoses for the musculoskeletal disorders discussed.

▼ Implement appropriate nursing interventions for the client with a musculoskeletal disorder.

▼ Evaluate the progress of the client with a musculoskeletal disorder for establishment of new nursing interventions based on evaluation findings.

KEY TERMS

Abduction	Moving a part of the body away from the midline of the body (think of abduction: moving people away from their home).
Adduction	Moving a part of the body toward the midline of the body (add to the body).
Mobility	The ability to move or have motion.
Paresthesias	Pins and needles or numb feeling in extremities.
Range of motion	Degree of movement of a joint.

CONTENT REVIEW

I. The musculoskeletal system is responsible for the support and movement of the body; the protection of the internal organs; the storage of minerals; the process of hematopoiesis

II. Structure and function
  A. Bones—total of 206; various sizes and shapes; outer layer called the periosteum
  B. Joints—formed where two bones touch each other
    1. Fibrous joints—no movement such as in suture lines of cranial bones
    2. Cartilaginous joints—small amount of movement such as between vertebrae
    3. Synovial joints—freely move, such as the elbow; articulating surfaces covered with hyaline cartilage
    4. Joint capsule is lined with synovial membranes and cavity is filled with synovial fluid to decrease friction
    5. Bones held in alignment by ligaments
  C. Muscles—muscle fibers are the actual working unit; skeletal muscle contraction and relaxation are accomplished by innervation by nerve impulses; skeletal muscles are commonly attached to two bones and cross a joint; some form sphincters, some connect bone with skin such as in the cheek; if the bone breaks, the muscle contracts and the extremity shortens

III. Targeted concerns
  A. Pharmacology—priority drug classifications
    1. Salicylates—inhibit prostaglandin synthesis; aspirin irreversibly inhibits platelet aggregation for the life of a platelet (7 to 10 days)

    a. Expected effects—antipyretic, analgesic, antiinflammatory, antiplatelet

    b. Commonly given drugs

       (1) Aspirin

       (2) Diflunisal (Dolobid)

       (3) Salicylate combination (Trilisate)

    c. Nursing considerations

       (1) Monitor for dizziness or ringing in ears (tinnitus)—may indicate toxicity

       (2) Do not give to children or teenagers; risk of Reye's syndrome

       (3) Do not give to clients with bleeding tendencies

       (4) Assess for bleeding

2. Nonsteroidal antiinflammatory drugs—inhibit prostaglandin synthesis

    a. Expected effects—antipyretic, antiinflammatory, analgesic

    b. Commonly given drugs

       (1) Ibuprofen (Motrin)

       (2) Naproxen (Naprosyn)

       (3) Sulindac (Clinoril)

       (4) Piroxicam (Feldene)

       (5) Ketorolac (Toradol)

    c. Nursing considerations

       (1) If client is unable to tolerate one NSAID, they may well tolerate another

       (2) Administer with food to decrease gastric distress

3. Prozalone derivatives—actions similar to NSAID

    a. Expected effects—potent analgesic and antiinflammatory actions; very high incidence of adverse reactions so therapy is limited to short term

    b. Commonly given drug

       (1) Oxyphenbutazone (Oxalid)

    c. Nursing considerations

       (1) Complete history and physical with CBC and urinalysis must be done before therapy begins

       (2) Instruct client to stop drug if any of the following occur: blurred vision, sore throat, mouth lesions, excessive bruising, bleeding, edema, weight gain, rashes

       (3) Instruct client to take with food or milk to reduce GI distress

4. Corticosteroids—(see Chapter 6 p. 158, Chapter 11 p. 357)

5. Central-acting muscle relaxants—mechanism of action unknown; possibly related to sedative effect
   a. Expected effect—relieves muscle spasm
   b. Commonly given drugs
      (1) Carisoprodol (Soma)
      (2) Cyclobenzaprine (Flexeril)
      (3) Methocarbamol (Robaxin)
   c. Nursing considerations
      (1) May impair mental functioning—evaluate carefully for lethargy
      (2) Instruct client to avoid alcohol, CNS depressing medications, hazardous tasks
6. Direct-acting muscle relaxants—act on a site within the muscle
   a. Expected effect—relaxation of tense skeletal muscles
   b. Commonly given drug— dantrolene (Dantrium)
   c. Nursing considerations
      (1) Instruct client to avoid concurrent use of CNS depressant drugs
      (2) Monitor liver function studies when ordered
      (3) Evaluate for findings associated with hepatotoxicity—rash, pruritus, bruising, tarry stools, jaundice
7. Acute antigout medication—specific action not understood
   a. Expected effect—decreases inflammatory response associated with acute gout
   b. Commonly given drug—colchicine
   c. Nursing considerations
      (1) Begin at first sign of gout attack, do not delay even an hour
      (2) For IV use dilute only in normal saline; give over 2 to 5 minutes
      (3) May also be given orally
      (4) Store in tight dark containers
8. Uricosuric drugs—increase renal excretion of uric acid
   a. Expected effect—prevents precipitation of uric acid in joints
   b. Commonly given drugs
      (1) Probenecid (Benemid)
      (2) Aulfinpyrazone (Aprazone)
      (3) Allopurinol (Zyloprim)
   c. Nursing considerations
      (1) Client must drink at least 2 to 3 liters of water a day to prevent formation of uric acid kidney stones

        (2) Aspirin reduces drug effectiveness

        (3) Allopurinol may cause drowsiness for as long as 12 hours after taken—instruct client to use caution when driving or using machinery

9. Gold compounds—mechanism unknown

    a. Expected effect—stops bone destruction and articular destruction in rheumatoid arthritis

    b. Commonly given drugs

        (1) Auranofin (Ridaura)

        (2) Aurothioglucose (Solganal), Gold sodium thiomalate (Myochrysine) deep IM

    c. Nursing considerations

        (1) Assess if client is pregnant—contraindicated in pregnancy

        (2) Evaluate for normal or near normal baseline—urinalysis, CBC, platelet count, liver function studies before beginning treatment

        (3) Avoid exposure to sunlight or ultraviolet light; use sunscreens

        (4) Report any skin or mucous membrane lesions

        (5) Instruct client that effects of drug may not be seen for 6 weeks to 6 months

10. Immunosuppressive agents (see p. 357 and p. 452)

11. Cytotoxic drugs—interferes with folic acid metabolism; used only in clients with severe cases of rheumatoid arthritis

    a. Expected effect—immunosuppression

    b. Commonly given drugs

        (1) Methotrexate (Rheumatrex)

        (2) Cyclophosphamide (Cytoxan)

    c. Nursing considerations

        (1) Monitor client carefully for findings associated with GI tract lesions and bone marrow suppression

        (2) NSAID should not be taken during this therapy

        (3) Monitor for symptoms of gout—severe pain in one joint; increase fluid intake to at least 2000 ml/day to reduce risk of gout

12. Gastric acid secretion inhibitor—inhibits gastric acid secretion

    a. Expected effect—prevention of gastric ulceration secondary to administration of NSAID and aspirin

    b. Commonly given drug—misoprostol (Cytotec)

      c. Nursing considerations
        (1) Must not be taken if pregnant
        (2) May decrease effects of aspirin

B. **Procedures**
1. Bone and joint x-rays—identifies irregularities in bones and joints
2. Magnetic resonance imaging (MRI)—produces body tissue images through the use of electromagnetic waves
3. Computed tomography (CT) scan—serial radiographic images of bone and tissue taken in cross sections
4. Bone scan—scanning of bones after an injection of radioisotope; evaluates its distribution throughout the bone
5. Arthroscopy—direct examination of a joint using a lighted, fiberoptic scope
6. Electromyography—evaluates nerve transmission; checks for muscle impulse response
7. Myelogram—injection of radiopaque solution into spinal canal; radiographic study to evaluate spinal conditions
8. Arthrography—injection of radiopaque solution into joint; radiographic study to evaluate joint integrity
9. Biopsies of bone, muscle, and synovium to evaluate for malignancies or other disorders

C. **Psychosocial**
1. Anxiety—uncomfortable feeling associated with an unknown direct cause; common in these clients related to the unknown outcome of the illness; threat to financial stability
2. Anger—related to forced changes in lifestyle; most often seen following trauma
3. Lifestyle changes—in response to changes in mobility or ability to continue working
4. Body-image change—usually related to structural changes as a result of trauma or malignancy
5. Isolation—may be related to decreased mobility or self-inflicted by client who is uncomfortable with new body image

D. **Health history**
1. What exactly is the problem you are experiencing?
2. Are you having pain? Point to the pain with one finger.
3. Describe the pain. Is it aching, throbbing, stabbing, or sharp?
4. Does anything make the pain worse or better?
5. Is your pain worse during rain or damp weather?
6. Does the pain wake you up at night?
7. Have you recently had an injury to the area?

8. Point to which joints are stiff. Are your joints always stiff? How long do they feel stiff each day? In the morning only?
9. Does your joint ever lock and not want to move?
10. Do you feel any weakness in your muscles? Which muscles?
11. How long have you had this swelling? Is there pain associated with the swelling?
12. Do you have any difficulty walking?
13. Do you have a loss of sensation, or burning and tingling in your extremities?
14. What past medical problems have you experienced?
15. Have you had any injuries or surgeries in the past?
16. What medical problems are you being treated for presently?
17. What prescription and over-the-counter medications are you taking presently?
18. Is there a family history of any bone, joint, or muscle problems?
19. Are you having any difficulties taking care of your personal hygiene?
20. Are you able to do the work of your occupation?

E. **Physical exam**
   1. Airway, breathing, circulation—vital signs
   2. Inspection and palpation of each body part—examine at rest and then while performing ROM exercises
   3. Observe general appearance
   4. Observe posture
   5. Observe gait
   6. Observe for any deformities
   7. Observe client in supine position for body alignment and deformity
   8. Inspect and palpate each muscle group
   9. Palpate each bone and joint
   10. Evaluate for crepitus in joints (grating sound or feeling in joint) with movement

IV. Pathophysiologic disorders

A. **Fractures (Figure 12-1)**
   1. Definition—a break in a bone; five categorizations
      a. Skin over fracture is open, open fracture, or intact, closed fracture
      b. Line of fracture—transverse, oblique, spiral, or linear
      c. Number of pieces—comminuted
      d. Position of distal fragment—displaced or angulated
      e. If fracture involves the joint—intraarticular or extraarticular

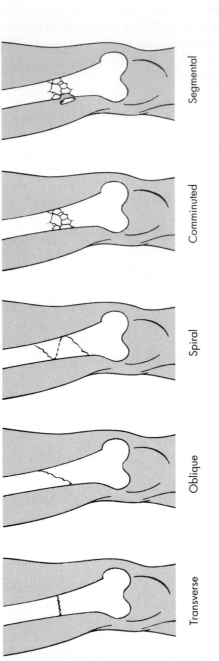

Transverse   Oblique   Spiral   Comminuted   Segmental

Figure 12-1. Five types of fractures. (From Beare PG and Myers JL: *Principles and practice of adult health nursing,* ed 2, St Louis, 1994, Mosby.)

2. Pathophysiology—stress placed on bone will result in fracture; stress includes direct blows, twisting, severe muscle contractions, or, as in a malignancy or severe osteoporosis, the bone will crumble

3. Etiology—usually a result of trauma in the workplace, sports, or in the case of older adult clients, osteoporosis and calcium loss from bones

4. Incidence—most commonly seen in young males or older adults

5. Assessment
   a. Ask the following questions
      (1) Do you have pain at the site?
      (2) Do you feel as if the area is swollen?
      (3) Can you move the area?
   b. Clinical manifestations—depend on cause, classification, type, and site
      (1) Pain with or without movement or weight bearing
      (2) Swelling
      (3) Inability to move
      (4) Discoloration at the area
      (5) Crepitus
      (6) Deformity
      (7) Hip fractures—affected leg is
         (a) Shortened
         (b) Abducted
         (c) Externally rotated
   c. Complications
      (1) Arterial damage—hemorrhage
      (2) Nerve damage—burning pain or loss of sensation or movement
      (3) Bleeding—hematoma
      (4) Avascular necrosis—loss of blood supply to bone results in death of bone; usually found at head of femur
      (5) Compartment syndrome—poor venous return in area results in edema which becomes so great in one of the compartments that arterial flow and nerve impulse transmission are impeded; absent or decreased pulses and paresthesia are common manifestations (Figure 12-2)
      (6) Fat emboli—usually with a femur fracture; fat globules enter vascular space and become emboli, eventually

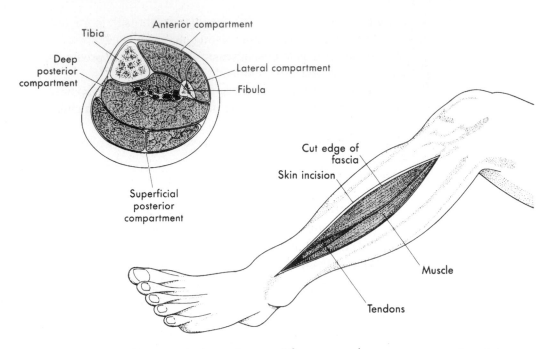

Figure 12-2. Compartment syndrome. Often more than one compartment is involved, and anterior compartment is especially vulnerable. Causes include trauma, severe burn, or excessive exercise. A single incision may open more than one compartment. (From Beare PG and Myers JL: *Principles and practice of adult health nursing,* ed 2, St Louis, 1994, Mosby.)

            entering the lung (see Chapter 6, Pulmonary embolism p. 195)

    (7) Osteomyelitis—infection of osseous tissue of the bone

  d. Abnormal diagnostic tests

    (1) Bone x-rays—show fracture

    (2) Arthroscopy—determines extent of joint involvement, if applicable

    (3) Bone scans—determine extent of pathologic fracture, if applicable

6. Expected medical interventions

  a. Closed reduction—bones manually manipulated back into alignment

  b. Open reduction—surgical incision; bone fragments held in place by plates, screws, pins, rods, and/or wires

  c. Casting once reduction is completed

d. Tractions
   (1) Skin traction—Buck's traction is used to decrease edema and muscle spasms before open reduction of a hip fracture (Figure 12-3)
   (2) Skeletal traction—uses pins, inserted through distal end of femur; traction is then applied to pins to pull bones back into alignment (Figure 12-4)
e. External fixation devices—metal frame with pins, inserted through the bone to hold the fracture in position; commonly used for multiple fractures in a long bone

7. Nursing diagnoses
   a. Pain related to injury of soft tissue and bone
   b. Impaired physical mobility related to restriction of cast, fixation device, or traction
   c. Risk for impaired skin integrity related to decreased mobility secondary to cast, traction, or fixation device application

8. Client goals
   a. Client will state pain is decreased or relieved
   b. Client will demonstrate appropriate mobility of extremities that can be moved and range of motion of joint that can be moved
   c. Client will not have skin breakdown at high risk areas

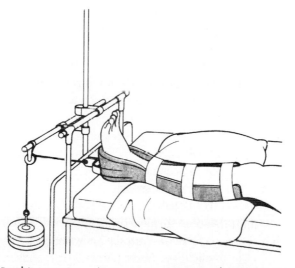

Figure 12-3. Buck's traction. (From Beare PG and Myers JL: *Principles and practice of adult health nursing*, ed 2, St Louis, 1994, Mosby.)

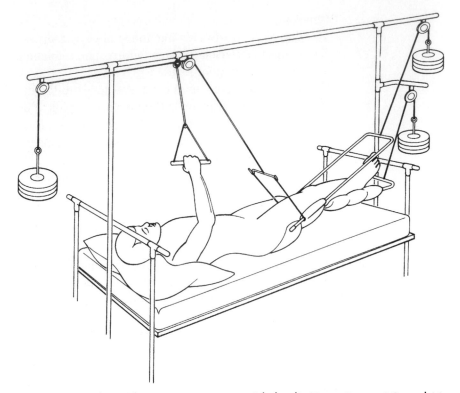

Figure 12-4. Balanced suspension traction (skeletal). (From Beare PG and Myers JL: *Principles and practice of adult health nursing,* ed 2, St Louis, 1994, Mosby.)

9. Nursing interventions
   a. Care of the client postoperative hip fracture repair (pinning or prosthesis)
      (1) Routine postoperative care
      (2) Assess the six Ps of neurovascular status with routine postoperative checks
         (a) Pain
         (b) Pallor
         (c) Paralysis
         (d) Paresthesia
         (e) Pulselessness
         (f) Polar
      (3) Assess surgical drainage devices—empty hemovac or Jackson-Pratt drains when half full or every shift, whichever occurs first
      (4) Notify physician if drainage >150 ml/hr
      (5) Monitor H&H for a further decrease, electrolytes for any change

      (6)   Antiembolism stockings or sequential compression device to nonaffected leg as per physician order

      (7)   Institute exercises

          (a)   Ankle rotations

          (b)   Dorsiflexion and plantar flexion of ankle

      (8)   Maintain abductor pillow while in bed (Figure 12-5)

      (9)   Turn every 2 hours to unaffected side and back only

   (10)   Do not allow hip flexion >35 to 40 degrees

  b.   Care of the client in a cast (plaster or synthetic—Table 12-1)

      (1)   Neurovascular checks every 30 minutes for 4 hours, then every 2 hours for 4 hours, then every 4 hours

      (2)   Evaluate for drainage through cast—circle with pen to evaluate size increase; include time with each circle

      (3)   Elevate casted extremity on a pillow to promote venous return and prevent edema

      (4)   Ice to cast, over affected area—protects cast from moisture

      (5)   Assess cast for area of increased heat—may indicate infection under cast

      (6)   Assess for foul odor from cast

      (7)   Do not handle cast with fingertips when wet—may cause indentation that could impair skin under cast; if it needs to be moved use palms of hands

      (8)   Do not cover cast—let air dry for first 24 hours

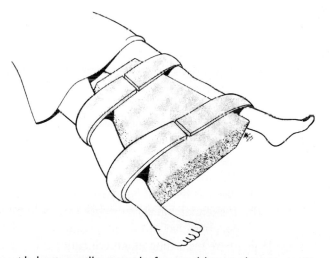

Figure 12-5. Abduction pillow used after total hip replacement. (From Beare PG and Myers JL: *Principles and practice of adult health nursing,* ed 2, St Louis, 1994, Mosby.)

Table 12-1. **Client Education Guide to Cast Care**

Plaster of Paris Cast

Do not wash the cast, because washing can weaken the cast and allow mildew to form. A slightly damp rag with cleanser may be used if moisture is wiped away afterward.

Protect the cast with a plastic wrap during bathing or if in rain or snow.

Remove loose plaster crumbs from under cast edges and brush them away from the area.

Synthetic Cast

Cover any rough edges by petaling, or smooth them by lightly filing with a nail file or emery board.

Use only a small amount of mild soap in the area of the cast if getting the cast wet is allowed; rinse the cast well after bathing.

Try to keep all particles, such as dirt or sand, out of the cast; rinse out any particles that may get into the cast.

After swimming in a chlorinated pool or lake, flush the cast thoroughly with water.

Thoroughly dry padding and stockinette each time the cast gets wet, so that skin maceration will not result:

1. Remove excess water by blotting cast with a towel.
2. Use a hand-held hair dryer (on cool or warm setting) in sweeping motion over cast surface to reduce drying time.
3. Continue drying cast for about 1 hour; the cast will be dry when it no longer feels cold and clammy.

From Beare P and Myers J: *Principles and practice of adult health nursing,* St Louis, 1990, Mosby.

        (9)   Petal edges of cast to prevent rough edges from breaking down skin

   c. Care of the client in traction (skeletal and skin)

        (1)   Use fracture bedpan for elimination

        (2)   Assess neurovascular status of the extremity q 1 to 2 hours

        (3)   Maintain body alignment

        (4)   Keep weights off floor, use correct weight size ordered

        (5)   If skeletal, pin care q 8 hrs with solution as ordered by physician

   d. Home care regarding client education

        (1)   Care of the cast (see Table 12-1)

            (a) Put nothing down cast

    (b) Weight bear when physician indicates it is safe

    (c) Call physician if area of cast feels warm or if odor comes from cast

  (2) Assistive device use

    (a) Crutch walking (Figure 12-6 for crutch walking gaits)

      (i) Non-weight-bearing using three-point gait

      (ii) Appropriate crutch fit—bottom of crutches, rubber tips, 6 to 8 inches from client's side or feet; top of crutch should be 2 inches below axilla crease

      (iii) Weight on hands not axilla

      (iv) Elbows slightly bent

    (b) Cane carried in hand opposite affected leg for greater support

    (c) Walker—with arms bent slightly position walker ahead of gait, to a comfortable length of the arms and walk into walker, repeat

  (3) Physician follow-up *very important*—first visit is usually within 1 week from traumatic event

10. Evaluation protocol

 a. How do I know that my interventions were effective?

  (1) Neurovascular status—palpable pulse, warm extremity with color equivalent to opposite extremity, appropriate sensation, movement, and brisk capillary refill <3 seconds

  (2) Pain is relieved

  (3) Cast is drying and intact

  (4) Skeletal traction is appropriate with correct body alignment

  (5) Traction pin sites are not infected; drainage, if any, is serous

  (6) Hip prosthesis is in appropriate alignment

  (7) Assessment findings do not indicate a tight cast or compartment syndrome

 b. What criteria will I use to change my interventions?

  (1) One aspect of neurovascular status has deteriorated

  (2) Increased pain

  (3) Cast is tight and skin is breaking down

  (4) Skeletal traction is out of alignment

  (5) Pin sites have purulent drainage

  (6) Hip prosthesis has left the acetabulum

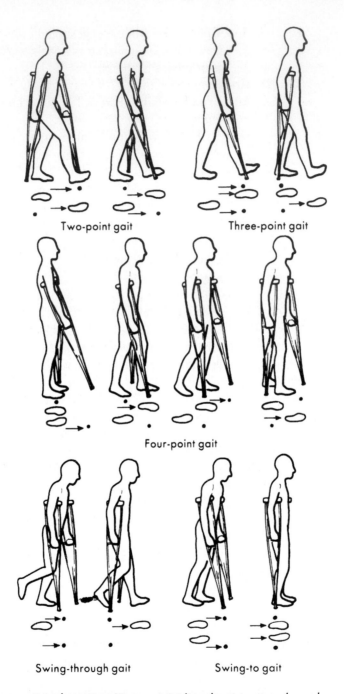

Two-point gait

Three-point gait

Four-point gait

Swing-through gait

Swing-to gait

Figure 12-6. Crutch gaits. (From *AJN/Mosby Nursing board review*, ed 9, St Louis, 1994, Mosby.)

        (7) Client assessment findings indicate possible complication—most often identified by a change in neurovascular status or increasing pain

    c. How will I know that my client teaching has been effective?

        (1) Cast has dried appropriately without any neurovascular impairment

        (2) Client can state symptoms that should be reported to the physician

        (3) Client demonstrates appropriate use of assistive device

11. Older adult alert

    a. The older adult client is more susceptible to fractures as a result of osteoporosis. Teaching should be aimed at preventing accidents.

    b. The older adult client who is bedfast will be at a much higher risk for complications than the younger adult

B. **Ruptured lumbar intervertebral disc (herniated disc)**

  1. Definition—displacement of intervertebral disc material

  2. Pathophysiology—most often occurs in back of disc where outer ring of tissue holding disc in place is the weakest; most often involves a tear in this outer tissue and the interior contents, the nucleus pulposus, bulges outward, putting pressure on the spinal nerve roots; pain and paresthesia result from compression of nerve roots

  3. Etiology—most clients report a previous back injury that involved flexion or rotation of the back in such a way to cause displacement of the disc

  4. Incidence—more than 10% of clients who seek medical advice for back pain have a herniated disc

  5. Assessment

    a. Ask the following questions

        (1) Where is your pain? Point to it with one finger.

        (2) Does the pain travel anywhere else?

        (3) Have you noticed any other feeling besides pain?

    b. Clinical manifestations

        (1) Lower back pain

        (2) Radiation of pain into posterior thigh

        (3) Muscle spasms

        (4) Decreased deep tendon reflexes

        (5) Numbness along nerve roots

    c. Abnormal diagnostic tests

        (1) Spinal x-rays—narrowed disc space

        (2) MRI—spinal stenosis, herniated material from disc

        (3)   Myelogram—narrowed disc space and herniation at a specific level

6. Expected medical interventions
   a. Antiinflammatory agents
   b. Muscle relaxants
   c. Analgesics
   d. Decreased activity, bedrest if necessary
   e. Pelvic traction
   f. Back brace
   g. Percutaneous lateral diskectomy
   h. Laminectomy and spinal fusion

7. Nursing diagnoses
   a. Pain related to pressure on nerve roots or to effects of surgery
   b. Impaired mobility related to lumbar pain secondary to pressure on nerve roots

8. Client goals
   a. Client will state pain is relieved or decreased
   b. Client will increase mobility by 10 to 20% each day

9. Nursing interventions
   a. Acute care—postoperative
      (1) Routine postoperative care
      (2) Neurovascular assessment with each set of vital signs
      (3) Empty and evaluate drainage from continuous portable suction device (hemovac or Jackson-Pratt drain) when half full or every shift, whichever occurs first
      (4) Logroll client every 2 hours
      (5) Evaluate lumbar incision and iliac incision if bone graft done
      (6) Out of bed to a straight back chair, with feet on floor, usually the evening of surgery, for 30 minutes to 1 hour as tolerated
      (7) If a spinal fusion was done, clients stay in bed for 24 to 48 hours, logrolled every 2 hours
      (8) Evaluate for urinary retention if indwelling urinary catheter not in place
   b. Home care regarding client education
      (1) All medication, when and how to take
      (2) Incision(s) should be cleaned with soap and water at least once a day; report redness, swelling, or drainage from incision to physician

          (3) Principles of correct body mechanics
              (a) Use leg muscles not back muscles when lifting
              (b) Always get help in lifting
              (c) Do not turn and lift at the same time
          (4) Do not twist back, especially when getting out of bed
          (5) Sleep on a firm mattress
          (6) Avoid sitting for longer than an hour at a time
          (7) Maintain or achieve ideal body weight
          (8) Do not climb steps for at least 2 to 3 weeks
          (9) Do not attempt any weight lift until first physician visit—at that time physician may tell client to lift only 5 lb at a time, slowly increasing by ½ pound at a time over the next 4 weeks
         (10) May be able to return to work in 3 to 4 weeks depending on the type of work

10. Evaluation protocol
    a. How do I know that my interventions were effective?
        (1) Neurovascular status is intact
        (2) Drains are intact with minimal drainage
        (3) Incisions are approximated, clean, and dry
        (4) Client is turned q 2 hours using logrolling technique
        (5) Client is OOB as ordered
        (6) No urinary retention
    b. What criteria will I use to change my interventions?
        (1) Neurovascular impairment
        (2) Drains are not intact or have increased bloody drainage
        (3) Client is trying to turn without logrolling technique
        (4) Urinary retention is identified
    c. How will I know that my client teaching has been effective?
        (1) Client correctly states medication regime
        (2) Client demonstrates correct body mechanics
        (3) Client indicates the sleeping on a firm mattress
        (4) Client indicates appropriate weight changes: has lost weight, is losing weight, or is maintaining ideal weight
        (5) Client follows regime for postoperative activity
        (6) Client indicates the incision is clean, dry, and edges are together

11. Older adult alert—older adult clients must be evaluated carefully for the complications associated with immobility during the recovery phase of this surgery

C. **Arthritis**
1. Definition
   a. Osteoarthritis—nonsystemic, degenerative disorder of the weight-bearing joints
   b. Rheumatoid arthritis—chronic systemic inflammatory disorder of the connective tissue; exacerbations and remissions are characteristic
   c. Gouty arthritis—inflammatory changes evident in one joint in response to high uric acid levels
2. Pathophysiology
   a. Osteoarthritis—wearing down and breakdown of the articular cartilage of the joints; cracks occur in the surface of cartilage; spurs form and pain is the result
   b. Rheumatoid arthritis—synovial lining of the joint becomes inflamed; granulation tissue forms; cartilage is destroyed; fibrous tissue is left in place of cartilage
   c. Gouty arthritis—increase in purine metabolism results in excess uric acid; uric acid crystals form in joints and connective tissue; most often affects the great toe; inflammation results and pain follows
3. Etiology
   a. Osteoarthritis—unknown; aging is considered a risk factor
   b. Rheumatoid arthritis—unknown; theories suggest autoimmune disorder and infectious agents
   c. Gouty arthritis—increase in purine metabolism, high purine diet, excess alcohol intake
4. Incidence
   a. Osteoarthritis—common after age 35; more common in females over age 55
   b. Rheumatoid arthritis—more common in female population
   c. Gouty arthritis—more common in male population
5. Assessment
   a. Ask the following questions
      (1) When does your pain occur?
      (2) Do you have swelling of your joints?
      (3) Does the weather make your pain worse?
      (4) What makes your pain worse?
      (5) What makes your pain better?
   b. Clinical manifestations (Table 12-2)
   c. Abnormal laboratory findings
      (1) Osteoarthritis—none specific for this disorder

Table 12-2. Comparison of Arthritis Types

	Osteoarthritis	Rheumatoid Arthritis	Gouty Arthritis
No. joints affected	1 or 2	Multiple	One
Joint deformity?	Yes	Yes	Possibly
Pain with movement?	Yes	Decrease with movement	Pain all the time
Morning stiffness?	Yes	Yes	No
Fever, increased WBC	No	Yes	Fever
Symptoms increase with humidity	Yes	Yes	No
Exacerbations and remissions	No	Yes	If medications and diet are not followed

      (2) Rheumatoid arthritis
         (a) Rheumatoid factor—positive
         (b) Sedimentation rate—elevated
      (3) Gouty arthritis
         (a) Serum uric acid—elevated
         (b) CBC—elevated WBC
         (c) Sedimentation rate—elevated
   d. Abnormal diagnostic tests
      (1) Osteoarthritis
         (a) Joint x-rays—narrowed joint space, bone cysts, sharpened articular surfaces
      (2) Rheumatoid arthritis
         (a) Joint aspiration—increased synovial fluid volume, cloudy
         (b) Joint x-rays—eroded joint surfaces, joint space narrowing, unstable joint
      (3) Gouty arthritis
         (a) Joint aspiration—presence of uric acid crystals
         (b) Joint x-rays—radiolucent urate tophi (nodules of urate)
  6. Expected medical interventions
   a. Osteoarthritis
      (1) Rest affected joints
      (2) Weight reduction if necessary
      (3) Moist heat
      (4) Intraarticular steroids

      (5) NSAIDs

      (6) Joint replacement

      (7) ROM, passive and active

   b. Rheumatoid arthritis

      (1) Rest, especially during exacerbations; splints may be used

      (2) ROM, passive and active

      (3) Cold therapy during acute exacerbations and moist heat for stiffened joints

      (4) Aspirin

      (5) Gold salts

      (6) Corticosteroids

      (7) Methotrexate

   c. Gouty arthritis

      (1) NSAIDs

      (2) Colchicine for acute episodes

      (3) Uricosuric agents, Allopurinol

      (4) Low purine diet

      (5) Gouty tophi excision if eroding through skin

7. Nursing diagnoses

   a. Acute pain related to inflamed joint spaces

   b. Impaired physical mobility related to joint pain

   c. Fatigue related to prolonged immobility and increased metabolic demands

8. Client goals

   a. Client will state pain has decreased or been relieved with the use of specified interventions

   b. Client will demonstrate active range of motion on all joints daily

   c. Client will state fatigue has decreased

9. Nursing interventions

   a. Acute care

      (1) Postoperative joint replacement—care will be the same as for the client following hip surgery (p. 404)

   b. Home care regarding client education

      (1) Medication regime

      (2) Need for daily activity, do not overexert

      (3) Application of heat for analgesia

      (4) Exercise joints to the point of pain but not past the point of pain

      (5) Use of splints on affected joints during acute exacerbations

   (6) Low purine diet for prevention of gout
   (7) Need for increased fluid intake to prevent uric acid urinary calculi with gout
   (8) Need for weight control if indicated
  10. Evaluation protocol
   (1) How will I know that my client teaching has been effective?
    (a) Client states performance of ROM three times a day
    (b) Client demonstrates correct medication regime and verbalization of side effects to relate to physician
    (c) Client loses weight with maintenance of appropriate weight
    (d) Client demonstrates correct procedure for moist heat application
  11. Older adult alert—this is a disorder of older adults and should be evaluated for when assessing older adult clients
 D. **Amputation**
  1. Definition—removal of a limb
  2. Pathophysiology—would be the pathophysiology of the disorder that led to the need for amputation
  3. Etiology—traumatic injury; surgical removal as a result of a gangrenous process, cancerous tumor, osteomyelitis, etc.
  4. Assessment
   a. Clinical manifestations
    (1) Traumatic
     (a) Discoloration of the limb
     (b) Muscle loss and vascular impairment
     (c) Neurovascular compromise
    (2) Surgical—(see Peripheral arterial occlusive disorders, Chapter 4, pp. 116)
   b. Abnormal diagnostic tests
    (1) Angiography—shows inadequate circulation
    (2) CT scan—evaluates for extensive neoplasm or osteomyelitis
    (3) Doppler ultrasound—indicates degree of inadequate circulation
  5. Nursing diagnoses
   a. Pain related to effects of trauma or surgical procedure
   b. Impaired physical mobility related to loss of lower extremity and the need to learn use of prosthesis

    c. Pain related to phantom limb sensation

    d. Body-image disturbance related to loss of a body part

6. Client goals

    a. Client will state pain is relieved or decreased

    b. Client will demonstrate ROM of remaining extremities

    c. Client will attempt an ability to maintain independence

    d. Client will state phantom pain is relieved

    e. Client will state feeling comfortable with change in body and adapting

7. Nursing interventions

    a. Acute care

        (1) Routine postoperative care

        (2) Maintain immediate postoperative prosthesis (IPOP) as ordered by physician—cast applied over postoperative dressing and prosthesis applied to cast; increases early ambulation and decreases edema; used until permanent prosthesis is ready

        (3) Air splints and ace wraps may be used to decrease stump edema

        (4) Elevate stump with physician order, for initial 24 hours to hasten a decrease in edema

        (5) After first 24 hours, assist client into a prone position if tolerated, for one hour, three times a day, to prevent hip and knee contractures

        (6) Treat phantom pain as needed

            (a) Physician may order beta blockers to increase serotonin level and decrease pain

            (b) Distraction therapy, massage therapy

            (c) Transcutaneous electrical nerve stimulation (TENS) units may be very helpful

            (d) Maintain epidural anesthesia postoperatively—very effective for reducing phantom pain

        (7) Encourage client to look at stump and touch it to begin acceptance

    b. Home care regarding client education

        (1) Stump care, before and after prosthesis use

        (2) Indicators of wound infection

        (3) Exercise regime

        (4) Ambulation with assistive devices

8. Evaluation protocol

    a. How will I know that my interventions were effective?

        (1) Stump does not become edematous

          (2) Hip and knee contractures do not occur

          (3) Phantom pain is controlled

          (4) Client is accepting of stump; looks at stump with beginning actions to care for incision

    b. What criteria will I use to change my interventions?

          (1) Edematous stump

          (2) Hip and/or knee contractures

          (3) Uncontrolled phantom pain

          (4) Client is unable to accept stump; refuses to look at or touch stump

    c. How will I know that my client teaching has been effective?

          (1) Client demonstrates correct technique for stump care

          (2) Client states findings associated with wound infection

          (3) Client demonstrates correct exercise regime

          (4) Client demonstrates correct technique for use of assistive devices

9. Older adult alert

    a. The older adult client will be more difficult to return to a preamputation mobility status because of joint changes in other extremities that may be present

    b. A prosthesis may be impossible to use for the older adult client as a result of impaired mobility in other extremities or difficulty on the client's part to place and remove the prosthesis due to decreased dexterity and/or vision

E. Osteoporosis

  1. Definition—metabolic bone disease that results in demineralization of the bone and subsequent fractures

  2. Pathophysiology and etiology—loss of bone density that starts in the third and fourth decade

    a. Due to aging, impaired osteoblasts are unable to form bone at the same rate as resorption of bone occurs

    b. Less vitamin D is available due to decreased estrogen, which results in an impaired calcium absorption

    c. Decreased intake of dietary calcium may also contribute

    d. Decreased weight-bearing exercise also contributes

    e. Smoking >10 cigarettes per day decreases serum estrogen

    f. Alcohol and caffeine intake can increase daily calcium loss

  3. Incidence—approximately 50 to 60% of women over age 65 have osteoporosis; more common in women

4. Assessment
   a. Ask the following questions
      (1) Do you ever have pain in your back or hip?
      (2) Have you noticed that your height has decreased over the past three years?
      (3) Do you have difficulty walking?
   b. Clinical manifestations
      (1) Unfortunately many clients are asymptomatic until a fracture occurs
      (2) Hump or kyphosis at top of spine
      (3) Shortened height
      (4) Pain, worsened by activity
   c. Abnormal laboratory findings
      (1) Serum calcium—high
      (2) Alkaline phosphatase—low
   d. Abnormal diagnostic tests
      (1) Bone x-rays—show demineralization, fractures
      (2) CT scan—demineralization in the cancellous bone, which can allow early diagnosis
      (3) Single-photon absorptiometry—measures skeletal density in two dimensions; shows a loss of density
5. Expected medical interventions
   a. Balanced diet with at least 1500 mg of elemental calcium per day
   b. Moderate daily exercise—walking, swimming
   c. Back or neck support to prevent fractures
   d. Calcium carbonate
   e. Vitamin D 1 to 2 times per week
   f. Estrogen-progestin combinations
6. Nursing diagnosis
   a. High risk for injury (fracture) related to falls, bumping into objects
   b. Impaired physical mobility related to change in vertebral column, decreased muscle tone
   c. Pain related to fracture
7. Client goals
   a. Client will not injure self, as evidenced by absence of bruises or fractures
   b. Client will demonstrate mobility as evidenced by walking for 10 minutes each day or swimming for 10 minutes each day
   c. Client will state pain has decreased to a 2 on a pain scale of 0 to 10

8. Nursing interventions
   a. Acute care—would be the nursing care of the client with fractures (p. 404)
   b. Home care regarding client education
      (1) Work with client to evaluate home for potential hazards
         (a) Use nonslip slippers
         (b) Remove throw rugs from floor
         (c) Have optimal lighting
         (d) Place handrails in bathroom near commode and in tub/shower
         (e) Use nonslip material on steps
      (2) Evaluate current drug therapy for any medications that may cause drowsiness or dizziness
      (3) Teach client about
         (a) Foods high in calcium
         (b) Avoiding caffeine and alcohol
         (c) Stopping tobacco use
      (4) Consult with physical therapy to devise an exercise program—deep water exercises with the use of flotation devices are excellent
      (5) Encourage assistive devices if necessary, such as a walker or cane
      (6) Pain control—medication if needed: narcotic or nonnarcotic, antiinflammatory drugs, moist heat
      (7) Assess fit of vertebral support—braces and neck supports
9. Evaluation protocol
   a. How will I know that my client teaching has been effective?
      (1) Client produces a food diary which indicates he or she is eating high calcium foods
      (2) Client states he or she is taking vitamins and calcium supplements
      (3) Client states he or she has stopped smoking, drinking caffeinated beverages and alcohol
      (4) Client states he or she has begun walking for 15 to 30 minutes at least once each day
      (5) Client demonstrates proper use of a cane
      (6) Client states that pain is controlled with NSAID and warm, moist compresses
10. Older adult alert—this is an illness found predominantly in the older adult population. This illness must be considered when treating an older adult client with new onset of skeletal pain or disability.

REVIEW QUESTIONS

1. The client who has a synthetic cast applied is permitted to swim or bathe with the cast, but must be given which of these instructions
    a. Blot cast dry on the outside, and allow to air dry
    b. Flush the cast with clean water, blot outside dry, use hair dryer on cool or warm setting to dry padding on inside
    c. Blot outside dry, use hair dryer on cool or warm setting to dry padding on inside
    d. Use hair dryer on cool or warm setting to dry padding on inside

2. A client calls the nurse and states that his cast feels warm in one spot. He is asking what he should do. The best answer will depend on an understanding of what is happening. The nurse knows a hot spot is an indication of
    a. Swelling under cast
    b. Inflammation under cast
    c. Cast tightness
    d. An object stuck under the cast

3. The purpose of the abductor pillow for the client who is postoperative for a total hip prosthesis is to
    a. Prevent mobility of the new joint until healed
    b. Prevent adduction
    c. Hold the prosthesis in the acetabulum until healing can begin
    d. Hold the prosthesis in the acetabulum and prevent slippage out of the acetabulum

4. A client experiencing compartment syndrome will exhibit which assessment finding?
    a. Paresthesia of extremity involved
    b. Increased redness of the extremity involved
    c. Warm then cold skin on the involved extremity
    d. Increased movement of the digits

5. The pain experienced by a client who is postoperative for a lumbar laminectomy with spinal fusion is commonly a
    a. Sharp quality that travels down one of the legs
    b. Dull ache in the area of the buttocks
    c. Sharp incisional pain
    d. Sharp incisional pain and muscle spasms around incisional area

6. An important assessment finding that can help distinguish between osteoarthritis and rheumatoid arthritis is
   a. Symptoms increase with increased humidity only in osteoarthritis
   b. Pain increases with use in both conditions
   c. Fever noted in both conditions during exacerbations
   d. Pain decreases with use in rheumatoid arthritis and increases with use in osteoarthritis

7. A food stuff that should be restricted on a low purine diet for gouty arthritis is
   a. Chicken
   b. Eggs
   c. Legumes
   d. Cereal grains

8. An understanding of phantom pain allows the nurse to explain to a client that it is caused by
   a. Nerves stimulated at the level of the surgical incision
   b. Nerves that have been cut but are still sending impulses from the severed limb
   c. Swelling around the nerves at the surgical site
   d. Bone nerves that have been cut

9. Clients with osteoporosis must be counselled to not only include high levels of calcium in their diet but also include
   a. Vitamin C
   b. Vitamin D
   c. Vitamin K
   d. Vitamins A and D

10. The therapy of choice for the client with rheumatoid arthritis in acute exacerbation is
    a. Hot compresses
    b. Warm, moist compresses
    c. Cold therapy
    d. Paraffin therapy

ANSWERS, RATIONALES, AND TEST-TAKING TIPS

Rationales	Test-Taking Tips

1. Correct answer: b

The cast must be flushed to remove traces of soap or chlorine. Blot the outside dry, and dry inside with a warm or cool hair dryer.

Clues in the stem are the words "swim" and "bath." Common sense reflects that in both of these situations the cast would need to be rinsed first then dried. Another approach is that response *b* is the most comprehensive.

2. Correct answer: b

The hot spot is typically caused by inflammation under the cast and should be evaluated by a physician.

The clue to selection of the correct response is the word "hot." Hot on the body typically indicates inflammation. Swelling would occur in more than just one spot.

3. Correct answer: d

Slippage of the head of the prosthesis, out of the acetabulum, is a very painful and dangerous complication. The abductor pillow will prevent this by holding the head of the prosthesis in correct position.

After narrowing the responses to *c* and *d,* reread *c* and note the clue "until healing can begin"; abductor pillows have no connection to the healing process.

4. Correct answer: a

Loss of sensation or altered sensation in the extremity is one of the more common assessment findings in the face of compartment syndrome.

Recall compartment syndrome results in compression of the arteries and nerves. Thus, deficits in these two areas are more likely.

5. Correct answer: d

The client feels sharp pain from the incision as well as muscle spasms from the procedure.

Eliminate responses *a* and *b* since they are general in focus and have nothing to do with surgery. Of the remaining responses *d* is more inclusive to expect after surgery.

6. Correct answer: d

Pain increases with use in osteoarthritis and decreases with use in rheumatoid arthritis. Symptoms increase with humidity in both; fever is noted only in rheumatoid arthritis during exacerbations.

The clue is that *osteo* = old, worn-out joint; it will hurt more if this type of joint is used. Remember: *osteo* = short word, therefore is a local condition; rheumatoid = long word therefore is a systemic condition and fever would be present, as well as anemia and the elevated labs of: sedimentation (sed) rates, rheumatoid factors.

7. Correct answer: c

Legumes, such as beans, mushrooms, are discouraged on a low purine diet, as well as organ meats, shellfish and alcohol.

The approach to correct answer selection is to "go with what you know." Eliminate chicken which is usually not restricted. Associate eggs restriction with clients having high cholesterol. Cereal grains are usually not restricted except when glutens are a problem. Select legumes—the only option left.

8. Correct answer: b

Phantom pain results from impulses sent from severed nerves, and does eventually subside.

Eliminate response *d*—there is no such thing as bone nerves. Responses *a* and *c* can be clustered to describe specific sites. Response *b* is the most comprehensive.

9. Correct answer: d

Vitamins A and D are required for appropriate absorption of calcium.

Cluster the first three responses since they have one vitamin. Then response *d* is correct.

10. Correct answer: c

Cold therapy is used to decrease inflammation during an acute exacerbation.

Use common sense that in any acute inflammation cold is used first.

The Integumentary System

STUDY OUTCOMES

After completing this chapter, the reader will be able to do
the following:

▼ Describe the function and structure of the integumentary system.
▼ Identify assessment factors common to clients who have disorders
of the integumentary system.
▼ Select appropriate nursing diagnoses for the client with a disorder
of the integumentary system.
▼ Identify appropriate nursing interventions for the client with a
disorder of the integumentary system.
▼ Evaluate outcomes of the client with a disorder of the integumentary
system to make appropriate changes to the care of that client based
on the evaluation.

KEY TERMS

Circumscribed	A specified area limited by a border.
Core temperature	Temperature of the body in the chest, abdomen, and head.
Ecchymosis	Discoloration of the skin as a result of blood extravasating into the area; bruise.
Erythema	Redness.
Eschar	Scab or dried crust resulting from burns, infection, or excoriation of the skin.
Indurated	Hardened raised tissue.
Lesion	Change in the normal skin structure.
Macule	A small, flat, discoloration of the skin, such as freckles or rashes.
Nodule	A small, rounded mass.
Papule	Lesion <1 cm, raised above the skin and solid.
Petechiae	Flat, tiny, red or purple spots that appear on the skin, usually upper anterior chest wall, as a result of tiny hemorrhages in the dermal or mucosal layer.
Pruritus	Itching.
Purpura	A bleeding disorder that results in bleeding under the skin or mucous membranes; produces ecchymosis or petechiae.
Sebum	Oil produced by the sebaceous glands.
Urticaria	Hives.
Vesicle	Small, thin-walled raised lesion filled with fluid, such as a blister.
Wheal	A raised, reddened, solid lesion of the skin, usually caused by an allergen.

CONTENT REVIEW

I. The integumentary system is responsible for protecting the body from pathogen invasion, fluid loss, chemicals, and ultraviolet radiation; also regulates heat loss from the body, excretes wastes, and synthesizes vitamin D

II. Structure and function
   A. Largest organ of the body

B. **Two layers to the skin—epidermis and dermis, joined together and situated above the subcutaneous layer**
   1. Epidermis
      a. Comprised of squamous epithelium divided into four or five layers
      b. Does not have its own blood supply
      c. Has a few nerve endings in layer found closest to the dermis
      d. New cells are formed in layer closest to the dermis and are pushed upward to the top of the epidermis
      e. Top layer of cells are dead and are eventually rubbed off the skin surface, either through friction or cleansing
      f. Melanin granules are found in the epidermis and are responsible for skin color
   2. Dermis
      a. Dense, fibrous, connective tissue with a considerable blood supply and lymph vessels
      b. Supplied with a group of sensory receptors
   3. Accessory structures
      a. Hair—protects scalp from heat and cold, protects nose and eyes from airborne particles
      b. Nails—found on tip of fingers and toes on the dorsal side; protects fingers and assists with picking up small objects
      c. Glands
         (1) Sebaceous—secretes sebum that keeps skin moist and supple
         (2) Ceruminous—secretes wax that lines ear canal and prevents drying of canal and eardrum
         (3) Sudoriferous—secretes sweat that assists in maintaining body temperature

II. Targeted concerns
   A. Pharmacology—priority drug classifications—commonly topical
      1. Antibacterial agents—alter chemistry of invading pathogen
         a. Expected effect—suppression of pathogen
         b. Commonly given drugs
            (1) Bacitracin ointment
            (2) Polysporin ointment
         c. Nursing considerations
            (1) Apply to skin as per order
            (2) Assess skin for redness
            (3) If break in skin integrity, may have systemic effects also

2. Antifungal agents—alter cell wall of fungus
   a. Expected effect—eradication of fungus infection
   b. Commonly given drugs
      (1) Nystatin (Mycostatin)
      (2) Clotrimazole (Lotrimin)
   c. Nursing considerations
      (1) Client must complete a 2- to 3-week course, twice a day, for effective treatment
      (2) Assess skin carefully for irritation from medication
3. Antiparasitic—Pediculicide
   a. Expected effect—eradication of parasites
   b. Commonly given drugs
      (1) Lindane (Kwell)
      (2) Permethrin (Nix)
   c. Nursing considerations
      (1) Caution client to avoid getting medication in the eyes
      (2) Assess client for successful removal of parasites
      (3) Repeat treatment after 48 hours to eliminate eggs
4. Antipruritics—block histamine and serotonin effect
   a. Expected effect—soothes skin
   b. Commonly given drugs
      (1) Calamine lotion
      (2) Aveeno bath
      (3) Burrow's solution wet dressing
      (4) Boric acid wet dressing
   c. Nursing considerations
      (1) Assess for sensitivity to solution
      (2) If solution contains an anesthetic; apply only as directed
5. Corticosteroids—reduce blood flow through their vasoconstrictive action
   a. Expected effect—decrease of redness and itching
   b. Commonly given drugs
      (1) Hydrocortisone (Hytone)
      (2) Triamcinolone (Kenalog)
      (3) Betamethasone (Diprosone)
   c. Nursing considerations
      (1) Apply evenly on skin
      (2) Assess use in clients with systemic infections carefully
      (3) Encourage short-term use only; long-term use tends to thin the skin and client may encounter systemic effects of steroids

B. **Procedures**
1. Skin biopsy—removal of a small piece of skin or a lesion to evaluate for cell makeup
2. Skin scrapings—skin can be scraped for evaluation of cell makeup; hair and nail scrapings can be taken also
3. Swab samples—usually of lesions; evaluated for pathogen and effective antibiotic therapy
4. Wood's light—high-pressure mercury light, also known as black light; used to visualize bacterial and fungal infections on the skin
5. Allergy skin testing
   a. Patch testing—an allergen is placed on the skin and covered with a nonabsorbent patch; skin area is assessed in 48 to 72 hours for erythema, vesicles, and induration
   b. Intradermal skin testing—allergen injected intradermally and a wheal produced; inspected in 48 to 72 hours to evaluate for allergic reaction
   c. Scratch test—allergen placed on an area of skin that has been scratched; if a wheal forms within 15 minutes the client is allergic to the allergen
C. **Psychosocial**
1. Anger—commonly associated with the client who has a skin disorder; a "why me?" response
2. Frustration—also commonly seen in the client with a skin disorder as a result of many different types of treatments that may have varying degrees of success
3. Anxiety—that uncomfortable feeling associated with an unknown direct cause; common in the client with a skin disorder because of the fear of what will happen
4. Embarrassment—common in skin disorders that are disfiguring or change the appearance of the client, especially in the face
5. Clients must have written instructions for skin care medications and treatments; anxiety and embarrassment may prevent the client from listening to directions and, therefore, not be able to perform them correctly at home
D. **Health history—question sequence**
1. Please describe the problem you have been experiencing.
2. When did you first notice your skin problem? How long have you had this skin problem?
3. Do you notice any new symptoms, such as nausea, vomiting, or diarrhea, which started since this skin problem started?

4. What symptoms are associated with the skin problem? Itching, pain, burning?
5. Can you associate the skin condition with anything new that you are eating, drinking, or using on your skin?
6. Have you been trying anything at home for this skin problem? Is it working? Did it make it worse?
7. Are you taking any medications for other problems, either ordered by a physician or purchased over the counter?
8. What medical problems and surgeries have you had in the past? Have you had the chicken pox?
9. Do you have any allergies to foods or medications?
10. Do you have new stresses in your life?
11. Are you following a new diet?
12. Have you been traveling lately? Where?
13. Is there any family history of any skin disorders?

E. **Physical examination—appropriate sequence**
   1. Airway, breathing, circulation—vital signs
   2. Total body skin evaluation—inspection, palpation, and olfactory evaluation
      a. Hair, scalp, nails
      b. Mucous membranes
      c. Skin—starting at head and working down to feet
      d. Evaluate for skin color, thickness, turgor, temperature
      e. Assess for purpura, petechiae
      f. General Considerations
         (1) Frequently the first organ to show signs of illness
         (2) With normal skin turgor, skin returns to baseline after being pinched up within 3 seconds
         (3) The elasticity of the skin decreases with age
         (4) Extremely important in the development of client's self-esteem and self-image
         (5) Skin color changes of the dark-skinned population are best observed in the sclera, conjunctiva, oral mucous membranes, tongue, lips, nail beds, palms, and soles
         (6) In clients with a brown tone to their skin, pallor will be seen as a yellow tint to the skin
         (7) In clients with a darker tone to their skin, pallor will be seen as an ashen gray color
   3. Complete assessment by evaluating heart, lungs, abdomen as previously discussed in other chapters

IV. Pathophysiologic disorders
A. Burn injury
   1. Definition—dermal injury as a result of skin contact with fire, hot liquids, chemicals, radiation, or electricity
   2. Pathophysiology and Etiology—burns cause destruction of the epidermis and in some situations the dermis of the skin
      a. Mechanism of injury
         (1) Electrical burns—create an entrance and exit wound and cause injury along the electrical path; often cause cardiac arrest; exit wound has typically more severe damage than the entrance site
         (2) Chemical burns—must be diluted and removed from the skin area or burning will continue
         (3) Thermal burns—flame or hot liquids
         (4) Radiation burns—caused by a radioactive source, radiation therapy, sunburn
      b. Burn categorization (Figure 13-1)
         (1) Superficial partial thickness (first degree)—sunburn; superficial epidermis; skin is pink, red, dry, and painful, slightly edematous

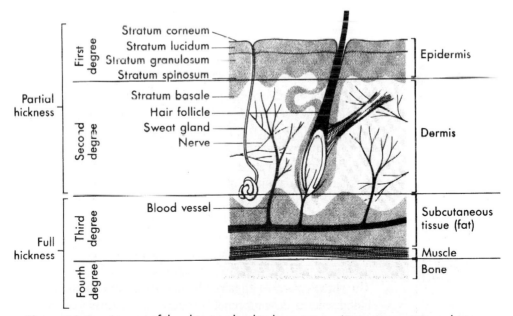

Figure 13-1. Layers of the skin involved in burn injury. (From Beare PG and Myers JL: *Principles and practice of adult health nursing*, ed 2, St Louis, 1994, Mosby.)

(2) Deep partial thickness (second degree)—epidermis and dermis are injured; skin is blistered and red, blanches appropriately; edematous and very painful

(3) Full thickness (third degree)—causes destruction of the epidermis and dermis; may include subcutaneous tissue as well; wound is dry and leathery, and may appear white or charred; does not blanch; wound itself may not be painful but surrounding tissue will be painful; will require skin grafting to cover area

(4) Fourth degree—same as full thickness but also involves fat, fascia, tendons, and bones

c. Phases of burn care

(1) Emergent phase—first 48 hours after burn; major concerns include shock, respiratory failure, hyperkalemia

(a) In initial stages of injury there is increased permeability of blood vessels allowing an outpouring of plasma and colloids into the interstitial space—this accounts for edema associated with burns; if burn injury is large enough, cardiac output can be significantly decreased due to fluid shift into the interstitial space

(2) Acute phase—from day 3 to several months; major concerns include fluid overload, CHF with pulmonary edema, hypokalemia

(3) Rehabilatation phase—from end of acute phase until several years; major concerns include attempt to regain near normal function, scar revision, contracture control, and body-image adjustments

d. The pulmonary system may be impaired if the client inhaled noxious fumes or heat, causing burn injury or inhalation injury to airways; airway obstruction can occur from airway edema associated with the burn; also inhalation may be impaired if there is sufficient burn injury to the chest wall such that inhalation is restricted by eschar or burned, noncompliant tissue

e. The renal system is impaired by decreased circulating blood volume causing renal shutdown; hematuria may be seen initially as a result of massive red blood cell destruction

   f. Burned body surface area (BBSA)
      (1) Rule of nines—rough estimate (Figure 13-2)
      (2) Lund and Browder burn assessment chart—accurate
           (Figure 13-3)
3. Incidence—over 2 million persons per year seek medical
   assistance in the United States for burn injury; of these over
   60,000 are hospitalized; burns are the third leading cause of
   accidental deaths
4. Assessment
   a. Ask the following questions
      (1) Are you having difficulty breathing?
      (2) Are you in pain? Where? On a scale of 0 to 10 how
           severe is your pain?
   b. Clinical manifestations—discussed in the pathophysiology
   c. Abnormal laboratory findings
      (1) Carboxyhemoglobin level—elevated, indicative of
           inhaled carbon monoxide and an inhalation injury
      (2) H&H—may be elevated as a result of
           hemoconcentration especially in the first 24 to 48 hours

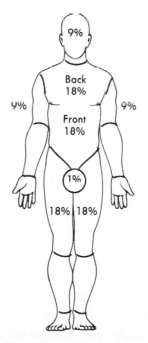

Figure 12-2.   Rule of nines. (From Beare PG and Myers JL: *Principles and practice of adult health nursing*, ed 2, St Louis, 1994, Mosby.)

AREA	AGE – YEARS					% 2°	% 3°	% TOTAL
	0 – 1	1 – 4	5 – 9	10 – 15	ADULT			
Head	19	17	13	10	7			
Neck	2	2	2	2	2			
Ant. Trunk	13	13	13	13	13			
Post. Trunk	13	13	13	13	13			
R. Buttock	2 1/2	2 1/2	2 1/2	2 1/2	2 1/2			
L. Buttock	2 1/2	2 1/2	2 1/2	2 1/2	2 1/2			
Genitalia	1	1	1	1	1			
R.U. Arm	4	4	4	4	4			
L.U. Arm	4	4	4	4	4			
R.L. Arm	3	3	3	3	3			
L.L. Arm	3	3	3	3	3			
R. Hand	2 1/2	2 1/2	2 1/2	2 1/2	2 1/2			
L. Hand	2 1/2	2 1/2	2 1/2	2 1/2	2 1/2			
R. Thigh	5 1/2	6 1/2	8 1/2	8 1/2	9 1/2			
L. Thigh	5 1/2	6 1/2	8 1/2	8 1/2	9 1/2			
R. Leg	5	5	5 1/2	6	7			
L. Leg	5	5	5 1/2	6	7			
R. Foot	3 1/2	3 1/2	3 1/2	3 1/2	3 1/2			
L. Foot	3 1/2	3 1/2	3 1/2	3 1/2	3 1/2			
					TOTAL			

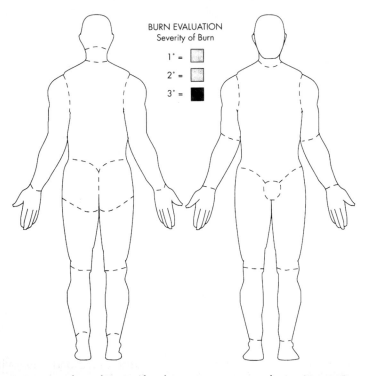

BURN EVALUATION
Severity of Burn

1° = ☐
2° = ☐
3° = ■

Figure 13-3. Lund and Browder burn assessment chart. (From Beare PG and Myers JL: *Principles and practice of adult health nursing*, ed 2, St Louis, 1994, Mosby.)

(3) ABG's—hypoxemia and metabolic acidosis with an inhalation injury

(4) Potassium—rises due to cell destruction especially in the first 24 to 48 hours

(5) Urinalysis—myoglobin, released from damaged muscles; damages renal tubules

(6) WBC—increased

(7) Platelets—decreased

d. Abnormal diagnostic tests

(1) Bronchoscopy—evidence of heat injury to the airways with resultant edema

(2) CXR—pulmonary edema as a response to an inhalation injury

5. Expected medical interventions

a. Airway maintenance—with endotracheal tube if necessary

b. Respiratory support with a ventilator if necessary

c. Fluid resuscitation—fluid administration is dictated by the percentage of burns and the client's weight; several formulas exist which establish calculations for fluid administration over the first 24 to 48 hours

d. Burn wounds

(1) Cleaned and debrided, blisters removed and any tissue that is not adherent is removed; hydrotherapy is most commonly used

(2) Topical antimicrobial agents are applied

(3) Wounds treated using a closed method of burn dressings or an open method, using only antimicrobial cream and no dressing

(4) If using tape, use paper tape as skin is much more likely to tear in surrounding area

(5) Biological dressings can also be used to cover wound until grafts can be placed

(a) Homografts come from another human

(b) Xenografts come from another animal

(c) Synthetic dressings can also be used

(6) Nutrition—burn clients require a large calorie intake, as high as 5000 calories per day; nutritional supplements may be required

(7) Skin grafts—most common method is removing pieces of skin from nonburned areas (donor sites), meshing the piece and placing it over the burn area; grafted tissue will grow over the cleaned burn site; initially donor sites may be quite painful

6. Nursing diagnoses
   a. Fluid volume deficit related to increased capillary permeability and fluid shift into the interstitial space
   b. Risk for infection related to loss of first line of pathogen defense (skin)
   c. Pain related to tissue effect of burn and exposed nerve endings
   d. Altered nutrition—less than body requirements related to increased metabolic demands of body

7. Client goals
   a. Client will have acceptable fluid volume as evidenced by balanced I&O and a CVP 5 to 15 mm Hg
   b. Client will have no infection as evidenced by clean burn wound and no exudate; clients are afebrile
   c. Client will state pain has decreased from a 10 to a 2 on a scale of 0 to 10
   d. Client will maintain preburn weight or gain ½ kg/wk

8. Nursing interventions
   a. Emergent phase—first 24 to 48 hours
      (1) Airway and ventilatory maintenance
      (2) Venous access for massive fluid resuscitation and pain medication
      (3) Pain management—usually morphine IV
      (4) Indwelling urinary catheter insertion to help monitor fluid volume and kidney function
      (5) Baseline and daily weights
      (6) Wounds bathed, debrided, and dressed
      (7) Family counseling begins at this phase
   b. Acute phase—begins third day after injury until several months later
      (1) Strict aseptic technique for care of burn wounds— may require isolation if wounds are infected
      (2) Pain management—IV narcotics, relaxation techniques, imagery and hypnosis are used
      (3) Severe pruritus requires management as well, usually with diphenhydramine (Benadryl)
      (4) Splinting and positioning of extremities to maintain function of extremity and prevent contractures
      (5) Active and passive range of motion
      (6) Nutrition—nutritional supplements to maintain high calorie needs; TPN discouraged because risk of infection

       (7) Prevention of stress ulcers—check pH of stomach and administer antacids as needed

       (8) Wound care—continue cleaning and debriding of wounds dressing with antimicrobial agents

  c. Home care or rehabilitation phase regarding client education

       (1) Bathing daily

       (2) Wound cleansing three to four times per day

       (3) How to dress wounds as per physician instructions

       (4) Elevation of limbs to prevent edema

       (5) Exercising affected limbs four times per day

       (6) Resumption of normal activities

       (7) Keeping physician appointments for follow-up

       (8) Maintaining nutritional balance

9. Evaluation protocol

  a. How do I know that my interventions were effective?

       (1) Vital signs are within 10% of baseline

       (2) Fluid balance I=O ± 300 ml

       (3) Urine output is ≥30 ml/hr

       (4) Wounds are clean and noninfected

       (5) Pain is manageable

  b. What criteria will I use to change my interventions?

       (1) Pain is not managed

       (2) Vital signs are not within desired parameters

       (3) Urine output is <30 ml/hr

       (4) Burn wound infection is apparent

  c. How will I know that my client teaching has been effective?

       (1) Burn wounds continue to heal without infection or severe contractures

       (2) Client reports increasing exercise daily

       (3) No evidence of edema in extremities

       (4) Client is maintaining adequate nutrition

       (5) Client returns to an acceptable normal daily routine

10. Older adult alert

  a. The older adult client has a higher mortality in burn injury than in the younger adult

  b. The older adult client is at higher risk for burn injury as a result of decreased reaction time, decreased mobility, and poor peripheral sensation

  c. The thinning of the older adult client's skin increases severity of burn injury

B. **Dermatitis**
  1. Definition—skin inflammation
  2. Etiology—allergy, stress, or unknown
  3. Pathophysiology—may be a response to something the skin has touched or an allergy to a known substance; the allergic response is a result of T cell sensitivity
  4. Assessment
     a. Ask the following questions
        (1) What symptoms are you feeling at the site of discomfort? Pain, itching, etc.?
        (2) Are there blisters? Are they open?
        (3) Is there swelling anywhere?
        (4) Are you having fevers?
     b. Clinical manifestations
        (1) Pruritus, pain, and burning at site
        (2) Reddened skin
        (3) Vesicles at site
        (4) Edema
        (5) Fever
        (6) Malaise
  5. Expected medical interventions
     a. Identify cause of disorder
     b. Lubricate and hydrate skin
     c. Topical corticosteroids
     d. Antibiotics
     e. Antihistamines
  6. Nursing diagnoses
     a. Pain related to skin response from causative agent
     b. Impaired skin integrity related to presence of allergic agent and itching
     c. Body-image disturbance related to presence of skin lesions
  7. Client goals
     a. Client will state pain has decreased to a manageable level
     b. Client will indicate skin is healing and lesions are decreasing in size
     c. Client will state feeling comfortable with the condition of the skin
  8. Nursing interventions—acute and home care
     a. Teach client to use soothing baths or solutions and how often to use them
     b. Teach client how to use topical steroids as ordered by physician

      c. Teach client how to use systemic steroids if ordered—to take with meals, not to miss a dose, and to take exactly as directed

9. Evaluation protocol
    a. How will I know that my interventions have been effective?
        (1) Client exhibits stable fluid volume with CVP 5 to 15cmH$_2$O
        (2) Client, afebrile, has absence of infection findings
        (3) Client verbalizes acceptable level of comfort
    b. What criteria will I use to change my interventions?
        (1) Incorrect technique of time span for baths and solutions
        (2) Incorrect technique for topical steroids
        (3) Incorrect statements regarding use of systemic corticosteroids
    c. How will I know that my client teaching has been effective?
        (1) Client reports the use of baths and solutions as per teaching
        (2) Client demonstrates how to place topical steroids
        (3) Client states precautions associated with oral corticosteroids

10. Older adult alert
    a. There is a decline in the number of sebaceous glands and as a result the amount of sebum. This means the older adult skin will be much drier and dermatitis will be much more difficult to control.
    b. Consider a drug interaction when observing dermatitis in the older adult taking multiple drugs
    c. The older adult client, in most instances, does not require a daily bath and should be discouraged from using hot water when bathing because of the fragility of the skin

C. **Pressure ulcers**
    1. Definition—tissue destruction as a result of prolonged pressure on an area of skin
    2. Etiology—commonly seen in areas of the body where bones are close to the skin; pressure on those areas pushes the bone against the tissues underlying the skin, beginning the breakdown process
    3. Pathophysiology—pressure on an area for a prolonged period of time causes decreased circulation to the area, tissue hypoxia, and death; shearing forces of the skin and skin that is moist, such as with incontinence, also contribute to ulcer formation

4. Assessment—see Table 13-1 for assessment factors associated with the stages of pressure ulcers
5. Expected medical interventions
   a. Wound debridement to allow healing
   b. Skin grafting for more severe wounds
6. Nursing diagnoses—impaired skin integrity related to prolonged pressure to an area
7. Client goal—Client will have pressure ulcers with a clean base and granulation tissue at edges
8. Nursing interventions
   a. Acute care
      (1) Wound management—follow physician orders for wound packing with wound cleansing agent
      (2) Nonabsorptive thin films and absorptive gel wafers work well on stage I and II ulcers

Table 13-1. Stages of Pressure Ulcers

Stage	Description	Goal of Intervention
I	A reddened area that returns to normal skin color after 15 to 20 minutes of pressure relief (e.g., turning to other side). The skin is intact, but the area may appear pale when pressure is initially removed.	To cover and protect
II	An area in which the top layer of skin is missing. The ulcer usually is shallow with a pinkish red base, and white or yellow eschar may be present.	To cover, protect, hydrate, insulate, and absorb
III	Deep ulcers that extend into the dermis and subcutaneous tissues. White, gray, or yellow eschar usually is present at the bottom of the ulcer and the ulcer crater may have a lip or edge. Purulent drainage is common.	To cover, protect, hydrate, insulate, absorb, cleanse, prevent infection and promote granulation
IV	Deep ulcers that extend into muscle and bone. These ulcers have a foul smell and the eschar is brown or black. Purulent drainage is common.	To cover, protect, hydrate, insulate, absorb, cleanse, prevent infection, obliterate dead space, and promote granulation

From Beare PG and Myers JL: *Principles and practice of adult health nursing,* ed 2, St Louis, 1994, Mosby.

      (3) Prevention techniques

         (a) All pressure points must be visualized for breakdown at least every 2 hours

         (b) Clients unable to do so on their own must be turned every 2 hours

         (c) Position client in bed at a 30 to 45 degree angle, propped with pillows

         (d) Support body parts with pillows

         (e) Use air mattresses or air fluidized beds to decrease skin pressure

         (f) Clean skin immediately after incontinence

         (g) Use turning sheet or pad to pull client up in bed and reduce sheering forces

         (h) Assess nutrition, ensure appropriate intake of vitamin C, zinc and vitamin E

  b. Home care regarding client/caregiver education

      (1) Teach caregiver specific strategies used prior to hospitalization

      (2) Teach caregiver findings of healing, poor healing, and when to notify physician

9. Evaluation protocol

  a. How will I know that my interventions have been effective?

      (1) Skin will remain clean and dry, without breakdown or redness

      (2) Wounds will have a clean base and show sign of granulation tissue at edges

      (3) Wounds will not enlarge but shrink in size at a slow, steady rate

  b. What criteria will I use to change my interventions?

      (1) New skin breakdowns

      (2) Wound base is covered with purulent drainage or necrotic tissue

      (3) Wounds are enlarging, no granulation tissue seen

  c. How will I know my client/caregiver teaching has been effective?

      (1) Client/caregiver reports diminished size or complete healing of pressure ulcer

      (2) Client/caregiver states finding of complications to report to physician

10. Older adult alert—as a result of the fragile nature of their skin, older adult clients are at great risk for pressure ulcers and must have optimal interventions to prevent them

D Skin cancer
1. Definition—malignancy of the skin
   a. Basal cell carcinoma—most common type; originates in the basal cell layer of the epidermis
   b. Squamous cell carcinoma—fast growing; found in previously damaged skin
   c. Malignant melanoma—cancer of the melanocytes of the skin; rapidly spreading cancer
2. Etiology—most common cause is overexposure to the rays of the sun
3. Incidence—most commonly seen cancer in the United States
4. Assessment
   a. Ask the following questions
      (1) How long have you had this growth?
      (2) How long has it had this appearance?
      (3) Are there other similar growths elsewhere on your body?
   b. Clinical manifestations
      (1) Basal cell carcinoma
         (a) Painless lesion
         (b) Usually found on areas of the body exposed to sun
         (c) A well-defined, dome-shaped papule with a pearl-like appearance; raised edges
         (d) Center may be ulcerated
         (e) Rarely metastasizes but will invade surrounding structures and destroy them
      (2) Squamous cell carcinoma
         (a) Thick, rough, shallow lesions with raised edges
         (b) May ulcerate in the center or have a gravel type center
         (c) Can metastasize at a rapid rate so diagnosis and treatment should be swift
      (3) Malignant melanoma
         (a) Superficial spreading melanoma—circle lesion whose borders are irregular
         (b) Nodular melanoma—berrylike nodules with a blue-black color
         (c) Lentigo melanoma—flat lesion that slowly turns black
         (d) Acral lentigious melanoma—irregular shaped macules, pigmented

    c. Abnormal diagnostic tests—incisonal biopsy or total excisional biopsy; positive for malignant cells

5. Expected medical interventions
    a. Excisional surgery; wide excision used for melanoma
    b. Cryosurgery—destroys tissue by freezing
    c. Mohs chemosurgery—removes tumor layer by layer until all tumor is gone
    d. Regional lymph node dissection—only used if nodes are involved but no metastasis
    e. External beam radiation therapy—not for melanoma
    f. Topical chemotherapy

6. Nursing diagnoses
    a. Fear related to beliefs about the diagnosis of cancer and of the possibility of death
    b. Anxiety related to unknown outcome, fear of disfigurement
    c. Body-image disturbance related to possibility of disfigurement

7. Client goals
    a. Client will state fear has decreased as more information is available
    b. Client will state anxiety is decreased as more information is learned about the body changes that will occur
    c. Client will state feeling comfortable with body changes that will occur as discussed with physician

8. Nursing interventions
    a. Acute care
        (1) Help reduce anxiety before surgery, reiterate plans for surgery with client and plans for grafting or reconstruction if applicable
        (2) Large postoperative wounds may require large dressings with care for drainage tubes and frequent changes
        (3) If skin grafting is required the graft site must be kept immobile and clean
        (4) Donor sites can be quite painful and may require analgesia
    b. Home care regarding client education
        (1) Need to perform monthly self-assessment of the skin for new lesions or changes in lesions
        (2) Need for any suspicious lesions to be seen by physician ASAP
        (3) Need for family members to watch for skin changes

            (4)   Client must use sunscreen >20 block when out in the sun

9. Evaluation protocol

    a.   How do I know that my interventions were effective?

        (1)   Does client feel less fearful since having discussed the surgical plans?

        (2)   Does client feel less anxious about the changes that will occur with treatments?

    b.   What criteria will I use to change my interventions?

        (1)   Increased fear

        (2)   Increased anxiety or body-image fear

    c.   How will I know that my client teaching has been effective?

        (1)   Client demonstrates appropriate technique for skin self-assessment

        (2)   Client states having purchased and used appropriate sunblock for times in the sun

        (3)   Client states the criteria for lesions that must be reported to physician

10. Older adult alert

    a.   Changes that occur in the skin of older adults make them especially prone to skin cancers

    b.   Many skin growths in older adults are benign. They should be encouraged to seek medical assistance especially if the lesion is creating distress in relation to their appearance.

REVIEW QUESTIONS

1. The client who has suffered burn injury may present with hematuria as a result of
   a. Bleeding of the internal structures related to the injury
   b. Massive red cell destruction from the intensity of the heat
   c. Heat injury to the kidney
   d. Heat injury to the ureters

2. The dehydration seen in a client with large surface area burns is related to
   a. Large amount of urine output
   b. Increased metabolic demands from the burns
   c. Fluid shift of plasma out of the vascular space and into the interstitial space
   d. Blood loss

3. A client with partial thickness burns over 30% of the body has entered the intermediate phase of care. In choosing a diet the nurse would suggest which items?
   a. Roast beef, green beans, rice, orange juice
   b. Salad, rolls, butter, soda
   c. Spaghetti, rolls, butter, milk
   d. Chicken noodle soup, salad, milkshake

4. Burn wound coverage may take the form of only antimicrobial creams or antimicrobial creams and bulky dressings. The bulky dressings would afford the client
   a. A cleaner method for wound coverage
   b. Coverage of the wound and better pain relief
   c. Better control of bacteria
   d. Better control of fluid loss

5. An older adult client is admitted to the emergency department with second and third degree burns from accidentally setting the clothes on fire while making dinner. This client's burns may be more severe than a younger adult client because
   a. Older adult clients have less pain receptors so they do not pull away from fire as quickly as younger adults
   b. Older adult clients are more prone to not move away from burning substances because they cannot respond quickly

    c. The skin of the older adult client tends to be thinner and there is less subcutaneous fat

    d. The older adult client wears less clothing in most cases than the younger adult

6. Teaching needs of the client with contact dermatitis who has been ordered a topical corticosteroid medication must include how to

    a. Apply the medication to the skin in a thick layer

    b. Cover the ointment once applied with a clean dressing

    c. Apply in a thin layer only as often as ordered by the physician

    d. Have awareness that the steroid is not absorbed by the skin, so there are no systemic effects of the steroid

7. The best defense against decubitus ulcers is

    a. Positive pressure mattresses

    b. Airflow beds

    c. Elbow and heel protectors

    d. Identifying high risk clients with incorporation of measures to prevent skin breakdown

8. An appropriate nursing diagnosis for a client with skin cancer would be

    a. Fear related to the diagnosis of cancer

    b. Anxiety related to an unknown outcome

    c. Body-image disturbance related to changes in appearance

    d. Body-image disturbance related to cancer

ANSWERS, RATIONALES, AND TEST-TAKING TIPS

Rationales	Test-Taking Tips

1. **Correct answer: b**

   Heat does cause a lysis of body and vascular compartment cells during a burn injury. Lysed cells will pass through the kidney with damaging effects and appear as hematuria.

   Cluster the responses *a*, *c*, and *d* under the category of larger structures of the body. Response *b* focuses on the cell rather than an organ.

2. **Correct answer: c**

   Following burn injury, fluid does shift from the intravascular space into the interstitial space.

   Select the response that provides a more comprehensive answer.

3. **Correct answer: a**

   A burn client needs high protein, such as that obtained from steak as well as vitamin C.

   To heal, one needs protein, vitamin C and A. Of the selections response *a* has the highest protein—roast beef, and the highest vitamin C—the orange juice.

4. **Correct answer: d**

   Fluid loss is controlled due to pressure exerted on the wound.

   Use common sense in that dressings are typically used to collect drainage.

5. **Correct answer: c**

   As a normal course of aging the older client has less subcutaneous tissue and thin skin, all of which burns easily.

   The question is asking about the reason for a "more severe burn." The only response that most closely addresses the burn site is response *c*. The other responses present information about reaction time or habits of dress.

6. **Correct answer: c**

A thin layer of antibiotic therapy is to be applied at the ordered intervals. A dressing would further irritate the area of the contact dermatitis.

Response *d* is not true. Response *a* is incorrect because of the word "thick"; typically substances applied to the skin should be in a thin layer—thicker isn't better.

7. **Correct answer: d**

Identifying the client at risk will allow the client to be treated before the decubitus begins to develop.

The key words in the question are "best defense." This leads to the selection of the most preventive action, response *d*. Note that this is the most comprehensive response also.

8. **Correct answer: c**

This client will have a body-image disturbance related to any changes that occur due to their illness.

Match the concern of skin from the question with the response that most closely relates to skin—body image and appearance.

The Immune System

STUDY OUTCOMES

After completing this chapter, the reader will be able to do the following:

▼ Describe the function and structure of the immune system.
▼ Identify assessment factors common to clients who have disorders of the immune system.
▼ Select appropriate nursing diagnoses for the client with a disorder of the immune system.
▼ Identify appropriate nursing interventions for the client with a disorder of the immune system.
▼ Evaluate outcomes of the client with a disorder of the immune system to make appropriate changes to the care of that client based on the evaluation.

KEY TERMS

Antibodies	Also known as **immunoglobulins,** responsible for the control or destruction of nonself antigens.
Antigens	Protein markers on cells that identify a cell as self or nonself.
B lymphocytes	Do not mature in the thymus; two varieties:
	1. Memory cells—responsible for storing information about nonself antigens and the appropriate response.
	2. Plasma cells—produce the immunoglobulins also known as antibodies.
Complement	A group of plasma proteins responsible for enhancing the initial steps of the inflammatory response and mediating the antigen-antibody response; also acts as an opsonin for phagocytosis.
Immunocompetence	Appropriate or intact functioning of the immune system.
Immunodeficiency	Incompetence of the immune system; inability to destroy or control invading organisms.
Leukocytes	White blood cells (WBC), active component of inflammatory and immune response (Table 14-1).
Nonspecific immune response	Immediate response to invading organisms with neutrophils and macrophages; result is inflammation.
Opsonins	Substances that coat nonself antigens making them more susceptible to phagocytosis.
Phagocytosis	Cells engulf microorganisms for destruction and cellular debris for removal.
Specific immune response	Response by lymphocytes programmed to respond to nonself antigens; also known as cell mediated immunity.
Stem cells	Also called **parent cells** in bone marrow; responsible for producing WBCs.
T lymphocytes	Lymphocytes that mature and establish various roles in the thymus; the varieties of T lymphocytes are helper cells, suppressor cells, natural killer cells, and cytotoxic cells.

CONTENT REVIEW

I. The immune system is responsible for protecting the body from invading organisms, providing homeostasis through the removal of defective cells,

and monitoring the body for the growth of abnormal cells; extremely important to the body is the immune system's ability to identify *self* and *nonself;* it is also activated when cells in the body are damaged

II. Structure and function

A. Bone marrow—produces competent WBCs

B. White blood cells (WBCs)—in adequate mature numbers are responsible for attacking any nonself antigen; an elevated level of WBC indicates infection and how high the WBC count rises is an indication of how severe the infection
   1. WBC >10,000 = leukocytosis = infection
   2. WBC <5000 = leukopenia = minimal defense against foreign growth

C. Lymphoid tissue—responsible for maturation and differentiation of the lymphocytes; also responsible for storing small collections of WBCs to interact with blood and lymph and quickly identify nonself antigens

D. Chemical mediators—histamine, kinins, complement, leukotrienes, prostaglandins and Interleukin-1, which is necessary to stimulate and enhance the activity of WBCs

E. Immunity—two types
   1. Innate—first defense; physical barriers, chemicals, and cellular defenses prevent invading pathogens from becoming rooted and multiplying

Table 14-1. Categories of White Blood Cells

Myeloid Stem Cell Produces:	Lymphoid Stem Cell Produces:
Granulocytes	T lymphocytes
Neutrophils	Helper/T_4 cells
Mast cells	Supressor/T_8 cells
Basophils (immature cells)	Natural killer cells
elevated in bacterial	Cytotoxic T cells
infections	B lymphocytes
Eosinophils (mature cells)	Plasma cells
elevated in pernicious	Memory cells
anemia, liver dysfunction	
Monocytes	
Macrophages	

From Beare PG and Myers JL: *Principles and practice of adult health nursing,* ed 2, St Louis, 1994, Mosby.

2. Adaptive—action of B and T lymphocytes against invading pathogen using memorized reactions to known pathogens and memorizing new pathogens; can be acquired actively or passively
   a. Active acquired—introducing an antigen into the body either intentionally or through exposure to the pathogen; the initial antigen will elicit a response creating a memorized response to this antigen if it is again introduced into the body; examples include vaccinations, hepatitis B vaccine, tetanus toxoid
   b. Passive acquired—antibodies passed from one person to another; mother to fetus transfer of antibodies is a good example; immunity is short lived as no memory is produced; immunity lasts only as long as antibodies are active; passive immunity in infant is 3 to 6 months; examples for injectable forms that have antibody action for 2 to 3 weeks: tetanus immune serum globulin which is given in multi-trauma victims, and Hyperab, a rabies immune serum globulin.

III. Targeted concerns

A. **Pharmacology—priority drug classifications**
   1. Immunosuppressants—block production of WBCs by the bone marrow
      a. Expected effect—inhibition of immune response
      b. Commonly given drugs
         (1) Azathioprine (Imuran)
         (2) Cyclosporin (Sandimmune)
         (3) Lymphocyte immune globulin (Atgam)
         (4) Muromonab-CD3 (Orthoclone OKT3)
      c. Nursing considerations
         (1) Monitor client carefully for signs of infection which will be masked by medication; temperatures of 99° F may be significant
         (2) Observe for anaphylaxis
   2. Antiinflammatory agents—block release of leukotrienes and prostaglandins
      a. Expected effect—decreased inflammatory response
      b. Commonly given drugs
         (1) Prednisone (Deltasone)
         (2) Hydrocortisone (Solu-Cortef)
         (3) Methylprednisolone (Medrol)
      c. Nursing considerations
         (1) Give medication with food to prevent GI distress

    (2) Never miss a dose; could cause adrenal crisis

    (3) Medication must be weaned because of the risk of adrenal crisis if stopped abruptly

    (4) Give IV push slowly to prevent a drop in BP and HR

  3. Drugs to treat AIDS—prevent replication of virus

   a. Expected effects—helps halt progression of AIDS

   b. Commonly given drugs

    (1) Zidouvudine (AZT, Retrovir)

    (2) Didanosine (Videx)

   c. Nursing considerations

    (1) Client must take medication around the clock; must wake to take medication

    (2) Teach client that these drugs do not eliminate the risk of HIV transmission

    (3) Teach client to avoid crowds and other people with infections

B. Procedures

  1. Complete blood count (CBC)—provides information about hemoglobin and hematocrit as well as the specific value for various white cells

  2. Immunodiffusion—detects antigen-antibody reactions

  3. Electrophoretic assays—measure serum immunoglobulins such as IgG, IgA

  4. Enzyme-linked immunosorbent assay (ELISA)—very sensitive in detecting antigens and antibodies

  5. Radioimmunoassay (RIA)—detects small amounts of antigens, antibodies, and antigen-antibody complexes

  6. Lymphocyte assays—determine absolute numbers of lymphocytes

  7. T cell and B cell surface markers—assist in diagnosing various immune disorders

  8. Bone marrow aspiration and biopsy—evaluation of cellular components of blood

  9. Lymph node biopsy—assess immunologic function and evaluate for malignancy of the lymph system

C. Psychosocial

  1. Stresses—in relation to illness or to lifestyle; overall can suppress immune response and raise glucose load

  2. Anxiety—uncomfortable feeling associated with an unknown cause; clients may be unable to discuss their feelings but are aware they are uneasy about what is going to happen

  3. Fear—uncomfortable feeling associated with real danger; clients' fear is of their death

    4. Social isolation—may be a result of the illness itself or in response to fear of contracting illness as a result of immunosuppression

    5. Changes in lifestyle and activities of daily living (ADL)—in response to illness

    6. Changes in work—is client able to work?

    7. Anger—clients may be angry about suffering from these types of illnesses

D. **Health history—question sequence**

    1. What problems have you been experiencing?

    2. Have you noticed frequent infections lately?

    3. Have you ever had any surgery or trauma to your extremities?

    4. Have you ever been treated for cancer? Where?

    5. Is your physician treating you for any illnesses at present?

    6. Do you have any food or drug allergies?

    7. Have you been more tired than usual?

    8. Have you noticed that you have had an elevated temperature frequently?

    9. Do you ever wake up at night covered with sweat?

    10. Have you noticed pain or swelling in your neck, underarms, or groin?

    11. Have you noticed a lack of appetite?

E. **Physical exam—appropriate sequence**

    1. Airway, breathing, and circulation—vital signs

    2. Inspect area over lymph node chain—compare sides (see Figure 4-1, p. 109)

    3. Inspect skin for lesions, color, rashes, temperature, and moisture

    4. Inspect hair for color, texture, and distribution

    5. Palpate superficial lymph nodes for size, shape, and tenderness

      a. Head and neck nodes

      b. Supraclavicular nodes

      c. Axillary nodes

      d. Upper extremity nodes

      e. Lower extremity nodes

    6. Inspect breathing pattern, effort, and rate

    7. Palpate chest for expansion and chest wall pain when pressure applied

    8. Auscultate breath sounds

    9. Auscultate cardiac rate and rhythm, abnormal sounds

    10. Inspect abdomen for lesion, nodules, or scars

    11. Auscultate for bowel sounds

12. Percuss abdomen for abnormal dullness
13. Inspect muscle areas for swelling, palpate for tenderness
14. Assess for gait, muscle strength, coordination, and range of motion

IV. Pathophysiologic disorders

A. Acquired immunodeficiency syndrome (AIDS)
1. Definition—a disorder associated with a deficiency of cell mediated immunity; characterized by development of opportunistic infections and cancers
2. Pathophysiology
   a. HIV invades the host cell, T_4, and uses genetic material of the cell to replicate itself
   b. Its own genetic code, carried on RNA instead of DNA, is transferred to the host's DNA and more will then be made with the genetic code of the HIV
   c. The virus can remain dormant for an unknown period of time, but will be stimulated to reproduce once the host T_4 cell has been stimulated to function immunologically
   d. More and more T_4 cells are infected and the total number is decreased
   e. The T_8 cells, or suppressor cells, now have a higher number than the T_4, or helper cells, and the suppressor cells dominate in immunologic action
   f. The client becomes immunosuppressed
   g. Pathogens and tumors are allowed to grow in the body unchecked, thus allowing opportunistic infections and cancers to become prominent
   h. HIV is found in all body fluids, but only semen, blood, vaginal secretions, and breast milk have been implicated in transmission (Figure 14-1)
3. Etiology—human immunodeficiency virus (HIV), a retrovirus responsible for destruction of T and CD4 lymphocytes
4. Incidence—majority of clients with HIV in the adult population are homosexual or bisexual males or clients who have abused IV drugs; the remaining population is comprised of clients who have obtained the virus through blood products, perinatally from their mother, or from infected sexual partners; incidence in the heterosexual population is increasing
5. Assessment
   a. Ask the following questions
      (1) Have you noticed swelling in your neck or groin?

SPECTRUM OF HIV DISEASE

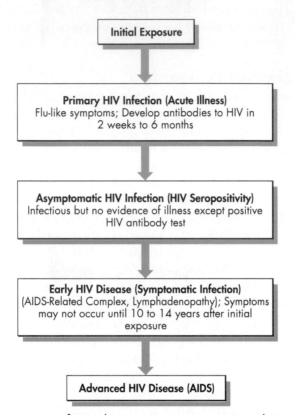

Figure 14-1. Spectrum of HIV disease. (From Beare PG and Myers JL: *Principles and practice of adult health nursing*, ed 2, St Louis, 1994, Mosby.)

      (2) Have you noticed bruising or purple areas on your skin?

      (3) Have you noticed a white buildup on your tongue?

      (4) Do you feel tired often?

      (5) Have you been losing weight?

      (6) Do you wake up sweating at night?

      (7) Do you suffer from frequent diarrhea?

  b. Clinical manifestations

      (1) HIV disease (previously known as AIDS related complex)

         (a) Generalized lymphadenopathy

         (b) Immune thrombocytopenia purpura

         (c) Hairy leukoplakia—raised white plaque on the tongue

    (2) AIDS

        (a) Severe fatigue

        (b) Malaise and weakness

        (c) Chronic weight loss

        (d) Chronic lymphadenopathy

        (e) Fevers

        (f) Joint pain

        (g) Night sweats

        (h) Chronic diarrhea

c. Abnormal laboratory findings

    (1) Enzyme linked immunosorbent assay (ELISA)—positive for antibodies against AIDS; usually repeated

    (2) Western blot analysis—positive for antibodies against AIDS; used to confirm ELISA

    (3) P24 antigen—positive for circulating antigen

    (4) CBC and differential—WBC, lymphocytes, neutrophils, platelets, RBC, hemoglobin and hematocrit; all are decreased

    (5) HIV culture—live HIV

    (6) T cell studies—analyze numbers and functions of the specific T cells; shows decreased T_4 and increased T_8 cells

d. Abnormal diagnostic tests—used primarily to confirm presence of opportunistic infections or cancers

    (1) Bronchoscopy—confirm cause of pneumonia

    (2) Pulmonary function tests (PFT)—used to assist detection of pneumonia

    (3) Electroencephalogram (EEG)—slowed activity as a result of encephalopathy

    (4) CT scan and MRI scan—used to evaluate a fever of unknown origin

6. Expected medical interventions

  a. The goal of medical management is to quickly diagnose the client and start him or her on the medication AZT, which is the best method known to date to assist in the repair of the immune system. Healthcare professionals usually work to quickly diagnose and treat opportunistic infections and cancers that occur.

  b. Common opportunistic infections and treatments

    (1) Pneumocystis carinii pneumonia (PCP)—Bactrim, Pentam 300

    (2) Toxoplasmosis—Fansidar, Cleocin

         (3)   Candida albicans—Mycostatin, Nizoral

         (4)   Histoplasmosis—Amphotericin B, Nizoral

         (5)   Tuberculosis—three-drug therapy: INH, Ethambutol, Rifampin

         (6)   Cytomegalovirus (CMV)—ganciclovir (Cytovene)

         (7)   Herpes simplex—acyclovir (Zovirax)

   c.   Common opportunistic malignancies

         (1)   Kaposi's sarcoma

         (2)   Lymphoma

         (3)   Non-Hodgkin's lymphoma

7.   Nursing diagnoses

   a.   Impaired gas exchange related to increased alveolar secretions secondary to pneumonia

   b.   Diarrhea related to inflammation of the intestinal tract secondary to viral infection

   c.   Altered nutrition—less than body requirements related to gastrointestinal inflammation secondary to viral infection

   d.   Fluid volume deficit related to anorexia, nausea and diarrhea

   e.   Altered oral mucous membranes related to oral infection

   f.   Fatigue related to altered nutrition and a wasting disorder

8.   Client goals

   a.   Client will exhibit a PO_2 and PCO_2 within normal baseline

   b.   Client will exhibit decreased episodes of diarrhea (two less per day) with a more solid consistency to stool

   c.   Client will demonstrate a stable weight with no further weight loss

   d.   Client will demonstrate a balanced I&O within 300 ml, with no further weight loss

   e.   Client will state mucosa of the mouth are less painful

   f.   Client will state feeling less fatigued

9.   Nursing interventions

   a.   Acute care

         (1)   Universal precautions as with all clients—assume all clients are infected; follow precautions

            (a)   Use barrier precautions to protect skin and mucous membranes from exposure to blood or body fluids—gloves, eyewear, gowns, and masks

            (b)   Wash hands before and after caring for every client; wash hands after removing gloves; always wash hands immediately after unexpected contact with body fluids

        (c)   DO NOT RECAP NEEDLES—place all sharp items in a sharps container for disposal

        (d)   Any healthcare worker with lesions or open areas should refrain from direct client care

    (2)   Balance client activity and rest to decrease fatigue

    (3)   Place client in position of comfort and for best respiratory effort

    (4)   Monitor for symptoms of respiratory illness

    (5)   Provide antidiarrheal agents as necessary to maintain appropriate fluid balance

    (6)   If client is tolerating oral intake, provide diet that will improve nutritional status

    (7)   If not tolerating oral intake, anticipate use of TPN

    (8)   Provide viscous lidocaine or similar agent to provide oral pain relief before client eats

  b. Home care regarding client education

    (1)   The syndrome and what complications clients should monitor

    (2)   Medications and possible side effects to report

    (3)   Symptoms of infection and to seek medical care immediately

    (4)   The avoidance of other people with illness as a result of the risk of contracting the illness

    (5)   How to avoid transmission of HIV to others

    (6)   Need to avoid sharing toilet articles and not to donate blood or organs

    (7)   Need to inform all appropriate health care personnel and sexual partners of illness

    (8)   Hospice intervention if necessary

10. Evaluation protocol

  a. How do I know that my interventions were effective?

    (1)   New infectious processes have been averted or decreased in intensity

    (2)   Respiratory status is stable with no increase or decrease of respiratory rate >10% of baseline; no findings of fluid-mucus accumulation in lungs

    (3)   Episodes of diarrhea have decreased

    (4)   Weight loss has stopped and/or client is gaining weight slowly

    (5)   Oral mucosa are showing signs of healing

    (6)   Level of fatigue has declined

      b. What criteria will I use to change my interventions?
- (1) New infections are apparent or present infections are becoming more intense
- (2) Respiratory function is more impaired; client has dyspnea at rest
- (3) More episodes of diarrhea are evident
- (4) Client is still losing weight at a steady pace despite increased nutrition efforts
- (5) Oral pain is worse making eating even more difficult
- (6) Client indicates fatigue is worse

      c. How will I know that my client teaching has been effective?
- (1) Client indicates having informed the physicians and dentist of illness as well as sexual partner
- (2) Client states side effects to be monitored each day in regard to medications and how to take medication
- (3) Client states symptoms to watch for regarding new infections and how to avoid them
- (4) Client states how to avoid transmission of the illness to others
- (5) Client states benefits of hospice and how to obtain the help when necessary

11. Older adult alert—this is a disorder to date found primarily in the younger adult. It is felt that if identified in the older adult client as a result of the normal changes of the older adult, client illness would progress rapidly.

B. Rheumatoid arthritis
1. Definition—chronic systemic inflammatory disorder of the connective tissue; exacerbations and remissions are characteristic
2. Pathophysiology—synovial lining of the joint becomes inflamed; granulation tissue forms; cartilage is destroyed; fibrous tissue is left in place of cartilage
3. Etiology—unknown; theories suggest autoimmune disorder and infectious agents
4. Incidence—more common in the female population
5. Assessment
    a. Ask the following questions
- (1) When does your pain occur?
- (2) Do you have swelling of your joints?
- (3) Does the weather make your pain worse?
- (4) What else makes your pain worse?
- (5) What lessens your pain?

    b. Clinical manifestations
      (1) Joint pain, warmth, edema
      (2) Joint motion limitation
      (3) Morning stiffness, fatigue
      (4) Proximal joints of hands and feet most commonly effected
      (5) Nodules over bony prominences
      (6) Hand deformity
      (7) Systemic findings—increased WBC, increased temperature
      (8) Anorexia, weight loss
    c. Abnormal laboratory findings
      (1) Rheumatoid factor—positive
      (2) Sedimentation rate—elevated
      (3) H & H—anemia
      (4) WBC—may be elevated
    d. Abnormal diagnostic tests
      (1) Joint aspiration—increased synovial fluid volume, cloudy
      (2) Joint x-rays—eroded joint surfaces, joint space narrowing, unstable joint

6. Expected medical interventions
    a. Rest, especially during exacerbations; possibily splints on effected joints during severe pain
    b. ROM passive and active
    c. Cold therapy during acute exacerbations and moist heat for stiffened joints
    d. Aspirin in high doses
    e. Gold salts
    f. Corticosteroids
    g. Methotrexate

7. Nursing diagnosis
    a. Acute pain related to inflamed joint spaces
    b. Impaired physical mobility related to joint pain
    c. Fatigue related to prolonged immobility and increased metabolic demands

8. Client goals
    a. Client will state pain has decreased or been relieved
    b. Client will demonstrate ability to perform active or passive range of motion on all joints every day
    c. Client will state fatigue has decreased

      9. Nursing interventions
         a. Acute care—postoperative joint replacement—care will be the same as for the client following hip surgery (see Chapter 12, p. 404)
         b. Home care regarding client education
            (1) Medication regime—when and how to take, side effects to report
            (2) Need to maintain a minimal activity level and not to overexert
            (3) Application of heat or cold for analgesia
            (4) Need to exercise joints to the point of pain but not past the point of pain
            (5) Splints on affected joints during acute exacerbations
            (6) Need for weight control to minimize stress on weight-bearing joints
    10. Evaluation protocol (Refer to Chapter 12, p. 407 for additional protocol)
         a. How will I know that my client teaching has been effective?
            (1) Client states performing ROM at least three times a day
            (2) Client demonstrates correct medication regime and has awareness of side effect to relate to physician
            (3) Client loses weight to within 4 to 8% of ideal body weight
            (4) Client demonstrates correct procedure for correct moist heat application
    11. Older adult alert—this is a disorder of the older adult and should be evaluated for when assessing older adult clients

C. **Lupus erythematosus**
    1. Definition—a widespread connective tissue disorder
    2. Pathophysiology—widespread destruction of collagen in the body; marked by exacerbations and remissions; leads to eventual destruction of organs and death
    3. Etiology—unknown; theorized as an autoimmune disorder
    4. Incidence—more common in females and younger adults or adolescents
    5. Assessment
         a. Ask the following questions
            (1) Do you burn frequently or easily when exposed to the sun?
            (2) Have you noticed a rash across the bridge of your nose?

          (3)   Have you noticed an increase in hair loss?

          (4)   Have you noticed any sustained fatigue?

  b. Clinical manifestations

          (1)   Symptoms which mimic arthritis

          (2)   Sun sensitivity

          (3)   "Butterfly rash" over the bridge of the nose

          (4)   Sustained fatigue

          (5)   Alopecia

          (6)   Symptoms indicative of organ involvement; renal impairment, cardiac dysrhythmias, etc.

          (7)   Inflammation of skeletal muscles—polymyositis

  c. Abnormal laboratory findings

          (1)   CBC—anemia

          (2)   Lupus erythematosus prep—positive

          (3)   ANA titer—positive

6. Expected medical interventions

  a. Plasmapheresis (plasma exchange) for exacerbations or preventive

  b. High dose steroids for exacerbation

  c. NSAID, aspirin in high doses for pain

7. Nursing diagnoses

  a. Pain related to inflammatory changes in the joint spaces

  b. Body-image disturbance related to butterfly rash

  c. Impaired mobility related to painful joints

8. Client goals

  a. Client will state pain is decreased or relieved

  b. Client will state feeling comfortable with facial or hair changes that have occurred

  c. Client will demonstrate ROM with participation in ADL with less fatigue

9. Nursing interventions

  a. Acute care—exacerbations

          (1)   Support before, during, and after plasmapheresis

          (2)   Treat pain

          (3)   Administer steroids as per order

          (4)   Teach client safe administration of steroids

  b. Home care regarding client education on remission

          (1)   Teach client safe administration of high doses of NSAID and aspirin with findings to report to physician

          (2)   Encouragement to stay out of sun and use high numbered sun block when in the sun

10. Evaluation protocol
    a. How will I know that my interventions were effective?
       (1) Client states pain has decreased
       (2) Client states desired effects from medication or plasmapheresis
    b. What criteria will I use to change my interventions?
       (1) Client states pain is increased or unrelieved
       (2) Client states plans to take steroids before meals or inbetween meals
       (3) Client reports severe fatigue that interfers with ADL or work
    c. How will I know that my client teaching has been effective?
       (1) Client indicates that NSAID or aspirin will be taken with food or milk
       (2) Client states plan to avoid being in sun or to wear high numbered sun block when in sun
11. Older adult alert—this disorder is uncommon in older adults

REVIEW QUESTIONS

1. Maintenance of the nutritional status of a client with AIDS is best accomplished by
   a. Providing for pain relief of mouth lesions, a diet high in calories and protein, and appealing food
   b. Starting total parenteral nutrition
   c. Starting enteral feedings with high calorie, high protein feedings
   d. Offering foods that the client finds appealing and small frequent meals

2. Client teaching regarding zidouvudine (AZT) must include that
   a. The medication will arrest the HIV virus
   b. The medication must be taken around the clock; the client must wake up at night to take the medication
   c. Medication dosages can be spread across the time the client is awake
   d. The medication kills the HIV virus

3. A common manifestation the nurse would expect to see in the client with AIDS is
   a. Constipation
   b. High fevers
   c. Night sweats
   d. Painful lymph nodes

4. The nurse must assist feeding a client who is HIV positive. Universal precautions that the nurse instructs the nursing assistant to take would consist of
   a. None needed
   b. Gloves
   c. Gown
   d. Mask

5. To plan care for a client with an acute exacerbation of lupus erythematosus, the nurse begins teaching the client about the appropriate administration of corticosteroids. The teaching must include that this medication
   a. Must be taken on an empty stomach for appropriate absorption
   b. Should be taken for only 10 days and then stopped
   c. Must be taken with food or antacids
   d. Must be taken with large amounts of water

6. The client with rheumatoid arthritis with an acute exacerbation must have the following interventions placed on the care plan
   a. Application of warm moist compresses to inflamed joints
   b. Institute range of motion exercises at least four times a day
   c. Splint affected joints with range of motion at least once a day
   d. Exercise affected joints just past the point of pain

ANSWERS, RATIONALES, AND TEST-TAKING TIPS

Rationales	Test-Taking Tips

1. **Correct answer: a**

   The pain of mouth ulcers must be attended to; diets should be high in proteins and calories, and should be food the client likes.

   The most comprehensive response is *a*. Responses *b* and *c* are interventions if the client cannot eat food by mouth; the stem gives no data to think this is the situation. Response *d* is fine but a less comprehensive answer.

2. **Correct answer: b**

   The client must wake up through the night to take the zidouvudine.

   The responses *a* and *d* are incorrect data. To be most effective any medication is best given around the clock; thus, response *b* is the best choice.

3. **Correct answer: c**

   Night sweats are a common manifestation; typically diarrhea, low grade fevers, and painless enlarged lymph nodes are seen also.

   The key word in the stem is "common" and this guides one to the choice of *c*. Note that night sweats most commonly are associated with four situations: TB, AIDS, Hodgkin's disease, and menopause.

4. **Correct answer: a**

   Unless contact with bodily fluids is a consideration then protective devices are not necessary. When one feeds a client usually there is no contact with body fluids.

   Be cautious in these types of responses where you know the answer is the first choice and you don't bother to read the remaining responses. This bad pattern of reading will commonly result in a wrong answer since the correct response may be included further on. However, in these options of question 4, luck helped and the correct response is *a*.

5. **Correct answer: c**

Corticosteroids are ulceragenic and must be taken with food or antacids. Steroids are not to be stopped abruptly.

Approach any exam with the thought that all medications need to be taken with food; the exceptions are tetracycline, carafate, and some sulfonamides which require a full glass of water when taken.

6. **Correct answer: c**

Affected joints should be splinted to prevent contractures; ROM must be done at least once a day.

In response *a* "compresses" aren't usually given. Compresses are more for pulled or strained muscles.

Comprehensive Exam

COMPREHENSIVE EXAM QUESTIONS

1. When planning care for a postoperative client following implantation of a hip prosthesis, the nurse must include
   a. Log-rolling the client
   b. Early ambulation to prevent pulmonary embolism
   c. Maintaining adduction of the legs to prevent dislocation of the prosthesis
   d. Maintaining abduction of the legs to prevent dislocation of the prosthesis

2. The client is just returning from the operating room following a partial gastrectomy. The student nurse working with the nurse has included the following interventions on the client's plan of care. Which of these will need to be discussed with the student regarding the need for change?
   a. Measure NG (nasogastric tube) output every 4 hours
   b. Reposition the NG if drainage decreases
   c. Check the pH of the NG drainage every 4 hours
   d. Irrigate with 30 ml of normal saline every 4 hours

3. Following instructions for combination insulin administration, the nurse evaluates that a 32-year-old client is using incorrect technique when the client
   a. Stretches the skin flat before administration
   b. Injects at a 90-degree angle
   c. Rubs the site following the insulin administration
   d. Shakes the vial to mix the insulin

4. A newly admitted client has a tentative diagnosis of tuberculosis. The client has been placed in respiratory isolation. What other measure must the nurse take to decrease the risk of transmission of the illness?
   a. Arrange for sterilization of the client's linen
   b. Give the client double-ply tissues for coughing and sneezing
   c. Arrange for the use of large amounts of bleach when the client's linen is laundered
   d. Have the client wear a mask when in contact with other individuals in the client's room

5. A client enters the emergency department complaining of severe substernal chest pain, unrelieved by 3 nitroglycerin tablets at home. The client now complains of pain radiation into the jaw. The nurse assesses vital signs, places the client on a cardiac monitor, and notes findings of diaphoresis, dyspnea, and whitish skin. What must the next action be?
   a. Call for a stat ECG
   b. Administer oxygen

    c. Administer sublingual nitroglycerin
    d. Start an IV of 5% dextrose in water at keep-vein-open rate

6. The client is started on heparin therapy following tissue plasminogen activator (t-PA) therapy. Teaching to the client and family regarding the heparin should include that this drug
    a. Is used to thin your blood
    b. Will slow the clotting of your blood
    c. Will dissolve the clot in your coronary artery
    d. Will prevent further clots from forming in your coronary arteries

7. Discharge teaching is begun on two clients with heart failure who will be taking Lasix at home. Which item should be included on the teaching plan?
    a. How to measure limb edema
    b. How to take their pulse daily
    c. How to measure urine output
    d. How to measure daily weight

8. The nurse is involved with cholesterol screening for the public. Clients identified with high cholesterol will be encouraged to eliminate which foods from their diets?
    a. Liver and onions
    b. Yogurt and strawberries
    c. Chicken and green beans
    d. Canola oil and lettuce salads

9. In caring for a client with left-sided heart failure, the nurse is aware that in the early stages of left-sided heart failure, the most commonly reported *first* symptom is
    a. Dyspnea
    b. Fatigue
    c. Pitting peripheral edema
    d. Enlarging abdominal girth

10. When instructing clients with Buerger's disease, the nurse warns that exacerbations may be noted in all of these situations except
    a. Stress
    b. Extreme cold
    c. Extreme heat
    d. Moderate, air-conditioned areas

11. A 54-year-old male with an acute exacerbation of chronic bronchitis has a history of smoking two packs of cigarettes a day for the past 30 years. When assessing the client, the nurse would anticipate that this acute episode might have been induced by which situation?
    a. The cold weather
    b. The flu that the client experienced a few days ago
    c. The clogged air filter in the client's home
    d. The client's increased cigarette use to two and one-half packs per day

12. A client has emphysema and is receiving oxygen at 1 liter per minute. His ABGs are are follows: PO_2—65, PCO_2—56, pH—7.34, Sat—91%, HCO_3—30. The best action would be to
    a. Call the physician
    b. Increase the oxygen
    c. Decrease the oxygen
    d. Do nothing at this time; the values are normal for the client

13. When educating a group of clients with bronchiectasis, the nurse is told that they are aware nutrition is important, but that they have no appetite. A suggestion should be for them to eat
    a. Six small, high-protein meals per day
    b. Carbohydrates (CHO) to increase energy levels
    c. Six small, high-carbohydrate meals per day
    d. Only proteins to ensure tissue-building capabilities

14. While caring for a client receiving a beta blocker for hypertension, the nurse is aware that the assessment finding of tiredness may be associated with a/an
    a. Decreased cardiac output
    b. Increased cardiac output
    c. Decreased blood pressure
    d. Increased intracranial pressure

15. A client admitted to the emergency department following a car accident is diagnosed with a left flail chest. The nurse would expect to see what type of chest movements?
    a. Paradoxical
    b. Labored
    c. Unilateral
    d. Bilateral

16. When evaluating a client's chest tube, the nurse identifies continuous bubbling in the water seal chamber. The correct intervention would be to
    a. Increase the suction
    b. Turn the suction off
    c. Clamp the chest tube
    d. Evaluate for an air leak starting at skin level

17. The nurse is aware that the suction in the chest tube canister is regulated by the amount of
    a. Suction on the wall regulator
    b. Water placed in the water seal chamber
    c. Bubbling in the suction control chamber
    d. Water placed in the suction control chamber

18. A postoperative client begins to complain of substernal chest pain radiating into the left lower chest border. The nurse is unsure if the client is suffering from an acute MI or a pulmonary embolism. Which diagnostic study report would the nurse check first to determine the cause of the pain?
    a. An ECG
    b. An ABG
    c. A chest x-ray
    d. A ventilation/perfusion scan

19. A 44-year-old client returned from the PACU 4 hours ago following a total hysterectomy. She has received medication for what she describes as severe pain. The nurse is still evaluating vital signs every 2 hours as ordered. The last set of vital signs indicates a BP of 80/50, a HR of 110 and irregular, which is a new onset, and an RR of 24. Her systolic BP has dropped 30 mm Hg. She complains of feeling dizzy and nauseated. Appropriate further evaluation at this point would be to
    a. Order an ECG
    b. Call the physician within 2 hours
    c. Order stat electrolytes
    d. Place her on a telemetry cardiac monitor

20. A client on a ventilator has been awake and responsive, but is suddenly unresponsive. When checked the monitor shows what looks like ventricular tachycardia. The first intervention must be to
    a. Order from the standing orders a stat ECG
    b. Deliver a precordial thump
    c. Assess for a carotid pulse
    d. Place oxygen on the client

21. When planning care for a right pneumonectomy client, the nurse is careful to include a turning schedule in the care plan with which format?
    a. Back, right, back, left
    b. Back, right, back, right
    c. Back, left, back, left
    d. Back, prone, back, supine

22. The murmur heard when listening to heart sounds of a client with mitral stenosis is caused by
    a. Valve protrusion
    b. Valve obstruction
    c. Turbulent blood flow in the aorta
    d. Turbulent blood flow in the ventricle

23. For a postoperative client following an abdominal aortic aneurysm repair, an assessment that is vital regarding the patency of the graft is
    a. Femeral pulses
    b. Abdominal girths
    c. Abdominal sounds
    d. Dorsalis pedis and posterior tibial pulses

24. A life-threatening complication associated with pericarditis is
    a. Hypertension
    b. Pleural effusion
    c. Renal insufficiency
    d. Pericardial effusion

25. A neighbor asks a nurse about a diagnosis of arteriosclerosis obliterans of the femoral artery. The nurse knows that it is most often first manifested by
    a. Terminal toe gangrene
    b. Intermittent thrombosis
    c. Intermittent claudication
    d. Pain in the affected extremity

26. The nurse is caring for an 8-hour, postoperative open cholecystectomy client who had a short episode of hypotension in PACU, but who has been quite stable since. Which one of the following would alert the nurse to continue to assess for the possibility of noncardiogenic pulmonary edema, also called ARDS (adult respiratory distress syndrome)?
    a. Auscultation reveals upper airway crackles
    b. The client is sleepy

c. The family tells the nurse that the client has been irritable this evening

d. The nurse notices that the client has a quarter-sized blood spot on the dressing

27. Nursing measures for the client with noncardiac pulmonary edema must be aimed at
    a. Reinflated alveoli
    b. Increased lung expansion
    c. Increased lung compliance
    d. Decreased oxygen consumption

28. In assessing a client who has just returned from surgery following a femoral-popliteal bypass to the left leg, the nurse must include an evaluation of
    a. The venous return in the left foot
    b. The color and temperature of both feet
    c. The color and temperature of the left foot
    d. The right and left dorsalis pedis (DP) and posterior tibial (PT) pulses

29. A common assessment factor the nurse would anticipate finding in the client with pericarditis is
    a. Pulmonary edema
    b. Adventitious lung sounds
    c. Pericardial friction rub
    d. Jugular venous distention

30. Positioning of the client with acute left upper lobe pneumonia should be aimed at
    a. Turning the client only to the back and left sides
    b. Turning the client to the back side and only slightly to the right side
    c. Keeping the client on the right side as much as possible to keep the affected lung well ventilated
    d. Keeping the client on the left side as much as possible to keep the unaffected lung well ventilated

31. A vital assessment factor to evaluate on a client in hypovolemic shock is
    a. Electrolytes
    b. Urine output
    c. Peripheral pulses
    d. Jugular venous distention

32. The nurse prepares an educational plan for a client with a deep vein thrombosis. When discussing the necessity of heparin therapy, the nurse is careful to include
    a. The necessity to increase green, leafy vegetables in the diet
    b. That the purpose of the heparin is to decrease the size of the clot
    c. That the heparin is used to prevent further emboli from occurring
    d. That the frequent prothrombin time evaluations are to evaluate the effectiveness of the heparin

33. When caring for a client with a radical neck dissection for laryngeal cancer, the nurse must include which of the following interventions?
    a. Suction airway every 2 hours
    b. Use only nonhumidified oxygen
    c. Keep the head of the bed in a low fowlers position to aid respirations
    d. Drain and resqueeze the Jackson-Pratt drains when half full or a minimum of every 4 hours

34. A priority for teaching clients who are newly diagnosed with glaucoma is
    a. How to give the eye drops without causing injury to the eye
    b. The need to wear protective glasses when engaging in sport activities
    c. The need to adjust the medication schedule according to lifestyle needs
    d. The importance of continuing the medication, even when the physician states that the glaucoma is under control

35. The activity that would be contraindicated for the client following cataract surgery would be
    a. Reading
    b. Wearing sunglasses
    c. Watching television
    d. Bending to pick up the newspaper

36. When being admitted with a confirmed retinal detachment, the client asks the nurse why both eyes must be patched. The best response would include the point that both eyes are patched
    a. To prevent further damage that may be caused by light
    b. To decrease ocular movement
    c. Because when one eye moves the other will, too, and the need is to decrease movement to decrease the risk of further retinal detachment
    d. To decrease ocular movement and decrease the pain associated with the retinal detachment

37. Clinical manifestations that may lead the nurse to identify a client's hearing loss are
   a. Slurred words and fatigue
   b. Self-confidence and an energetic attitude
   c. Showing interest in what is going on around and changing direction of the head with conversation changes
   d. Placing themselves in situations where they must interact and engaging in solitary activities

38. An expected assessment finding for the client who has suffered a cerebral vascular accident (CVA) is
   a. Diarrhea
   b. Hemiparesis
   c. Urinary continence
   d. Fixed and dilated pupils

39. An appropriate nursing goal for a postoperative craniotomy client would be to
   a. Open eyes on command
   b. Have decreased lower airway sounds
   c. Demonstrate a weight gain of ¼ kg per day
   d. Make needs known by way of effective verbal communication

40. Bed rest should be discouraged in the client with multiple myeloma due to the higher risk for
   a. Hypobilirubinuria and subsequent liver failure
   b. Hypercalcemia and subsequent renal failure
   c. Hypoproteinuria and subsequent kidney infection
   d. Hypouricemia and subsequent urinary tract infection

41. A nursing measure that may effectively treat urinary incontinence is
   a. An indwelling urinary catheter
   b. Frequent toileting of the client
   c. The use of pubococcygeal exercises
   d. The use of a protective device such as a diaper

42. An appropriate nursing diagnosis for the client suffering from hyperthyroidism would be
   a. Altered nutrition: less than body requirements related to increased metabolic functions
   b. Altered nutrition: more than body requirements related to decreased body metabolism
   c. Hypothermia related to increased metabolic rate
   d. Ineffective breathing pattern related to increased metabolic rate

43. Due to a decreased metabolic rate, the client with hypothyroidism should be cautiously given which of the following drugs?
    a. Vitamins
    b. Diuretics
    c. Sedatives
    d. Potassium supplements

44. A clinical manifestation that can indicate the onset of osteoporosis is
    a. Fractures
    b. Kyphosis
    c. Bone cracking
    d. Lengthening of the lower limbs

45. When educating a client about mammography, the nurse tells her that the benefit of the test is to
    a. Pinpoint the position of a breast mass
    b. Identify a breast mass and its size
    c. Identify a breast lesion before it is palpable
    d. Identify the metastatic nature of a breast mass

46. During the assessment of a client with a full-thickness burn injury, the nurse identifies a decrease in urine output to less than 25 ml/hour, and that the urine now looks like wine. The nurse is aware that these findings are most likely due to
    a. Injury to the kidneys from blunt trauma
    b. Edema surrounding the kidneys, causing decreased kidney perfusion
    c. Increased circulating blood volume and removal of the burn tissue through the kidneys
    d. Decreased circulating blood volume and removal of damaged RBCs through the kidneys, causing kidney damage

47. The nurse is aware that the burn client most likely to require considerable pain medication would have
    a. A sunburn
    b. A third-degree or full-thickness burn
    c. A first-degree or superficial-thickness burn
    d. A second-degree or deep, partial-thickness burn

48. When assessing a client with acquired immunodeficiency syndrome (AIDS), the nurse anticipates that the most common clinical manifestation is
    a. Pneumonia
    b. Diarrhea

    c. Constipation

    d. Urinary infection

49. Patient education about preventing skin cancer must include information regarding
    a. Sunscreen use whenever skin is exposed to the sun
    b. The type of tanning bed to use if you burn easily
    c. How to tan if you have a history of tanning poorly
    d. The fact that moles with a brown tint and irregular edges are unlikely to be malignant

50. The nurse would discuss with a student that the most important drug classification used in the treatment of lupus erythematosus is
    a. Vitamins
    b. Diuretics
    c. Corticosteroids
    d. The digitalis preparations

51. A client, following a transurethral prostatectomy, complains of a feeling that he must void, as well as a feeling of pressure and fullness in his bladder. The nurse thinks that this is most likely bladder spasms, and that these spasms must be controlled to prevent which of the following complications?
    a. Bleeding
    b. Indwelling urinary catheter displacement
    c. Indwelling urinary catheter obstruction
    d. Decreased urine formation

52. A client with cancer of the prostate is voiding 30 to 40 ml of urine at a time and at frequent intervals. The nurse suspects
    a. Urine retention
    b. A urinary tract infection
    c. Epididymitis
    d. Urine retention with overflow

53. The nurse working in a clinic must complete teaching for a client with a history of recurrent urinary tract infections. What point must be included in the teaching session?
    a. Wear only satin underwear to repel organisms from the urethral meatus
    b. Drink only cranberry juice during the treatment of an acute infection
    c. Urinate immediately after sexual intercourse to flush bacteria out of the urethra
    d. Abstain from intercourse for 1 week after the last dose in the drug therapy for an acute infection

54. An important question the nurse would ask when evaluating a newly admitted client following head trauma is
    a. "Do you hear ringing in your ears?"
    b. "Do you have an ache in your neck?"
    c. "Did you lose consciousness?"
    d. "Are you taking any aspirin-like drugs?"

55. The admitting nurse in the emergency room for a client with suspected spinal cord injury expects the client to manifest spinal shock. The nurse anticipates finding which assessment variable in the face of spinal shock?
    a. Tachycardia
    b. Hypertension
    c. Lack of diaphoresis below the level of the injury
    d. Normal bladder tone

56. A student writes the following as nursing goals for the client with multiple sclerosis. Which of these goals needs no correction by the supervising nurse?
    a. The client will have no changes in the retina
    b. The bladder is emptied with no residual with each voiding
    c. The client can bathe upper half of body without assistance
    d. The client's legs are less spastic and painful in the evening hours

57. A client admitted for a workup of syncope fell in a mall and lost consciousness for several minutes. The client's general appearance denotes a lack of nutrition—pale, waxy skin color, poor skin turgor, and weight 20 pounds less than normal for height. As the nurse reviews the chart, particular attention would be given to what laboratory study to help explain the client's condition?
    a. Electrolytes
    b. Hemoglobin/hematocrit
    c. BUN/creatinine
    d. Albumin

58. When assessing a client admitted for severe anemia, the nurse would anticipate which of the following findings with the acquired vital signs?
    a. Hypertension, tachycardia
    b. Hypotension, tachycardia
    c. Hypertension, bradycardia
    d. Hypotension, bradycardia

59. In caring for a client with acute nonlymphocytic leukemia (ANLL), the nurse noticed an increase in the client's temperature to 38.8 degrees Celsius. The

nurse called the physician, who has ordered the client placed in reverse isolation. The nurse is aware that isolation intervention is aimed at
a. Prevention of a contagious spread of the leukemia
b. Isolation of the organism that caused the fever
c. Protection of the client from any viruses the staff may have
d. Protection of the client from further infection, to which he/she is susceptible due to ineffective WBCs

60. A client is admitted due to weakness, fatigue, and weight loss. The nurse is concerned because the client believes that the symptoms are caused by arthritis. The nurse becomes convinced that the client's illness is not arthritis. In fact, the nurse thinks it may be chronic leukemia when he/she sees which of the following assessment findings and associates it with the admitting clinical manifestations?
a. Jugular venous distension
b. Decreased peripheral pulses
c. Lymphadenopathy
d. Diarrhea

61. An important home teaching need of the client with nonHodgkin's lymphoma is
a. How to take the medication
b. How to cleanse the radiation area with soap and water
c. The importance of using antiemetic drugs before chemotherapy *only*
d. The need to hold tight pressure over any bleeding wound and seek medical help

62. A client with Hodgkin's disease has returned from the operating room after a staging laparotomy. An appropriate, specific nursing goal would be
a. Airway will remain clear at all times, as evidenced by clear upper airway sounds
b. Client will be afebrile with no signs of redness, swelling, or exudate in the surgical incision
c. Pain will be relieved to a level of 0 on a scale of 0 to 10 within 30 minutes after the pain medication
d. Breathing pattern will be effective, as demonstrated by a respiratory rate of 18 to 20 and normal depth for the client

63. An appropriate nursing diagnosis to include in the clinical pathway of a client with asbestosis in its acute stage is
a. Activity intolerance related to hypoxemia and fatigue
b. Impaired gas exchange related to alveolar collapse

    c.   Ineffective airway clearance related to bronchial secretions
    d.   Ineffective breathing pattern related to asbestos in the bronchial tree

64. An important nursing evaluation action to include when caring for a client who is receiving multiple or long-term antibiotics is
    a.   Serum creatinine
    b.   Stool for guiac
    c.   Urine specific gravity
    d.   Oral mucous membranes for white patches

65. A nurse visits a client in the home for a leg ulcer dressing change. The client also has a history of gastroesophageal reflux. The nurse should be sure to encourage elimination of which of the following food stuffs from the diet?
    a.   Orange juice
    b.   Skim milk
    c.   Bananas
    d.   Green beans

66. A client with a confirmed hiatal hernia is taught how to take the medication. Which schedule indicates that the client's knowledge of antacids is adequate—1 to 3 hours
    a.   After meals
    b.   Before meals
    c.   Before bedtime
    d.   Before and after meals and at bedtime

67. A priority of care for the client who is 22 hours post-operative for a classic cholecystectomy would be
    a.   Meticulous skin care surrounding the T-tube
    b.   Dressing changes to prevent incisional infection
    c.   Antibiotic therapy to prevent incisional infection
    d.   Pain relief to improve turning, coughing, and deep-breathing efforts

68. A client is admitted with acute pancreatitis. The physician gives orders to keep the client NPO and to place an NG tube attached to low, continuous suction. The family asks the nurse the purpose of the NG tube and NPO status. The nurse should include that the NG tube is used for the prevention of
    a.   Stimulation of and spasm of the duodenum
    b.   Regurgitation of pancreatic juices
    c.   Increased infection in the pancreatic area
    d.   Stimulation of the pancreas to produce more pancreatic enzymes

69. Important nursing assessment criteria that must be included for the client suffering from ascites are
    a. Lung sounds, heart sounds
    b. Daily weight, abdominal girths
    c. Daily weight, lung sounds
    d. Lung sounds, abdominal girths

70. An important nursing intervention in the plan of care for a client who has reached the icteric stage of hepatitis is
    a. Mild exercise to increase stamina
    b. Frequent baths with a mild soap to decrease skin irritation
    c. Skin lotions to decrease itching associated with this stage
    d. Increased carbohydrates and fats in the diet to ensure sound nutrition

71. An appropriate nursing goal for the client with ulcerative colitis is
    a. Intake will balance with output within ± 600 ml per day
    b. Episodes of constipation will reduce to 2 times per month
    c. Episodes of diarrhea will decrease to 2 bowel movements per day
    d. Client will gain 2 kg per week and not lose the gained weight within 6 months

72. At a home follow-up visit with a client who was hospitalized for an acute episode of diverticulitis, the nurse would be concerned if the client were eating which foods?
    a. Peanuts and cashews
    b. Salad with ranch dressing
    c. Pork barbecue with french fries
    d. Peanut butter and jelly sandwich

73. A neighbor has come to a nurse to discuss various assessment findings. The neighbor asks if there should be concern about any of the following findings. Which of these would lead the nurse to suspect colon cancer and kindly tell the neighbor to see a physician soon?
    a. Weight loss
    b. Change in bowel habits
    c. Abdominal pain
    d. Family history of cancer

74. The nurse is assigned to a client who was involved in a motor vehicle accident a week earlier and sustained multiple injuries. The physicians now believe the client is in acute renal failure. The physicians have

ordered Mannitol to be given. The family asks why. The nurse would include which reason?
a.   To increase urine output
b.   To decrease fluid volume and edema
c.   To increase renal perfusion
d.   To increase renal filtration

75.   A client with newly diagnosed chronic renal failure has asked how long it will take for the kidneys to "get better." The nurse is aware that the physician has discussed this thoroughly with the client. The nurse's response must be as follows
a.   "You may not see improvement in your kidneys for about a year"
b.   "We have no idea how long it will take for the damage to reverse"
c.   "This illness is not reversible. Your kidneys will not get better"
d.   "Your kidneys will not get better, but your body will allow a new kidney to grow"

76.   A client has been admitted to the unit with a renal calculus, which has lodged in the right ureter. The client is in extreme pain in the right flank area and has been vomiting. The client voids after admission to the room and states that the pain is relieved. The best intervention at this point would be to
a.   Call the physician
b.   Strain the urine and evaluate for a stone that has passed
c.   Decrease the pain medication, as the client obviously had received enough
d.   Increase the IV rate because the stone must be moving down the ureter and must be flushed out

77.   In the emergency room the nurse is triaging a client who is complaining of pain at the costovertebral angle (CVA), "stinky" urine, and a fever for 24 hours of 39° C. The nurse suspects
a.   Pyelonephritis
b.   Renal calculus
c.   Diverticulitis
d.   Urinary tract infection

78.   A client is admitted with gross hematuria. Diagnostic studies indicate a renal carcinoma, and the physician has advised a nephrectomy. Changes in assessment for which area would be extremely important to expediently inform the physician?
a.   The lungs
b.   The bladder

    c. The kidneys
    d. The heart

79. An appropriate nursing diagnosis for the client with bladder cancer who has undergone a radical cystectomy and ileal conduit formation would be
    a. Body-image disturbance related to change in the manner of urinary elimination
    b. Pain related to cancer metastasis
    c. Altered urinary elimination related to ileal conduit
    d. Impaired gas exchange related to a flank incision

80. The purpose of a scrotal support following an orchiectomy for testicular cancer is to
    a. Decrease pain
    b. Decrease edema
    c. Hold the dressing in place
    d. Prevent twisting of the remaining testicle

81. A client, following a total abdominal hysterectomy for cervical cancer, has a PCA (patient-controlled analgesia) pump ordered for pain management. She is worried about the possibility of overdosing herself on the morphine in the PCA pump. What should the best response be?
    a. "The pump won't allow you to overdose yourself"
    b. "The PCA pump is set up with safety features, which prevent you from overdosing yourself"
    c. "The physician has a timed lockout, which will prevent you from receiving too much medication in an hour"
    d. "There is a period of time called a lockout, which is preset by physician's order and set on the pump, during which time no medication can be received. This prevents an overdose."

82. The nurse home-visits a client following a hospitalization for intracavitary radiation. Her husband looks very nervous, and the nurse is aware that he has a question that he is uncomfortable to ask. In private he tells the nurse that he is worried about the effects of the radiation treatment on him, so he has been hesitant to initiate sexual intercourse. The best response would be what?
    a. "Your wife is only radioactive for a week after the treatment is stopped"
    b. "Once the radioactive implant has been removed, you are safe to have sexual relations"

    c. "Once the radioactive implant is removed, your wife is no longer 'radioactive.' You should feel comfortable to initiate sexual intercourse a week after the therapy has stopped."

    d. "You should avoid sexual relations for at least a month following the treatment. After that time, it will be perfectly safe to have sexual relations."

83. When talking with clients in a screening clinic for ovarian cancer, the nurse is aware that one of the most important questions to ask them is

    a. "Have you had children?"

    b. "Has your mother, sisters, grandmother, or aunts been diagnosed with ovarian cancer?"

    c. "Did you breast-feed your children?"

    d. "Have you gone through menopause?"

84. When preparing a teaching plan for the client diagnosed with hyperparathyroidism, the nurse is sure to include which of the following points?

    a. Increase fluid intake to 2000 to 3000 ml per day to prevent renal calculi

    b. Follow a high-calcium diet to force calcium into the bones

    c. Get as much rest as possible, as this allows time for calcium to transport back into the bones

    d. Decrease fiber and bulk in your diet to prevent constipation

85. The nurse is aware that a client in acute Addisonian crisis will manifest complete vascular collapse. The treatment regime should include

    a. Intravenous calcium

    b. Intravenous dexamethasone

    c. Controlled fluid administration

    d. Frequent blood pressure monitoring

86. When counseling the client with Cushing's syndrome (after the client's surgery has left an adrenal insufficiency), the nurse makes it very clear that the client *must*

    a. Monitor daily weights

    b. Follow a high-sodium diet

    c. Protect himself/herself from viruses

    d. Be aware of the need for more steroids during times of stress or illness

87. A nursing intervention that must be included for the client who is 8 hours postoperative for a lumbar laminectomy is

    a. Do a neurovascular assessment every 2 hours

    b. Move client out of bed to an easy chair the night of surgery

c. Evaluate for urinary retention if an indwelling urinary catheter is not in place

d. Elevate the head of the bed 30 degrees and turn every 2 hours

88. The nurse is teaching a client being discharged with a cardiac condition and also suffering from rheumatoid arthritis. An important item to include would be for the client to
    a. Exercise joints just past the point of pain
    b. Keep joints still or rested to prevent pain
    c. Exercise joints to the point of pain and no further
    d. Wear splints only after acute exacerbations are resolved

89. A client is received from the recovery room following an above-the-knee amputation of the right leg. Appropriate positioning of the stump at this time should be
    a. Flat on the bed
    b. Elevated 30 to 40 degrees for 24 hours only
    c. Elevated 10 degrees for 3 days only
    d. Flat with restraints to hold the stump against the bed

90. An understanding about the formation of pressure ulcers allows nurses to incorporate into the plan of care preventative measures. These measures should include which item?
    a. Reposition clients every 2 to 4 hours
    b. Visualize pressure points every 4 hours
    c. Cleanse the skin immediately after incontinence occurs
    d. Avoid the use of turning sheets to pull up or reposition clients in bed

ANSWERS, RATIONALES, AND TEST-TAKING TIPS

Rationales	Test-Taking Tips

1. Correct answer: d

The legs are abducted to prevent the head of the prosthesis from moving out of the acetabulum. This is usually accomplished with the aid of an abduction splint or pillows. Log rolling is not necessary in these clients, and ambulation is typically not early in their postoperative course. Log rolling is most frequently done with postoperative spinal surgery clients.

Tip to remember: to abduct is to move from—in this case to move from the midline of the body. Recall that *Logroll* is done for the *Laminectomy.*

2. Correct answer: b

A nasogastric tube (NG) is never repositioned following gastric surgery. The possibility of pushing the NG tube through the gastric incision line is too great a risk. All the other interventions are appropriate.

If you have no idea, use the strategy to cluster the three responses that have 4 hours in them and select the response without the time frame.

3. Correct answer: d

Insulin should never be shaken, but instead should be rolled between the hands. Shaking can cause a breakdown of the insulin. All the other options are correct techniques.

As a rule of thumb in medication mixing, the action is typically done by rotating the container, not by shaking it. If you have no idea, try clustering responses *a, b,* and *c* under the category of "actions taken for administration to the client." Select response *d,* which is an action for the medication mixture.

4. Correct answer: b

Double-ply tissues that are then burned after use will offer the best containment of the bacilli during coughing and sneezing. Sterilizing the linen and using large amounts of bleach are not necessary, as a hot water wash is sufficient to kill the bacilli. The client need not wear a mask in respiratory isolation. This is suggested only if the client must leave the room. The staff members wear masks while caring for a client in respiratory isolation.

If you have no idea, cluster the two responses that deal with linen and eliminate these. Of the remaining responses, common sense eliminates *d,* since usual protocol dictates that the visitors wear the mask.

5. Correct answer: b

Placing oxygen on the client may relieve the chest pain by delivering more oxygen to the myocardium. After placement of oxygen on the client, start an IV, then call for a stat ECG. Start the IV first in case of dysrhythmias, which are most common in the initial hours of an MI. At this point try one sublingual NTG. A possibility exists that the NTG the client had at home was out-of-date.

The primary need for the heart tissue at this point is to increase oxygen delivery. This action is also the most likely to be completed in a few seconds, whereas the others may take minutes. Lastly, protocol suggests using a heparin lock type of IV access instead of the KVO-with-fluids approach.

6. Correct answer: d

The use of heparin following thrombolytic therapy is to prevent further clot formation in the coronary arteries.

Responses *a* and *b* are correct, but they are both too general—specific questions like this usually need specific answers.

7. Correct answer: d

Daily weight is a vital assessment tool for the physician to determine if therapy is effective. The client must be taught correct technique to make this an effective evaluation tool. Measuring urine output and limb edema is not as helpful to the physician. Education about how to take their pulse is provided if clients are sent home on digitalis preparations.

Think *Daily* weights for *Diuretic* therapy. Also, the clustering technique can be used to cluster responses *a* through *c*—"how to."

8. Correct answer: a

Organ meats are very high in cholesterol and should be eliminated from the diet if the cholesterol reading is high. The others are low in cholesterol. Yogurt is high in fat unless described as low-fat yogurt.

Organ meats are typically correct choices when the question asks for foods to avoid. They have higher amounts of cholesterol as well as purines, which are restricted in clients with gout.

9. Correct answer: b

The majority of clients will first report overwhelming fatigue. As the left-sided failure progresses, more lung involvement occurs, and the client will experience dyspnea. The fatigue is a manifestation of the decreased cardiac output.

If you have no idea of the correct option, use common sense to cluster from the most to the least noticeable—responses *b, a, c,* and *d*—then select response *b*. Note that options *c* and *d* are later findings.

10. Correct answer: d

Stress and temperature extremes can cause an acute exacerbation of Buerger's disease.

Use common sense to cluster from most severe to least severe, which is how they are listed. Select the least severe, option *d,* to answer the question. Read carefully to avoid missing "except."

11. **Correct answer: b**

Clients with COPD very often have acute exacerbations following an upper respiratory infection or flu. In contrast, cold weather can cause bronchospasm. The increased inhalants from the clogged air filter or the increase in cigarettes would not likely be a cause of the exacerbation.

Focus on the key words "exacerbation . . . bronchitis" and not on "chronic." Recall that "itis" = inflammation from a bacteria, fungus, or virus.

12. **Correct answer: d**

The client with COPD most often will be stable in a near-compensated respiratory acidosis. This is related to the longstanding CO_2 retention.

Recall that COPD clients include those with asthma, chronic bronchitis, and emphysema. In the COPD clients the PO_2 and the PCO_2 are nearly the same for both of these parameters—50 to 60s. Associate that 50 to 60 is the age that most of these clients reach before dying.

13. **Correct answer: c**

Clients are encouraged to eat small, frequent meals to prevent overdistention of the stomach, which would impede inhalation. Meals high in carbohydrates are encouraged, since the large number of calories are consumed by COPD clients from just the effort needed with breathing. Caution clients not to eat large amounts of high CHO at one setting, since the breakdown of CHO releases more of CO_2 than other types of food.

Recall that CHO are needed for energy and protein production, and vitamin C and zinc are needed for healing after any tissue trauma.

14. Correct answer: a

One of the expected effects of beta blockers is the decrease in myocardial contractility. This leads to a decreased cardiac output. Ultimately this will also lead to a decreased blood pressure, but the actual cause of the fatigue is related to the decreased cardiac output. Similarly, fatigue is commonly an initial complaint of a client with congestive heart failure.

Associate fatigue with decreased cardiac output.

15. Correct answer: a

When a client sustains a flail chest, the flail section is separated from the rib cage and moves independently of the attached rib section. This will cause the flail section to bulge on exhalation and sink in on inspiration.

Paradoxical breathing is when the lung deflates during inspiration and inflates during exhalation.

16. Correct answer: d

Continuous bubbling in the water seal chamber means there is air leaking into the system. Checking for this leak, beginning at the level of the skin and working down the tube to the chamber system, will identify the site of the leak. The bubbling will stop when the clamp is just below the air leak. In this situation, without a physician's order the nurse cannot turn off the suction, increase it, or clamp the chest tube.

In the given situation, cluster the first three options under "the need for an order," since how the options are worded gives no time for how long to do each of these. Select the action that requires no order.

17. Correct answer: d

The suction control chamber is filled with sterile water to the level of suction the physician has ordered; usually it is 20 cm H_2O. The chamber tubing is then attached to wall suction and turned on so that the chamber continuously, gently bubbles. The other options have no effect on the amount of suction.

If you have no idea of the correct response, use common sense to narrow the responses to the two that give information on "suction control," options c and d. Then use common sense to establish that the amount of water is better controlled than the amount of bubbling which cannot be measured in any manner—select option d.

18. Correct answer: d

The ventilation/perfusion scan will actually allow visualization of impaired blood flow to an area of the lung, which gives a diagnosis of pulmonary embolism. The ECG may indicate changes with either problem. ABGs and a chest x-ray may be abnormal with either problem.

Cluster responses a, b, and c as general and response d as specific, for identification of clots in the lungs

19. Correct answer: d

The assessment of a rapid, irregular pulse that is a new onset, along with the BP that is 30 mm Hg lower than it had been, is a clear indication that the client is experiencing a dysrhythmia. Placing the client on a cardiac monitor is the only way of determining this. The physician will want to know this information when the nurse calls.

Use common sense—if the client has an irregular heart rate, the telemetry is the best method to evaluate the situation. An ECG is correct but not the best method, since it captures the electrical activity as a snapshot in time does, whereas the telemetry offers more continuous monitoring, as with a video camera. Also note that from the given options, eliminate a and c since the nurse cannot order independently; eliminate option b since waiting 2 hours is inappropriate.

20. Correct answer: c

The nurse must establish that the client is pulseless before giving a precordial thump. Actions such as an ECG and oxygen therapy can be done if the client has a pulse.

Use the steps in the nursing process: further assessment is the best choice before interventions. Note that as written about the dysrhythmia, there was not a witnessed cardiac dysrhythmia.

21. Correct answer: b

Pneumonectomy clients should be positioned only on the back and operative side. This prevents mediastinal shifting and allows optimal ventilation of the remaining lung.

Note that the time frame is not immediate post-op which is when there is a highest risk of a mediastinal shift. With the removal of one lung, recall that the total blood volume now is delivered to just one lung. Therefore, ventilation is a priority for the remaining lung which should be kept up. This position also helps to drain any secretions that may have accumulated.

22. Correct answer: d

When a mitral valve is stenosed or stiff, some of the blood will be propelled forward into the left ventricle and some will be shunted backward into the left atrium. This will cause turbulent flow as the forward-flowing blood meets the backward-flowing blood. This causes the murmur.

Remember that a murmur typically results from turbulent flow. Narrow the responses to either *c* or *d*. Then recall normal anatomy, with the mitral valve located between the left atria and ventricle. Select response *d*.

23. Correct answer: d

If the graft is patent, the client will have appropriate dorsalis pedis and posterior tibial pulses. The Doppler pressures in the lower extremities will be close to

Important to this question is the focus on the vessels. Thus the better options will contain a response about vessels, which are options *a* and *d*. Of these two choices, response *d* is best

the same pressure as in the arms. The femoral pulses are not assessed, since the more distal pulses are better to check.

because these pulses are more distal to the surgical site.

24. Correct answer: d

A pericardial effusion forms due to the friction between the layers of the pericardial sac. The friction forms fluid in response to inflammation and begins to build up in the pericardium. The fluid buildup will eventually constrict the heart and prevent it from filling and contracting appropriately. This can lead to pericardial or cardiac tamponade. Heart sounds become muffled and distant on auscultation. If caused from a bacterial infection, a high fever, sweating, chills, and prostration also occur (Prostration is a condition of extreme exhaustion and inability to exert oneself further).

These suggestions can be used if you have no idea of the correct response. One approach is to match a similar word in the stem (pericarditis) with one in the options (option *d*, pericardial). A second approach is to note that the question is about the heart— so cluster responses *a*, *b*, and *c* into "noncardiac" and select response *d*, the only one with a reference to "cardiac."

25. Correct answer: c

Intermittent claudication, or pain on walking, will usually be the first manifestation of arteriosclerosis obliterans. Pain at rest will be manifested as the obstruction increases. Response *d* is correct but is too general to be the best answer. Gangrene, from complete arterial occlusion, is the most severe result to occur.

If you have no idea of the correct response, use common sense to narrow the responses to intermittent versus an ongoing problem. Then recall that thrombus typically form in the low pressure system, the veins; select response *c*.

26. **Correct answer: c**

Unusual interpersonal interactions are one of the first clues that the client may be slightly hypoxemic and may be advancing into ARDS. Lower airway crackles would be more typical of the client in ARDS. Sleepiness may be indicative of increased CO_2. Increased CO_2 occurs later in ARDS and is not a reliable indicator of early ARDS, or early hypoxemia client.

It is important to note that the question is asking about the earliest sign of a lack of oxygen rather than a CO_2 problem. Recall that a change in the level of consciousness is a first finding in a decreased oxygen level. The initial change of level of consciousness for hypoxemic and the hypoglycemic clients is irritably, restlessness or agitation.

27. **Correct answer: d**

It may not be possible to deliver more oxygen to the tissues due to the damaged lungs, so the nursing measure must decrease oxygen consumption by the body to prevent cellular hypoxia.

The critical point is to note that the question is asking about a "nursing measure," not medical goals, which are options *a, b,* and *c.*

28. **Correct answer: d**

Evaluation of the DP and PT of the affected leg and the nonaffected leg are required for the comparison of perfusion of both extremities. The color and temperature of both extremities are also important, but the pulses are more of a priority.

Narrow the responses to *b* and *d,* since these are most specific and comprehensive. Then select *d,* since the pulses are prioritized over color and temperature, both of which are influenced by the external environment; this fact makes these assessments less reliable.

29. **Correct answer: c**

The client with pericarditis will commonly exhibit a pericardial friction rub caused by the two inflamed layers of the pericardium

Note that options *a* and *b* indicate heart failure, which has nothing to do with the question. In choosing between responses *c* and *d,* select *c,* since it is most aligned to

rubbing together. Jugular venous distention (JVD) may occur if the pericarditis evolves into a constrictive pericarditis.

pericarditis; or think in terms of anatomy, that it is more anatomically near than the neck veins; or match the similar themes or words.

30. Correct answer: c

The need is to keep the "sick" lung in the up position as much as possible. This will ensure optimal ventilation and drainage of secretions. If the lung is well ventilated, secretions will be more easily loosened and removed from the lung.

For positioning questions, the best approach is to visualize by drawing a picture on paper or to close your eyes and do a mental visualization with minimal movement of your own body as you go through each given option. After going through all of the options, reread the question and think of one priority need for the given situation. For example, in this situation of pneumonia it is critical to get the infected secretions out of the lung.

31. Correct answer: b

Urine output can accurately indicate the cardiac output of the client. Peripheral pulses do indicate peripheral perfusion but are not reliable indicators of adequate cardiac output. A client in hypovolemic shock will not have jugular venous distention. Electrolytes have no connection with the given situation.

There are two ways to approach this question. The first is to simply use common sense and basic, normal body physiology: "hypovolemic" is decreased volume, which leads to decreased blood to the organs and most frequently the kidney, which then conserves water with the result of a decreased urine output. A second approach is to cluster responses *a, c,* and *d* as parameters used to evaluate various body functions, whereas the urine output is typically specific to evaluate renal function; select the option outside of the cluster, *b.*

32. Correct answer: c

Heparin will prevent further clot formation and prevent an increase in the size of the clot already present. Green, leafy vegetables, which contain higher amounts of vitamin K, should not be eaten when a client is taking oral anticoagulants. The increased amounts of vitamin K may decrease the effectiveness of the anticoagulant. Activated partial thromboplastin times (aPTT) are used to evaluate the effectiveness of the heparin.

Eliminate responses *a* and *d,* since they relate to oral anticoagulants such as coumarin, not heparin. Eliminate response *b,* since the only drugs that "decrease" clots are streptokinase or activase.

33. Correct answer: d

Jackson-Pratt drains are emptied every 4 hours or when half full. When they are half full, they have lost the suction effectiveness. The head of the bed is kept in high fowlers to aid respirations. Oxygen must be humidified, and suctioning should occur only when the client requires suctioning: the client frequently has findings of a congested cough, or upper airway congested sounds.

Common sense will help you select the correct option. Ask yourself: if you only suction every 2 hours, what happens if the client needs it between that time? Be sure to slow down and see the "non" humidified oxygen—air into the respiratory passages needs humidification, with the exception of emergency resuscitation situations. Lastly, low fowlers is a 20- to 30-degree elevation of the head of the bed, not high enough to facilitate respirations.

34. Correct answer: d

The client with glaucoma must understand that medication is a lifelong need. This is a priority for inclusion in a teaching plan.

Response *a* is correct; however, it is not the priority focus. For this and similar situations such as hypertension, hypothyroidism, and other hormonal replacement, the education about the lifelong need for medication takes precedent over teaching the steps for administration.

35. Correct answer: d

A postoperative client with cataracts must not bend, sneeze, cough, or lift heavy objects.

After surgery to the eye or brain, a need is to prevent increased pressure in these areas, intraocular and intracranial. Remember that the top of the body, the head, is similar to the top of the volcano; the pressure at the top should not be increased or dysfunction will occur, with potential for permanent damage.

36. Correct answer: c

This is the most complete and informative answer. Eye movement must be minimized to prevent further detachment.

Light has nothing to do with the detached retina. The retina does not contain sensory nerves, so the condition is painless. Both options *b* and *c* are correct; however, *c* is the most complete answer.

37. Correct answer: a

Slurred words and fatigue would not be unusual in the deaf client. It would be unusual for such clients to appear energetic, self confident, interested in what is going on around them, or to put themselves in situations where they must interact.

Cluster the responses into positive actions—options *b, c,* and *d.* Select response *a,* the negative type of information.

38. Correct answer: b

The CVA client may manifest hemiparesis, loss of feeling or sensation, or hemiplegia, loss of movement. Constipation, urinary incontinence, and

Recall that effects from a CVA are one sided. Thus eliminate response *d,* since it is bilateral; the pupil will be dilated on the same side as the infarct in the brain. Response *c* is a

unequal pupils would be other manifestations of a CVA, since there may be a loss of muscle tone internally in the stomach, intestine, and bladder similar to the loss in muscle function of the extremities.

normal finding; be careful not to read too quickly and misread this as incontinence. Of the two responses left, use common sense to eliminate option *a,* since diarrhea is usually the result of a local irritant, intestinal infection, the types or amounts of food eaten, or a medication side effect. Since there is no data in the stem to support any of these, select option *b.*

39. Correct answer: d

The best choice is *d,* since it offers the most detailed, complete, and measurable outcome.

There is no data in the stem to support the selection of responses *b* and *c.* While option *a* looks like the answer, it is too narrow of a choice for the general or broad question about a goal. Option *d* is more general and encompassing.

40. Correct answer: b

Bed rest can encourage the movement of calcium out of the bones, causing hypercalcemia. This can ultimately lead to kidney failure by damaging kidney structures as the blood with high levels of calcium is filtered through the kidneys; this also may cause formation of renal calculi.

If you have no idea of the correct response, cluster the three "hypo" options. Select hypercalcemia as the correct answer.

41. Correct answer: c

Pubococcygeal exercises (Kegal) can increase muscle tone and allow for normal urination without incontinence.

The question is asking for a "nursing" measure; an indwelling urinary catheter is a prescribed treatment. Diapers are protective to the sheet and bed but not to the client. Toileting frequently is appropriate; however, the better action is to increase bladder muscle tone first.

42. Correct answer: a

The client with hyperthyroidism is in a hypermetabolic state and thus requires a high-calorie intake.

Careful reading is a must for these type of questions and responses. "Hypothyroidism" is commonly misread as "hyperthyroidism," leading, incorrectly, to selection of response *c*.

43. Correct answer: c

The client who is hypometabolic should be given sedatives cautiously, as the medication will be slowly metabolized. The sedative effect could last much longer than anticipated. There are no contraindications for the other drug classifications.

Remember that with slow metabolism poor liver of renal function, give with caution any medications for sedation or the narcotic analgesics.

44. Correct answer: b

Kyphosis, or a hump at the base of the neck, is often the first indication that osteoporosis is occurring.

The key word in the stem is "onset" of osteoporosis. Responses *a* and *c* are more likely to occur after the condition has been present for awhile. Response *d* is incorrect, since limbs do not lengthen.

45. Correct answer: c

The major benefit of mammography is that visualization of a lesion can occur before the client palpates it during the self-breast exam. This allows for optimal treatment in a timely manner, and a far better prognosis.

Remember that a mammogram is included in secondary health prevention for early diagnosis. The only option that suggests early detection is *c*.

46. Correct answer: d

Unfortunately, the wine-colored urine indicates massive RBC destruction, and the filtering of these damaged RBCs

Eliminate response *a*, since there is no data to suggest blunt trauma. Eliminate response *b*, since it only focuses on the decreased urine

through the kidneys will damage the renal tubules.

output; it does not address the urine color change. Eliminate response *c*, since it is in conflict with the given data of decreased urine output. The only response left is *d*.

47. Correct answer: d

The deep, partial-thickness or second-degree burns are the most painful, especially if blisters have broken and the skin underneath is exposed. Third-degree burns are not painful, since the nerves are destroyed. Sunburns or first-degree burns are painful, but not as painful as second-degree burns.

Eliminate response *b*—remember, no nerves in third-degree burns = no pain. Cluster responses *a* and *c*, since both are first-degree type of burns. Select the second-degree burn. However, remember that the tissue around the third-degree burn may be painful for clients.

48. Correct answer: b

Diarrhea is the most commonly reported clinical manifestation of AIDS. It is also one of the more difficult to control.

Pneumonia, an opportunistic infection, in AIDS clients is a complication of the disease, not a usual finding with AIDS.

49. Correct answer: a

Sunscreen must be included in all educational endeavors regarding skin cancer. If a person burns easily, tanning beds should not be used. If clients have a history of poor tanning, it would be best for them to stay out of the sun. Brown moles with irregular edges are most often malignant.

Read carefully on these type of questions and responses. Option *d* is a correct statement for early detection; however, it does not answer the question for "prevention" of skin cancer.

50. Correct answer: c

Corticosteroids are imperative to decrease the inflammatory process of connective tissue associated with the illness.

Note that this is a more difficult question, since all of the responses are correct. The question asks for the most important. In prioritizing the options, it is identified that the other given medications might be used to treat specific problems that arise from lupus.

51. Correct answer: a

Bleeding can occur if bladder spasms are not controlled in the post-TURP client. The spasms are not strong enough to cause a urinary catheter obstruction or dislodgement. Since urine is formed in the kidney, it is impossible for bladder spasms to cause a decreased urine formation.

One approach is to cluster options *b, c,* and *d* under the common umbrella that if these occurred, there would be a decreased urine output. A second approach is to select the most severe situation, which is option *a.*

52. Correct answer: d

This client is not emptying his bladder; he is only voiding overflow of what the distended bladder cannot hold. Retention with overflow is best identified by a post-void, straight catheterization with a return of >100 ml.

There is no specific data in the stem to support an inflammation, epididymitis, or infection. Frequency is not a definitive finding only a suggestive finding of inflammation or infection in the urinary tract. Eliminate options *b* and *c.* Responses *a* and *d* are both correct; however, response *d* is most correct and related to the given situation. Also, with only urine retention there would more likely be no urine output.

53. Correct answer: c

Voiding immediately or shortly after intercourse will flush out any bacteria that may have been introduced due to the friction of intercourse. Clients with frequent urinary tract infections should wear only cotton underwear. An

Eliminate responses *a* and *b,* which have the absolute "only" in them; absolutes such as "only," "never," "always" are commonly indications that the option is the incorrect one. Of the remaining responses, *c* is correct, even though you may not agree with "immediately." Be

increased fluid intake is appropriate, but it does not have to be only cranberry juice. Intercourse can be resumed at the client's choice and comfort.

cautious of your emotional reactions from personal experiences and biases.

54. Correct answer: c

The loss of consciousness for any length of time indicates a more severe injury and requires more extensive evaluation. Questioning an ache in the neck or upper back would be a second priority because many head injuries are accompanied by neck injuries.

Ringing in the ears is more typical of medication overdosage such as aspirin or Lasix. Another approach is to associate head trauma with the priority of level of consciousness.

55. Correct answer: c

The client will have a lack of diaphoresis below the level of the injury, because of autonomic disruption. The client in spinal shock would manifest bradycardia, hypotension, and lack of bladder tone with urinary retention from autonomic disruption.

Remember that spinal shock is like other shocks in that the blood pressure decreases; however, it is different in that the heart rate "decreases" bradycardia, rather than the classic tachycardia, with shock. The normal reflexes to empty a full bowel and bladder are also lost in spinal shock, which may last from 3 days to 3 weeks. Thus all the responses can be eliminated except c.

56. Correct answer: c

This is the only nursing goal. The lack of changes in the retina, the bladder-emptying, and the less leg pain and spasticity are medical goals. The physician would order medication in hopes of relieving these problems.

Careful reading, then differentiating between nursing and medical goals are important for the correct selection of option c.

57. Correct answer: b

You suspect anemia because of assessment findings, especially the pale, waxy skin and the poor nutritional status. The hemoglobin and hematocrit would need to be low to substantiate the suspicion of anemia. A low albumin may suggest poor nutritional intake of protein; however, it may also reflect poor liver function or loss of protein in the interstitial space or through the kidneys.

Creatinine is specific to glomerular function. BUN (blood urea nitrogen levels) are commonly elevated in severe dehydration, kidney failure, or excess breakdown of protein in the body. Refer to the rationale.

58. Correct answer: b

The client would manifest shocklike symptoms with hypotension and tachycardia.

Remember that with decreased hemoglobin and hematocrit there is a lack of oxygen delivery to the tissues, which then manifests the body's response to that of shock, cellular hypoxia.

59. Correct answer: d

These clients are very susceptible to any and all infections due to poor WBC effectiveness, and they must be protected from infection.

Responses *a* and *b* have nothing to do with this condition. Option *c* sounds like a correct answer, but it is too restrictive in that it only includes "staff" (the client will also come in contact with visitors). Thus response *c* is the most comprehensive answer.

60. Correct answer: c

One of the classical manifestations of chronic leukemia is bone pain, which is often mistaken by older adults for arthritis. One of the factors that helps differentiate between the

Cluster options *a* and *b* under "cardiac" and eliminate, since they have nothing to do with the body's defense system. Associate that leukemia affects the WBC defense for the body, and that the lymph system plays an important part in

two illnesses is the finding of lymphadenopathy, which is any disorder of the lymph nodes or lymphatic system.

the fight against foreign substances in the body. Of the options *c* and *d* that remain, *c* is the most reasonable selection over diarrhea. Remember, *Leukemia* with *Lymphatic*.

61. Correct answer: d

The client with nonHodgkin's lymphoma must be taught how to treat bleeding as an emergency, since bleeding is a usual problem. Antiemetics are given as needed, and often before chemotherapy. Radiation areas are never cleansed with soap and water due to the drying effect of the soap.

Eliminate option *a*, since it is too general and the question is asking specifics related to a specific disease. Eliminate response *b*—the word "soap" is the clue that this is an incorrect answer, since soap is irritating to the skin. Eliminate response *c,* since it contains the absolute "only"; common sense dictates that the client might need antiemetics at other times.

62. Correct answer: b

This nursing goal is most specific to this client, as the client's immune system is impaired and infection would be a common finding.

All of the responses are correct, which makes this a more difficult question. After rereading the stem and responses, note that the question is asking for specifics. Then associate that Hodgkin's disease is associated with a lymphatic system disease. Reread the responses with the focus of prevention and the identification of infection; option *b* would be chosen.

63. Correct answer: a

The client with asbestosis will resemble the client with COPD. They will be hypoxemic and fatigued. Alveolar collapse is not common in this client. The breathing pattern is not impaired due to asbestos in

There is not enough data in the stem to support the selection of options *b*, *c*, or *d*. If you have no idea, another approach is to cluster these responses under "lung or pulmonary" and select response *a*, since it is different and deals with activity.

the bronchiole, but rather to smaller airway and alveolar changes and increased secretions.

64. **Correct answer: d**

Clients receiving multiple or long-term antibiotics are very likely to develop oral candidiasis due to normal oral flora disruption. This would be manifested by white patches on the tongue and oral mucous membranes. This may be called a superinfection.

The question is too general to select responses *a, b,* and *c.* If the question had asked about specific drugs such as aminoglycosides, options *a* or *c* would be better selections; with steroid or aspirin use, response *c* is best. One general effect of long-term antibiotic use not given as a choice is diarrhea.

65. **Correct answer: a**

Foods high in acid, such as orange juice, are more likely to cause belching and exacerbate the reflux.

The use of common sense to select the foodstuff that is most irritating to the upper gastrointestinal tract will lead to selection of option *a.* Avoid reading into the options; for example, do not think of the green beans as being cooked with grease.

66. **Correct answer: d**

Antacids are taken optimally 7 times a day: 1 to 3 hours before and after meals and at bedtime.

Use knowledge recall that the purpose of antacids is to neutralize the acid to prevent the irritation of the hiatal hernia. The most likely times the acid is present in the stomach are before and after meals and during sleep at night.

67. **Correct answer: d**

The classic cholecystectomy incision is found at the border of the right rib cage. Deep-breathing will cause the rib cage to descend on top of

All of the responses are correct. The priority is to maintain pulmonary and cardiac function. Thus the ABCs (airway, breathing, and circulation) principle could be

the incision, causing pain. Pain medication will allow more effective turning, coughing, deep-breathing and incentive sperometer use.

applied here for the correct selection of the answer.

68. Correct answer: d

When food or fluid travels through the duodenum, the pancreas is stimulated to produce more pancreatic enzymes. The NPO status and NG suction from the stomach will prevent gastric juices from flowing into the duodenum.

Remember the normal anatomy and physiology for the movement of gastric contents into the small intestine. Then use common sense to eliminate responses *a, b,* and *c.*

69. Correct answer: b

Daily weight will identify if fluid is being retained or lost. The abdominal girths will identify an increase in the ascites.

If you have no idea of the correct response, cluster responses *a, c,* and *d* with the similar term—lung sounds. Select response *b.*

70. Correct answer: d

A major problem in clients with hepatitis is nausea and subsequently anorexia. Nutrition is a priority concern in their care. By offering small, frequent feedings higher in carbohydrates (CHO) and lower in fat than the usual diet with the largest meal in the morning, nutrition may be improved. The client is very fatigued, so exercise is not an option. Baths with soap and lotions may only complicate the pruritus.

Oatmeal baths may diminish itching. Protein would be more restricted than CHO in clients with liver inflammation. Fats are limited in these clients and in persons with acute pancreatitis. The icteric stage of hepatitis is the most contagious stage; this is another reason to avoid contact with others and not institute mild exercise. The use of "soap" is not usually a correct choice. Lotion is preferred if the skin is dry, but not for itching from the deposition of bilirubin with liver failure.

71. **Correct answer: c**

    The most feasible nursing goal for this client is to decrease the diarrhea episodes. Constipation is not seen in this client.

    Note that in option *a* the balance is too wide of a range. In response *d* the weight gain or loss will vary depending on the frequency of remissions and exacerbations.

72. **Correct answer: a**

    Clients with diverticulosis should not eat nuts because they may lodge in the diverticula and initiate diverticulitis.

    Recall that anatomy of large intestinal diverticula is the outpouching of the intestinal wall. Approach the options with common sense and ask yourself which of the foodstuffs would most likely get lodged in the sacs. Option *a* is most likely.

73. **Correct answer: b**

    This assessment finding is most indicative of possible colon cancer. Abdominal pain and weight loss could indicate many problems. A family history of cancer predisposes the client to cancer but does not indicate colon cancer.

    If you have no idea of the correct response, match the problem in the stem, colon cancer, with the specific area or system in the options, bowel.

74. **Correct answer: d**

    The diuretic effect of Mannitol, a hypertonic solution, will increase renal filtration and help maintain renal function by osmotic effects. It increases urine output and decreases fluid volume. In the given situation, it is used by the physician to increase renal filtration. Mannitol may be given in acute head injuries to decrease cerebral edema.

    Response *a* can be subsumed under the correct response *c*, since an increase in renal filtration will increase urine output. Renal perfusion is increased by increasing cardiac output. Eliminate option *b*; there is no information in the stem about too much volume or edema.

75. Correct answer: c

It is best to be honest to help the client adjust to the diagnosis. Knowing what the physician has told the client about the prognosis, the nurse can now help the client understand and adjust. A better response but not a choice is, "Tell me what the physician has talked with you about," or "Tell me what you have heard."

In these types of questions, read slowly and carefully. Be tuned in to your biases and personal experiences, which may lead to the selection of the incorrect response. Response *c* may sound harsh, yet it is the most accurate of the choices.

76. Correct answer: b

Renal stone pain is typically relieved when the stone is passed. All urine of the client with a renal calculus must be strained. If the pain is relieved, the nurse must look for the stone.

The next best action after straining the urine is to call the physician to convey the information that the pain is gone and to indicate if a stone was strained from the urine.

77. Correct answer: a

The pain at the costovertebral angle is more indicative of pyelonephritis than of a urinary tract infection. The foul-smelling urine rules out diverticulitis and a renal calculus. Fever may be found in all of the listed conditions.

The identification of the location for the typical pain with each of the conditions is most important to answering this question correctly: pyelonephritis and renal calculus are at the CVA angle; diverticulitis is in the lower left quadrant; urinary tract infections are suprapubic from bladder spasms or urethral meatus from the burning.

78. Correct answer: c

Since the physician is preparing to remove one kidney, it would be prudent to ascertain that the other kidney can handle the function required of the two kidneys.

If you have no idea of the correct response, match the system in the stem with the system in the options for the correct selection of response *c.*

79. **Correct answer: a**

This diagnosis is most complete and specific for this client and the supporting data given in the stem.

There is no data in the stem to support the selection of options *b*, *c*, or *d*.

80. **Correct answer: b**

Keeping the scrotum elevated will decrease edema following the surgery. Twisting of the remaining testicle would be unlikely, since it is stabilized within the scrotum.

Use the common rationale to support anything after surgery, such as an extremity; this is usually to decrease edema.

81. **Correct answer: d**

This response is most therapeutic, as it gives the client the best and most complete information.

Note that all of the responses are correct, so careful reading and rereading of the question and the responses are indicated in this type of question.

82. **Correct answer: c**

This response gives the client and her husband the most informative and therapeutic answer. Intracavitary therapy is a kind of radioactive therapy in which one or more radioactive sources are placed, usually with the help of an applicator or holding device, within the body cavity to irradiate the walls of the cavity or adjacent tissue.

If you have no idea of the correct answer, eliminate option *a* with the absolute, only. Use common sense to eliminate option *b*. With any kind of radiation therapy the site will be inflamed after therapy. So it would be safest to allow the site to recover for about a week. Eliminate option *d* since waiting a month is too long after the treatment. Select option *c* which is the most comprehensive reply.

83. **Correct answer: b**

It is well accepted that there is a familial tendency for ovarian cancer. For this reason we must evaluate family history of ovarian cancer when screening clients.

If you have no idea of the correct response, cluster responses *a*, *c*, and *d* under the category of "directly related to the client." Response *b* deals with relatives.

84. Correct answer: a

Fluid intake must be increased to prevent renal calculi due to resorption of calcium from the bones. The client with increased parathyroid has a high-serum calcium, so calcium must be restricted in the diet. Sleeping too often will not encourage transport of calcium into the bones, but instead impair that transport. Weight-bearing exercises such as walking increase calcium deposition in the bones. Fiber and bulk need to be increased in the diet to prevent constipation.

Cluster responses *b, c,* and *d* under "incorrect facts." Select option *a.*

85. Correct answer: b

Intravenous corticosteroids are imperative, as this client has a major lack of steroids. Calcium administration will not be helpful. Fluids must be infused rapidly to help stabilize the vascular status. Frequent blood pressure monitoring will not be enough. This client will require invasive hemodynamic monitoring.

If you have no idea of the correct response, cluster *a, c,* and *d* under "nonmedications"; select *b,* the only medication.

86. Correct answer: d

This client must be aware that he/she will require more steroids in situations of illness, stress or surgery. This information has a higher priority than teaching about daily weights. In addition,

Associate that an increased need for steroids is similar to the increased need for insulin—it occurs in all situations in life; however, with insulin an increase in exercise may decrease a need for insulin.

education about daily weights should include tracking/calculating the daily and weekly gain or loss. This client should follow a low-sodium diet due to the tendency for salt and water retention from steroids and the loss of potassium. The client should protect himself/herself from all infections.

87. **Correct answer: c**

Evaluate neurovascular status with *every* set of vital signs, not every 2 hours. The client should get out of bed and sit in a straightback chair. The client should be kept flat and log-rolled every 0 hours. Urinary retention must be evaluated due to the possibility of neurovascular impairment preventing normal urinary patterns.

There are clues in the options that help eliminate them as correct answers. In option *a,* "every 2 hours" for neurovascular assessment is inappropriate since the client is already 0 hours postop. In option *b,* "an easy chair" is not appropriate for clients with back problems or surgery. In option *c,* "turn" is too general of a description and the "head elevated 30 degrees" usually results in increased pressure or strain on the lower back.

88. **Correct answer: c**

They should be exercised only to the point of pain and no further. Joints should be rested with splinting only during acute exacerbations.

Eliminate option *a* based on common sense—don't exercise anything beyond to point of pain. Eliminate option *b* since no time period or frequency is given for the joint being still. Eliminate option *d* based on your knowledge that during exacerbations of illness rest is recommended. Select option *c.*

89. **Correct answer: b**

The stump must be elevated for 24 hours to prevent stump edema. After the first

Apply knowledge from basic post-surgical care. The surgical site is usually elevated for

24 hours, the stump should be maintained in an extended position as much as possible to prevent hip contractures, the most common complication.

24 hours to decrease as well as prevent further edema.

90. **Correct answer: c**

Clients must be turned and pressure points visualized every 2 hours. Turning sheets should be used to pull clients up and reposition clients in bed to prevent shearing of the skin. The skin should be cleaned immediately after incontinence occurs.

Eliminate options *a* and *b* with the maximum time of 4 hours for turning. Be sure to read option *d* carefully to note the word "avoid." If you are tired especially at this question no. 90, you may tend to read quickly to "get done" and miss easier types of questions. Remember to stop about every 20 to 25 questions, close your eyes, take 3 SLOW deep breaths, and then get back to the task of test completion.

BIBLIOGRAPHY

Beare, PG and Myers, JL: *Principles and Practice of Adult Health Nursing,* ed 2, St Louis, 1994, Mosby.

Belcher, A: *Blood Disorders,* St Louis, 1993, Mosby.

Belcher, A: *Cancer Nursing,* St Louis, 1992, Mosby.

Black, JM and Matassarin-Jacobs, E: *Luckman & Sorensen's Medical-Surgical Nursing: A Psychophysiologic Approach,* ed 4, Philadelphia, 1993, W.B. Saunders Co.

Brundage, DJ: *Renal Disorders,* St Louis, 1992, Mosby.

Canobbio, MM: *Cardiovascular Disorders,* St Louis, 1990, Mosby.

Chipp, E, Clanin, N and Campbell, V: *Neurologic Disorders,* St Louis, 1992, Mosby.

Degen, JH and Vallerand, AH: *Davis's Drug Guide for Nurses,* Philadelphia, 1993, F.A. Davis Co.

Doughty, DB: *Gastrointestinal Disorders,* St Louis, 1993, Mosby.

Eliopoulous, D: *Gerontological Nursing,* ed 3, Philadelphia, 1993, J.B. Lippincott Co.

Fischbach, F: *A Manual of Laboratory and Diagnostic Tests,* Philadelphia, 1992, J.B. Lippincott Co.

Gahart, BL: *1995 Intravenous Medications,* ed 11, St Louis, 1995, Mosby.

Gray, M: *Genitourinary Disorders,* St Louis, 1992, Mosby.

Grimes, D: *Infectious Diseases,* St Louis, 1991, Mosby.

Ignatavicius, DD and Bayne, MV: *Medical-Surgical Nursing: A Nursing Process Approach,* Philadelphia, 1991, W.B. Saunders Co.

Kestel, F: *Are You Up to Date on Diabetes Medications? American Journal of Nursing,* pp 48-52, July 1994.

Mosby's Medical, Nursing & Allied Health Dictionary, ed 4, St Louis, 1994, Mosby.

Mourad, L: *Orthopedic Disorders,* St Louis, 1991, Mosby.

Mudge-Grout, CL: *Immunologic Disorders,* St Louis, 1992, Mosby.

Pagana, KD and Pagana DJ: *Mosby's Diagnostic and Laboratory Test Reference,* ed 2, St Louis, 1995, Mosby.

Rollant, PD: *Acing Multiple Choice Exams,* American Journal of Nursing Career Guide for 1994, pp. 18-21, 36, Jan. 1994.

Swearinger, P: *Manual of Medical-Surgical Nursing Care,* ed 3, St Louis, 1994, Mosby.

Wilson, SF and Thompson, JM: *Respiratory Disorders,* St Louis, 1990, Mosby.

INDEX

Instructions for Disk Start-Up

DOS Version
System Requirements

A computer with at least 324K of RAM (Random Access Memory) available is needed for this program. This computer must be IBM PC or 100% compatible.

For these examples we assume that your A drive is your floppy drive, and your C drive is your hard drive. Please substitute the letter of your floppy drive for A if your floppy drive letter is different. Substitute the letter of your hard drive for C if your hard drive letter is different.

Start-up (floppy drive):

1. Turn your computer on
2. At the prompt, insert the disk into your A drive
3. Type A: and press <Enter>
4. Type MOSBY and press <Enter>
5. Follow the instructions on the screen

Start-up (hard disk):

1. Turn your computer on
2. At the prompt, insert the disk into your A drive
3. Type C: and press <Enter>
4. Type MD\MOSBY and press <Enter>
5. Type CD\MOSBY and press <Enter>
6. Type COPY A:*.* and press <Enter>

The software is now installed on your hard drive. Once the software is installed, start the software by following these directions:
1. Type CD\MOSBY and press <Enter>
2. Type MOSBY and press <Enter>
3. Follow the directions on the screen

MAC Version
System Requirements

Mac 68XXX or Power Mac with a total of at least 1 MB of RAM is needed for this program.

Start-up:

1. Create a new folder on your hard disk called MOSBY.
2. Insert the disk into your floppy drive and open it.
3. Drag all items from the disk to the new folder.

The software is now installed on your hard drive. Once the software is installed, start the software by following these directions:
1. Open the MOSBY folder.
2. Select the MOSBY program.
3. Follow the directions on the screen.

WRITE DOWN THE PASSWORD THAT YOU HAVE SELECTED.
YOUR DISK WILL BE BRANDED WITH THIS INITIAL ENTRY.